Clinical Retinopathies

Clinical Retinopathies

Paul M. Dodson MD FRCP, FRCOphth
Consultant Physician
East Birmingham Hospital
Birmingham, United Kingdom
and Honorary Senior Clinical Lecturer
University of Birmingham
Honorary Consultant Physician
Birmingham and Midland Eye Hospital
Examiner for FRCOphth, final fellowship

Jonathan M. Gibson MD, FRCS, FRCOphth
Consultant Ophthalmologist
East Birmingham Hospital
Birmingham and Midland Eye Hospital
Birmingham, United Kingdom
and Honorary Senior Clinical Lecturer
University of Birmingham
Examiner for fellowship examinations (FRCS/FRCOphth) in ophthalmology

Erna E. Kritzinger MSC, FRCS, FRCP, FRCOphth
Consultant Ophthalmologist
Birmingham and Midland Eye Hospital
Birmingham, United Kingdom
and Honorary Senior Clinical Lecturer
University of Birmingham
Examiner for FRCOphth, final fellowship

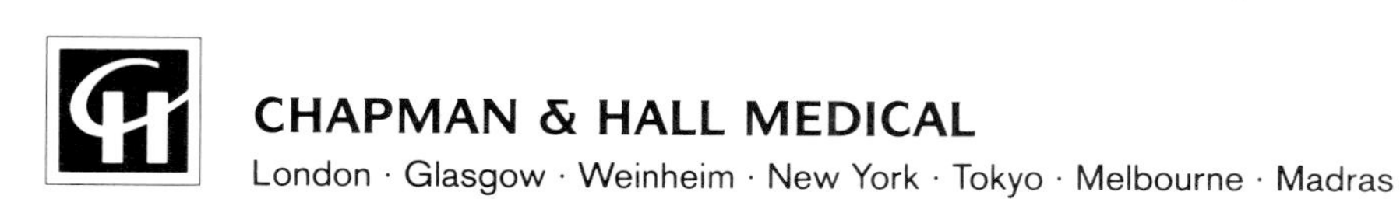
CHAPMAN & HALL MEDICAL
London · Glasgow · Weinheim · New York · Tokyo · Melbourne · Madras

Published by Chapman & Hall, 2–6 Boundary Row, London SE1 8HN, UK

Chapman & Hall, 2–6 Boundary Row, London SE1 8HN, UK

Blackie Academic & Professional, Wester Cleddens Road, Bishopbriggs, Glasgow G64 2NZ, UK

Chapman & Hall GmbH, Pappelallee 3, 69469 Weinheim, Germany

Chapman & Hall USA , One Penn Plaza, 41st Floor, New York NY 10119, USA

Chapman & Hall Japan, ITP-Japan, Kyowa Building, 3F, 2-2-1 Hirakawacho, Chiyoda-ku, Tokyo 102, Japan

Chapman & Hall Australia, Thomas Nelson Australia, 102 Dodds Street, South Melbourne, Victoria 3205, Australia

Chapman & Hall India, R. Seshadri, 32 Second Main Road, CIT East, Madras 600 035, India

---

First edition 1995

Designed by Geoffrey Wadsley

Typeset in 10/12pt Palatino by Keyset Composition, Colchester, Essex

Printed in Hong Kong by Thomas Nelson

ISBN 0 412 35930 8

A catalogue record for this book is available from the British Library

Library of Congress Catalog Card Number: 93-74901

∞ Printed on acid-free text paper, manufactured in accordance with ANSI/NISO Z39.48-1992 (Permanence of Paper).

Contents

Authors

P. M. Dodson MD, FRCP, FRCOphth
Consultant Physician
East Birmingham Hospital
Bordesley Green East
Birmingham
B9 5ST

Honorary Senior Clinical Lecturer
University of Birmingham

and

Honorary Consultant Physician
Birmingham and Midland Eye Hospital

J. M. Gibson MD, FRCS, FRCOphth
Consultant Ophthalmologist
East Birmingham Hospital
Bordesley Green East
Birmingham
B9 5ST

and

Honorary Senior Clinical Lecturer
University of Birmingham

Erna E. Kritzinger MSC, FRCS, FRCP, FRCOphth
Consultant Ophthalmic Surgeon and Honorary
Senior Clinical Lecturer
Birmingham and Midland Eye Hospital
Church Street
Birmingham
B3 2NS

WITH CONTRIBUTIONS FROM

D. G. Beevers MD, FRCP (Chapter 5)
Reader in Medicine
and Honorary Consultant Physician
Dudley Road Hospital
Birmingham
B18 7QH

S. Eames, MRCOphth (Chapter 5)
Staff Ophthalmologist
East Birmingham Hospital
Bordesley Green East
Birmingham
B9 5ST

M. Wood MA, FRCP (Chapter 10)
Consultant Physician
Department of Communicable and Tropical Diseases
East Birmingham Hospital
Bordesley Green East
Birmingham
B9 5ST

Note: East Birmingham Hospital has now become Birmingham Heartlands Hospital.

Preface

The eye is the only organ in which both vascular and neural tissue can be directly viewed. In particular, the retina gives many clues to the nature, diagnosis and course of underlying systemic disorders.

Experience has shown that physicians find the principles of ophthalmology difficult, even though most regularly use ophthalmoscopes. Equally, ophthalmologists find the ever expanding literature on the management of common medical disorders daunting. This book is intended for physicians and ophthalmologists in training, and other health workers within medicine and ophthalmology, including GPs, optometrists, internal medicine and ophthalmology nurses. It concentrates on common retinopathies confronting both the physician and ophthalmologist, although rarer conditions that may be encountered in practice and conditions that are difficult to classify, are covered in Chapter 13.

Three sections have been written describing the basic principles of retinal disease (anatomy, physiology, physical signs and investigations). Specific common disease states are described in the context of their retinopathy and each chapter contains an ophthalmologist's as well as a physician's viewpoint. It is hoped this text highlights new areas of interest. A detailed discussion and description of every related ocular and systemic disease with detailed medical management would make this work an encyclopaedic volume. Key areas of medical management and common retinopathies are the emphasis of this overview with the intention of presenting updated modern aspects of this multi-disciplinary subject. There are extensive illustrations to enable pattern recognition, as well as tables to identify important medical points. We hope this book will assist doctors in preparation for both MRCP and FRCOphth examinations.

We are indebted to our contributors and to Professor S. Lightman, who contributed slides on inflammatory eye disease and diabetic macular oedema, without whom this text would not have been achieved. The extensive secretarial assistance needed to create this book was provided by the hard labours of Catherine Rushton and Joanne Tolley and moral support was always given by Lynne Dodson and Jennifer Gibson.

Paul M. Dodson
Jonathan M. Gibson
Erna E. Kritzinger

1 *Practical anatomy and physiology of the eye*

Clinical Retinopathies. Paul M. Dodson, Jonathan M. Gibson and Erna E. Kritzinger.
Published in 1995 by Chapman & Hall, London. ISBN 0 412 35930 8

1.1 INTRODUCTION

In this chapter the structure and function of the important component parts of the eye will be discussed. In considering diseases primarily affecting the retina, it is nevertheless helpful for non-ophthalmologists to have a working knowledge of other parts of the eye. In addition it is important to consider the retina and choroid, with their differing vascular supplies, in some detail and these are described.

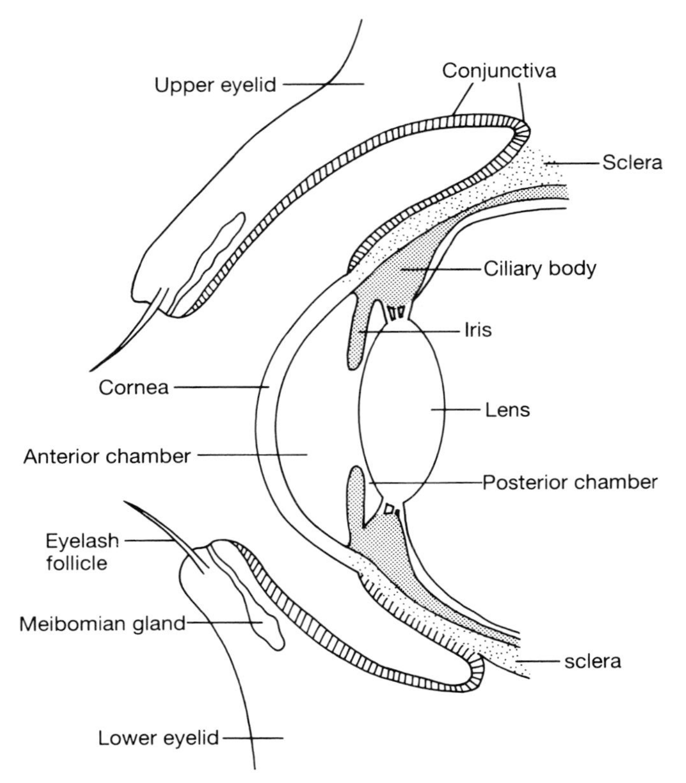

Fig. 1.1 Diagram of cross-section of conjunctival sac and globe of the eye.

1.2 THE CONJUNCTIVA

The conjunctiva is a mucous membrane which lines the inner side of the eyelid and is reflected on to the globe of the eye. It is composed of an epithelial layer and an underlying stroma. The epithelium is 2–5 layers in thickness and near the edge of the eyelid, in the tarsal conjunctiva, surface layers are formed by skin-like, stratified squamous epithelium. The stroma, underlying the epithelium, is a layer which is rich in connective tissue and is also vascular. The conjunctiva lining the inside of the eyelids is termed the tarsal conjunctiva, and is quite firmly attached to the inside of the eyelid, in comparison to the bulbar conjunctiva, which is a loose transparent layer overlying the sclera. This is continuous at the limbus with the cornea.

Throughout the conjunctiva goblet cells are present. These are particularly numerous in the lower and upper fornices and produce mucus which is an important constituent of normal tears.

The conjunctiva literally joins the eyelids to the eyeball and the epithelium, which is a continuation of the corneal epithelial, forms a lining to the conjunctival sac, whose opening is the space between the eyelids, the palpebral aperture (Fig. 1.1). The main role of the conjunctiva is in protection of the surface of the eye and the mucus that is produced promotes wetting of the cornea and normal tear function. Since the conjunctiva has a rich vascular supply, it is an important source of immunological protection to the front of the eye.

1.3 THE CORNEA

The cornea is the transparent window of the anterior part of the eyeball and is approximately 11.5 mm in diameter. It is customary to divide the cornea into five layers in a cross-section (Fig. 1.2).

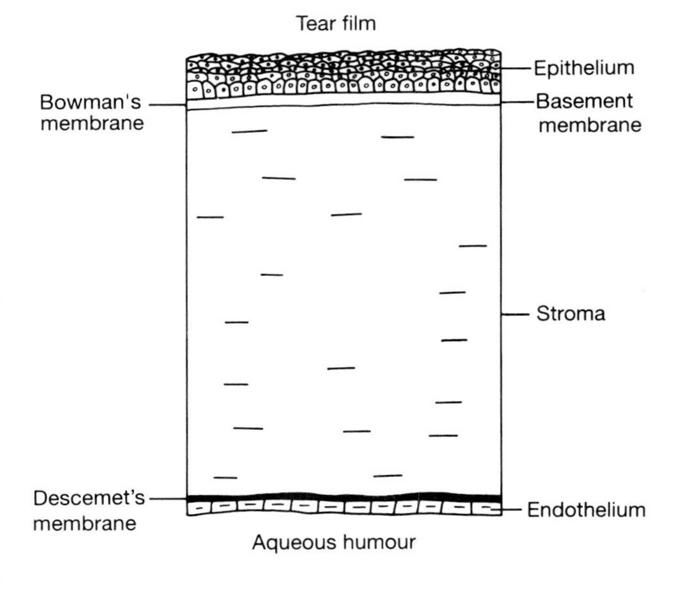

Fig. 1.2 Cross-section of the cornea.

1. The corneal epithelium, which is a layer of 5–6 cells deep, composed of a columnar basal cell layer with wing cells in the intermediate layers and a surface layer of unkeratinized flat cells. The surface of the epithelium is extremely smooth and flat and this is important for refractive properties.
2. Bowman's membrane, which is the basement membrane of the epithelial cells and is transparent.
3. The stroma, which comprises about 90% of the corneal thickness and consists of layers of fibrous lamellae, which are composed of collagen fibrils. These are arranged in such a way that the stroma transmits light readily and remains transparent. Scattered in the stroma, between the lamellae, are the keratocytes.
4. Desçemet's membrane, which is the basement membrane of the endothelium, situated in the posterior aspect of the stroma.
5. The endothelium, which is a thick single layer of flattened polygonal cells with central nuclei, continuous with the endothelium on the anterior surface of the eyelid. The endothelium has only limited powers of regeneration compared to the epithelium, which can repair itself very readily.

1.3.1 Function

The main function of the cornea is to remain transparent and act as the main refractive surface of the eye and accordingly the healthy cornea is avascular. The endothelial layer is extremely important in maintaining normal corneal hydration and produces a relative dehydration of the cornea by actively pumping out fluid from the stroma. The failure of this pump, which is sometimes seen following damage to the endothelium by trauma or surgery, results in corneal oedema with increasing thickness of the cornea, loss of the regular arrangement of the collagen fibrils and inevitable loss of transparency, with visual deterioration.

To maintain the optical refraction of the eye, a tear film is essential and this is composed of a superficial lipid layer, an underlying aqueous phase and an inner mucous layer which spreads over the surface of the cornea to form a lining. In this tear film are dissolved immunoglobulins, in particular IgA, IgG and IgM and antibacterial enzymes such as lysozyme, which help to protect the surface of the eye from infection.

1.4 THE SCLERA

The sclera is the tough, fibrous white outer coat of the eye, which is clearly visible beneath the transparent conjunctiva. It is continuous anteriorly with the cornea, but unlike the cornea it is not transparent and this is due to the apparently haphazard manner in which the collagen fibrils are arranged. This has the benefit of providing enormous strength to the sclera, which is important for it to maintain its main function, which is to help keep the integrity of the shape of the globe of the eye. The sclera probably has other properties, such as the transfer of some substances into and out of the eye. The sclera is between 0.3 mm and 1 mm thick.

1.5 ANTERIOR AND POSTERIOR CHAMBERS OF THE EYE

The anterior chamber of the eye is the space between the cornea anteriorly and posteriorly the anterior surface of the iris and lens. In the peripheral part of the anterior chamber is the anterior chamber angle. This is the site of the trabecular meshwork, through which about 80% of the total outflow of aqueous humour from the eye occurs. The posterior chamber is much smaller and is the space bounded anteriorly by the iris and posteriorly by the front surface of the zonular fibres, the lens and the ciliary process. Its volume is extremely small and it is important because aqueous humour is secreted by the ciliary processes and flows from the posterior chamber, through the pupil, into the anterior chamber. These are shown in Fig. 1.3.

1.5.1 The anterior chamber depth

From the clinical aspect it is important to estimate the depth of the anterior chamber and hence from this the narrowness of the anterior chamber angle of the eye, so that the pupil can be dilated. There is a risk in patients who have a shallow anterior chamber and a narrow anterior chamber angle, that dilatation of the pupil can cause obstruction of the outflow of aqueous humour and hence acute glaucoma. In practice this appears to occur quite infrequently but nevertheless general practitioners and physicians are naturally apprehensive about the risk of it if they do dilate the pupils. An easy way of assessing whether the pupil is safe to be dilated is shown in Fig. 1.4, using a pen torch or ophthalmoscope. A light source is shone from the side of the eye parallel to the iris plane and if the anterior chamber is deep, the surface of the iris will be illuminated on both sides of the pupil. If on the other hand the anterior chamber is shallow, then the nasal part of the iris will not be illuminated and this will appear as a dark crescentic shadow.

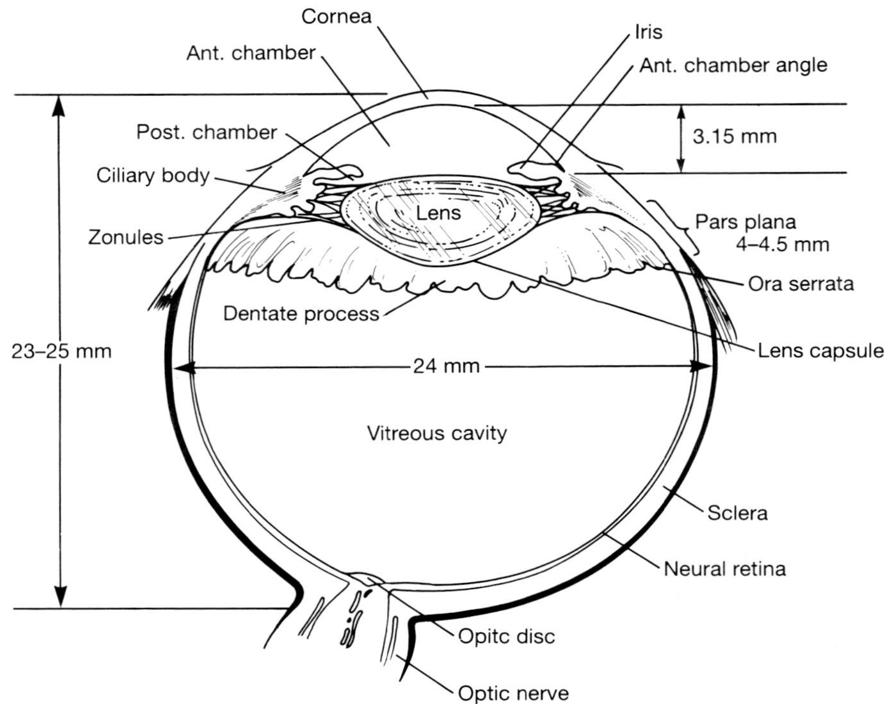

Fig. 1.3 Cross-section of the eye. Dimensions are approximate and are the average dimensions in the normal adult eye. From Ryan, S.J. (1989) *Retina*, vol. 1, C.V. Mosby Company, St Louis, p 12.

1.6 AQUEOUS HUMOUR

The aqueous humour contributes to the normal maintenance of intraocular pressure and supplies the metabolism of the lens, which itself is avascular. The aqueous humour also contributes to the nutrition of the endothelial layer of the cornea. Aqueous humour is produced by a combination of active filtration, secretion and diffusion in the epithelium of the ciliary processes. The fluid flows through the posterior chamber, around the margin of the pupil, and into the anterior chamber. The majority of aqueous humour drains out from the eye via the trabecular meshwork into the Canal of Schlemm, but a small but significant part does flow directly via the so-called uveoscleral outflow path and into the potential space between the sclera and the ciliary body.

The blood aqueous barrier prevents a free exchange of substances between the plasma and the aqueous humour: the site of this barrier is in the ciliary body and in the vessels in the iris. The aqueous humour is similar to plasma in many respects, but it has several important differences, notably that it contains chloride and ascorbate, far in excess of plasma.

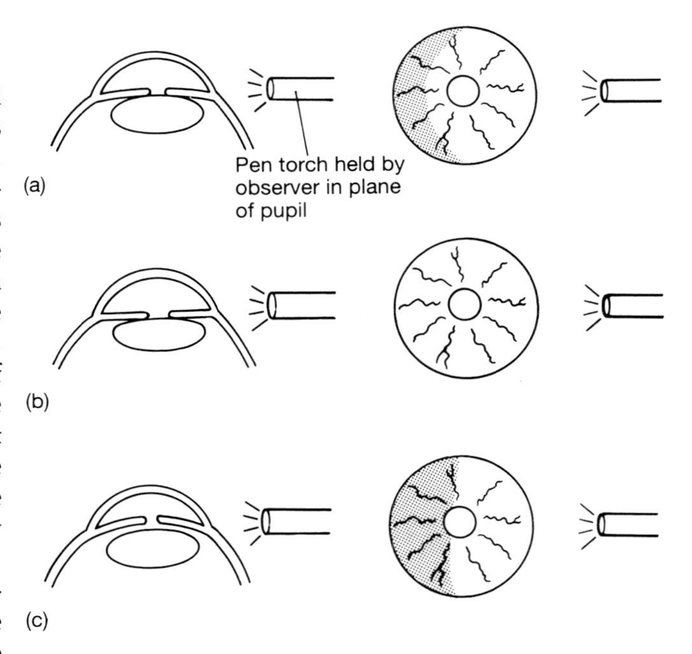

Fig. 1.4 Testing the anterior chamber depth. (a) Normal depth: small crescent in shadow. (b) Deep anterior chamber: all of iris surface illuminated. (c) Shallow anterior chamber: large shadow over distal iris.

The normal intraocular pressure is between 10 and 20 mmHg, but it is affected by a number of factors. There is a pulsatile variation with each heart beat, due to fluctuations in the intraocular vascular volume and also there may be a slow variation with respiration. The most important variation is the diurnal variation that occurs in normal individuals. Other factors which increase intraocular pressure are increased venous pressure, as occurs in the Valsalva manoeuvre, and decreased outflow of aqueous humour through the trabecular meshwork. Factors which decrease intraocular pressure are decreased production of aqueous humour, such as occurs with drugs that are used in the treatment of glaucoma.

1.7 THE LENS

The human crystalline lens is derived embryologically from the ectoderm. It comprises a homogeneous capsule that has a lens epithelium only beneath the anterior capsule. The lens contains a central nucleus that is surrounded by cortex and throughout life new cells are formed at the equator and migrate inwards towards the nucleus. The lens is held in position behind the pupil by means of zonular fibres, which transmit contractions of the ciliary muscle that will result in changes to the shape of the lens, which occurs during accommodation. The lens is transparent and this is partly achieved by the fact that it is acellular and that most of the layers of the lens have the same index of refraction. The lens is composed almost entirely of protein and it is dependent on glycolysis and the pentose phosphate shunt for its metabolism and energy production.

1.8 THE UVEAL TRACT

The uveal tract is the main vascular coat of the eye and comprises the iris, ciliary body and the choroid, as shown in Fig. 1.3. The iris is a delicate structure which acts as a diaphragm and it surrounds the central aperture, the pupil. The iris is formed from anterior and posterior leaves. The anterior leaf is coloured whilst the posterior surface is deeply pigmented. The posterior layer also contains an epithelial layer and the sphincter pupillae, which is supplied by the parasympathetic nervous system, from the third nerve. Posterior to this in the posterior layer, is the dilator pupillae muscle, which is supplied by the sympathetic nervous system. The function of the iris is to regulate the amount of light which is entering the eye via the pupil. Optically, as the pupil constricts, it increases the depth of focus of the eye and minimizes spherical and chromatic aberrations of the eye and oblique astigmatism. The iris has a very rich blood supply from the major and minor arteriolar circles and the vessels of the iris form with the ciliary body the blood aqueous barrier. Breakdown of the blood aqueous barrier occurs in conditions such as iritis, where there is leakage of protein, leucocytes and other substances into the anterior chamber. That is clinically seen on the slit lamp as flare (protein) and cells (leucocytes).

1.9 CILIARY BODY

The ciliary body is a ring of tissue about 6 mm wide situated between the base of the iris and the choroid. It is divided anatomically into uveal and epithelial portions. The uveal portion is adjacent to the sclera and contains a ciliary muscle and the vessel layer. The epithelial portion comprises the pars plicata and the pars plana.

The ciliary muscle is situated in the uveal part of the ciliary body and is made up of longitudinal, circular and radial fibres, which arise from the ciliary body and are inserted into the zonule in the lens. In accommodation, when the ciliary muscle contracts, there is relaxation of the zonule, permitting the lens to become more convex. When the ciliary muscle relaxes, there is contraction of the zonule, permitting the lens to become less convex.

The pars plicata is an important part of the epithelial portion of the ciliary body and contains about 60–70 ciliary processes. These processes are the site for the formation of aqueous humour. The pars plana forms the junction of the ciliary body with the anterior part of the retina and this represents the most peripheral part of the fundus that can be viewed with the indirect ophthalmoscope. The pars plana appears to have a toothed or scalloped margin and its practical importance lies in the fact that the vitreous base is inserted straddling the ora serrata, the toothed area of the pars plana.

The production of aqueous humour is a complex process requiring active transport of solutes against an electrochemical gradient.

Ultrafiltration from highly specialized vascular networks and intercellular movement of small molecules and ions across tight junctions in the ciliary epithelium, play a part in separating the blood effectively from the aqueous. The ciliary processes are important because they affect the way in which drugs are transported across the blood aqueous barrier and into the eye.

1.10 THE CHOROID

The choroid is composed mainly of a large number of blood vessels arranged roughly in layers, according to their size. The choroid extends from the optic nerve posteriorly to the ciliary body anteriorly. It has an important function as it acts as the blood supply for the outer half of the sensory retina, and in fact the outer retina is totally dependent on the blood circulation in the choroid for its metabolic needs. The choroid consists of three main layers of blood vessels with the larger vessels being situated near the sclera and the smaller capillary layer, the so called choriocapillaris, consisting of fenestrated capillaries, which form a dense network adjacent to the retina. The blood supply to the choroid is derived from the short posterior ciliary arteries and the two long posterior ciliary arteries, which are derived from the ophthalmic artery. Blood drains away from the choroid via the vortex veins, of which there are four, one in each quadrant.

The choroidal blood flow seems to be higher than in any other tissue in the body and it has been postulated that the blood supply is greatly in excess of the metabolic requirements of the retina. The blood vessels in the choroid are very wide bore compared with retinal capillaries and they are permeable without tight junctions in the vessels. Various explanations have been given as to why the choroidal circulation seems to be so well developed and perhaps surplus to retinal metabolic requirements and it has been postulated that an important function of this very rich blood supply is maintenance of temperature of the retina either by cooling or warming. Metabolites from the choroid must pass through Bruch's membrane, the retinal pigment epithelium and the interphotoreceptor space to get to the retinal photoreceptor layer. There is a now evidence that the retinal pigment epithelium actively and selectively transfers molecules to and from the retina and also is involved in the continuous outward movement from the vitreous cavity and subretinal space of water and other molecules.

1.11 THE RETINA

1.11.1 Practical Anatomy (Fig. 1.5)

The retina forms the inner layer of the eye and comprises two layers with a potential space in between. The outer layer is the retinal pigment epithelial layer, the inner layer is the neuro-sensory layer, which contains the photoreceptor cells and neuronal connections. The retina extends from the optic disc posteriorly to the ora serrata anteriorly. On ophthalmoscopy several distinct landmarks can be seen, which help to orientate the observer. The

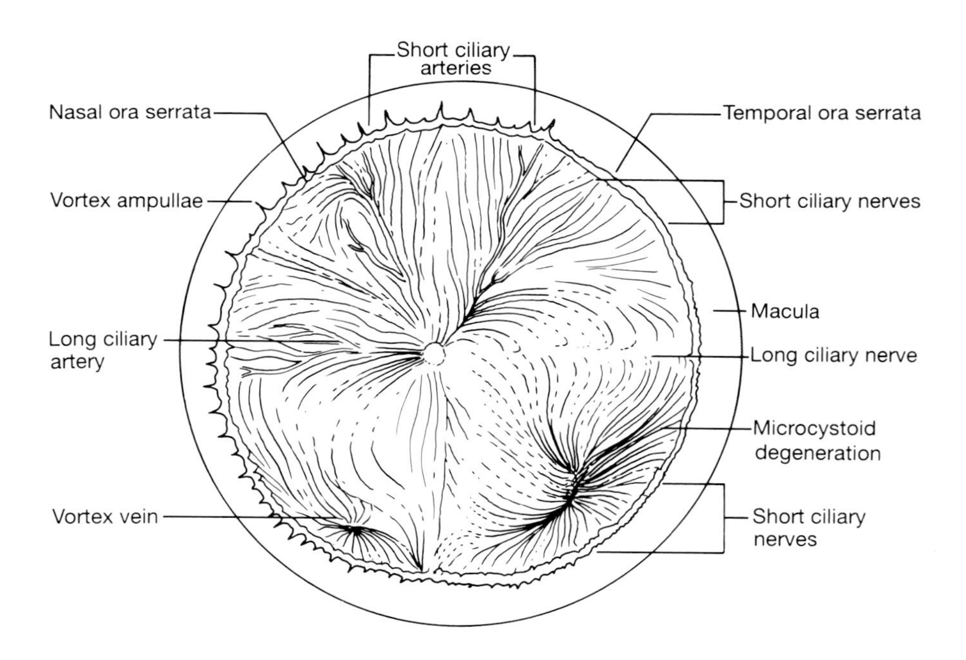

Fig. 1.5 Normal anatomical landmarks of the retina. From Kanski, J. (1988) *Clinical Ophthalmology*, Butterworth and Co., London, p 263.

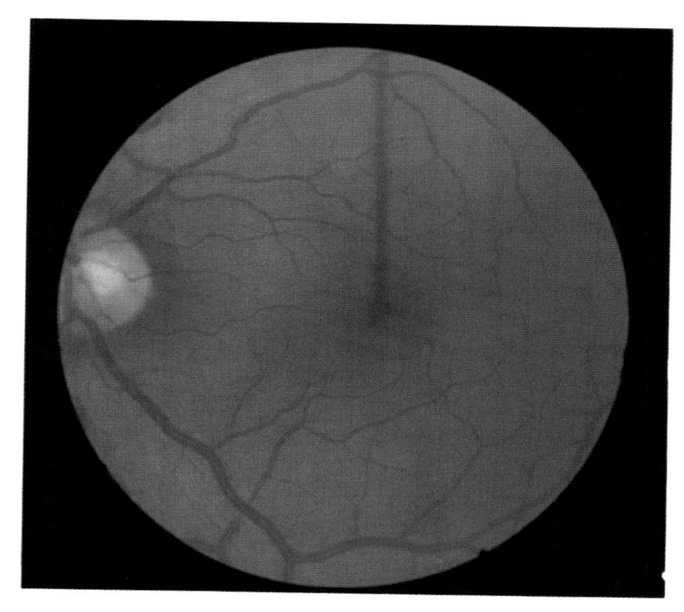

Fig. 1.6 Fundus photograph of the normal macula (with fixation marker).

most obvious landmark is the optic disc, which is about 1.5 mm in diameter and situated temporal to this is the macular lutea. This appears as a darker area than the surrounding retina and the fovea in the central part of the macula appears yellow, due to the luteal pigment, xanthophyll. Fig. 1.6 is a fundus photograph of the normal macula.

The vortex veins are visible in the four quadrants of the fundus and their ampullae mark the inner position of the equator of the eye. This is an important landmark when examining the retina from the point of view of retinal detachment. On either side, at 3 o'clock and 9 o'clock, are the long posterior ciliary nerves and vessels. These can be seen as yellow streaks. This is of practical importance when carrying out laser pan-retinal photocoagulation, as these areas are quite tender when heated by laser burns and may cause patient discomfort.

1.11.2 Morphology of the Retina

The neuro-sensory retina can be divided into three layers:

1. The most external layer is the photoreceptor layer, which includes the outer and inner segments and the layer of photoreceptor cell bodies, which is sometimes called the outer nuclear layer.
2. The second layer is that of intermediate neurones or the inner nuclear layer.
3. The third layer consists of ganglion cells.

The axonal processes of the photoreceptor cells synapse in the outer plexiform layer with processes of the bipolar cells and the horizontal cells and these cells have their cell bodies located in the inner nuclear layer. The horizontal cells form a means of lateral communication between the photoreceptor cells amongst which they send processes. Bipolar cells synapse with amacrine and/or ganglion cells. Amacrine cells are located primarily in the inner portion of the inner nuclear layer. The axons of the ganglion cells converge to form the nerve fibre layer, which is the most superficial layer of the retina and they exit the eye via the optic nerve. The outer limiting membrane of the retina is formed between cell membranes of the major glial cells, the Muller cells and the photoreceptor inner segments. The inner limiting membrane, which separates the retina from the vitreous, is a surface modification of the vitreous body and is probably partly formed by the processes of the Muller cells.

The photoreceptors comprise the rods and cones, which are so called because of their microscopic shape and appearance. Cone density is maximal in the fovea and decreases towards the periphery. Rods are distributed unevenly across the retina and there seems to be a rod-free area in the foveola. The highest concentration of rods is seen about 20° eccentrically from the fovea, after which the concentration decreases gradually into the periphery.

1.11.3 Function of the photoreceptors

The outer segment of the photoreceptors is the site of phototransduction, where light energy is converted into electrical signals. Both rods and cones contain an elaborate system of stacked membranous discs and these discs undergo a continuous process of phagocytosis by the retinal pigment epithelial cells and renewal. It seems that this degradation and phagocytosis of the outer segments of the rods and cones follows a diurnal rhythm.

Rod cells are sensitive to light because they contain a visual pigment, rhodopsin, which is capable of trapping photons. Rhodopsin is composed of vitamin A aldehyde, or retinal, and this is attached to a second molecule called opsin. In the cone cells the visual pigments are very similar, but slightly different from rhodopsin, and unlike rod cells they are sensitive either to blue, green or orange-yellow light. These three types of cone pigment are sensitive to different wavelengths of light and this is the basis of colour vision.

1.11.4 Retinal pigment epithelium

The retinal pigment epithelium is situated between the photoreceptors and their blood supply, the choriocapillaries (Fig. 1.7). The retinal pigment epithelium consists of a single layer of epithelial cells, which are hexagonal shaped, the cells having tight junctions between them. They have apical villi on the aspect which is in contact with the photoreceptors with the basement membrane, Bruch's membrane. The retinal pigment epithelium is involved in the renewal of the photoreceptor outer segments and in the phagocytosis and removal of waste products from them. In addition to this the important function of the retinal pigment epithelium is to act as a blood retinal barrier and this is achieved by the tight junctions between the retinal pigment epithelium cells, which prevent the ingress of outside molecules. The retinal pigment epithelium thus forms the outer blood retinal barrier, the inner blood retinal barrier being formed by the retinal vessels themselves. A further important function of the retinal pigment epithelium appears to be its role in maintaining the attachment between the neurosensory retina and the retinal pigment epithelium.

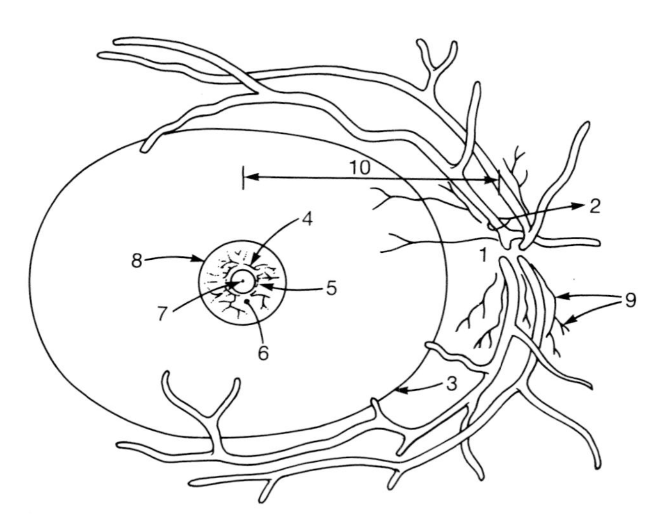

Fig. 1.7 Landmarks and dimensions of the macula and posterior pole of the eye as photographed by the standard fundus camera. Details of special interest in fluorescein angiography: (1) Disc (1500 μ). (2) Vein width at disc (150 μ). (3) Clinical macula (area centralis), an oval area enclosed by the major temporal vessels. (4) Innermost layer of the perifoveal capillary net, within which is the avascular zone of the retina (usually 300 to 500 μ). (5) Fovea (350 μ area of high cone density). (6) Small retinal capillary (6 to 8 μ lumen). (7) Fixation, a tiny area of sharp central acuity (<1°), at approximately the same location as the foveal reflex. (8) Reflex at thickest layer of retina as the slope of the fovea begins (1500 μ), marking the anatomical macula. (9) Fine, long, superficial radial peripapillary capillaries. (10) Distance from the centre of the fovea to the centre of the disc (about 4 mm or 15°). From Berkow, J.W., Orth, D.H., and Kelley, J.S. (1991) *Fluorescein Angiography*, Academy of Ophthalmology, San Francisco, p 6.

1.11.5 The macula

The macula consists of the central area of the retina at the posterior pole and it is approximately 5 mm in diameter. The centre of the macula, the foveola, is situated approximately 4 mm temporally and 0.8 mm inferior to the centre of the optic disc.

The important clinical landmarks within the macula are the fovea, the foveola and the foveal avascular zone and are shown in Fig. 1.7. The fovea is the central pit in the inner retinal surface at the centre of the macula, which is about 1.5 mm diameter. By ophthalmoscopy, it can be seen as a light reflex arising from the central area and with the red free filter on the ophthalmoscope the yellow xanthophyll pigment can be seen clearly, especially in younger patients. The foveola is the central pit floor and it has a diameter of only 0.35 mm. This is the thinnest part of the retina, has the highest cone density and serves fine discriminatory vision and colour vision. The foveal avascular zone is the central area where there are no retinal capillaries. This measures 0.5 mm in diameter. It is of practical importance in fluorescein angiography, where the fovea avascular zone (FAZ) is an important landmark in deciding whether to treat or not to treat subretinal neovascular membranes.

1.11.6 The retinal circulation and autoregulation

The retinal circulation consists of the retinal arterioles, veins and capillaries. In the normal anatomical distribution there is a single central retinal artery and central retinal vein and these branch into four main trunks supplying the four quadrants of the eye. The temporal vessels arch above and below the macula, while the nasal vessels radiate from the optic nerve head. The main layer of capillaries in the retina are found in the nerve fibre ganglion cell layers and are therefore very superficial. However, an additional deep capillary network is found in the very superficial nerve fibre layer, particularly in the area around the optic disc. There is no nervous system control of the retinal circulation as there is no sympathetic nerve supply to the vessels in the retina. Regulation is by non-nervous mechanisms intrinsic to the retina, called autoregulation.

Autoregulation is a physiological phenomenon which results in the maintenance of a constant blood flow in the presence of a variable perfusion pressure. Autoregulatory responses are triggered by acute changes in oxygen tension or perfusion pressure. High oxygen levels in the tissues leads to vasoconstriction, whilst raised intraocular pressure causes vasodilatation. Retinal autoregulation appears to be extremely efficient and adjusts the retinal blood flow and tissue oxygenation to changes in retinal perfusion pressure and oxygen tension. The system seems to be less effective with ageing and in disease processes and also is probably immature in the premature infant.

1.12 THE VITREOUS HUMOUR

The vitreous body occupies 80% of the globe of the eye and has an average volume in the adult eye of 4 ml. The peripheral area of the vitreous is known as the vitreous cortex and comprises a high density of collagen fibrils. The vitreous cortex is firmly attached along the vitreous base which is a circular band straddling the ora serrata and varying in width from 2 to 6 mm. Traction on this area would be transmitted to the peripheral retina and pars plana, which is a common site of retinal hole formation. A weaker attachment of the vitreous occurs in the circular zone at the margin of the optic nerve head and with age this attachment weakens which may cause a posterior vitreous detachment, which is not uncommon in the elderly.

The vitreous has a complex structure of collagen fibrils, together with molecules of a high molecular weight, which are glycosaminoglycans. The most important of these is hyaluronic acid and this imparts on the vitreous gel its properties of being highly viscous but also being elastic (visco-elasticity). The vitreous gel therefore has remarkable water binding properties and this partly gives it its great optical clarity, but also may prevent rapid movement of water into and out of the vitreous body, thus maintaining the volume of the globe.

2 *The basis of ophthalmological physical signs*

Clinical Retinopathies. Paul M. Dodson, Jonathan M. Gibson and Erna E. Kritzinger.
Published in 1995 by Chapman & Hall, London. ISBN 0 412 35930 8

2.1 INTRODUCTION

The basis of diagnosis of any medical condition depends on eliciting the patient's history and interpreting the physical signs that are present. The eye is unique in this respect because of its transparent media, which allows the direct visualization and examination of abnormalities occurring in the retina and posterior segment of the eye.

Physical signs in the anterior segment of the eye that are important in relation to the retina are described, but the majority of this chapter is devoted to abnormalities occurring in the posterior segment.

2.2 ANTERIOR SEGMENT OF THE EYE

Opacities in the optic media of the eye, particularly in the cornea and lens, can be readily assessed by using the direct ophthalmoscope and examining the eye from a distance of about a foot (30 cm). These opacities show up as dark areas against the red reflex and can be particularly useful in assessing the degree of cataract that is present.

2.2.1 Anterior chamber and iris

If a pen torch or a bright ophthalmoscopic light is used, the anterior chamber of the eye can be inspected. This is important when assessing the depth of the anterior chamber and making sure that the pupil is safe to dilate. One of the best ways of performing this is to examine the anterior chamber with a pen torch and shining it in parallel to the iris (section 1.5).

The anterior chamber can also be inspected for the presence of blood in the anterior chamber (a hyphaema) and white cells in the anterior chamber (a hypopyon). Details of the iris itself, such as the presence of rubeosis iridis, are difficult to see unless they are particularly gross, without using some form of magnification such as with a slit lamp.

2.2.2 The pupil

The pupil reactions are extremely important to test for in cases of retinopathy. The direct and consensual test should be performed to light and to accommodation. When carrying out pupil reactions a bright light is essential and it is important to get the patient to look into the distance at a fixed object. This is because if he attempts to look directly at the pen torch or ophthalmoscope light, the pupils will tend to constrict due to the near reflex (accommodation).

One of the most important tests in the clinical examination of the eye for any condition is to look for an afferent pupil defect. This is a very subtle sign of disease affecting the visual pathway, particularly lesions in the retina and optic nerve. It is particularly useful in the assessment of patients with optic nerve conditions, such as demyelinating disease, but also has an important part to play in the assessment of patients with ischaemic retinopathy, such as following a central retinal vein occlusion, where the presence of an afferent pupil defect is an indication that the eye is at risk of developing neovascular glaucoma at a later date.

The afferent pupil defect can be detected even when it is quite subtle, by using the swinging torch test and the basis of this is shown in Fig. 2.1.

2.3 THE VITREOUS

The vitreous humour is an inert, transparent gel, which fills the majority of the posterior segment of the eye. On normal ophthalmoscopy, it is easy to overlook abnormalities in the vitreous as they can be quite subtle, but small opacities within the vitreous cavity can be focused with the direct ophthalmoscope and particularly in the elderly where they give rise to the common symptom of floaters. These small opacities move around across the visual axis and because they are opacities in the gel, they do tend to move around very readily. This can be seen during examination. They represent small degenerative changes within the structure of the vitreous humour and are usually not serious.

A more important physical sign is the presence of a posterior vitreous detachment, which occurs when the vitreous humour loses its rather loose attachment with the optic disc and macula and comes loose, but maintaining its very strong attachment with the peripheral retina at the ora serrata. In this situation it is usually possible to see a ring opacity on the posterior face of the vitreous, where it was previously attached to the optic disc. This opacity can be noticed by the patient and is called Weiss's ring. Generally posterior vitreous detachments are harmless and they are common, but nevertheless they can be associated with the formation of peripheral retinal holes.

If haemorrhage occurs into the vitreous humour, the patient will complain of a sudden onset of floaters and may lose vision completely. If this

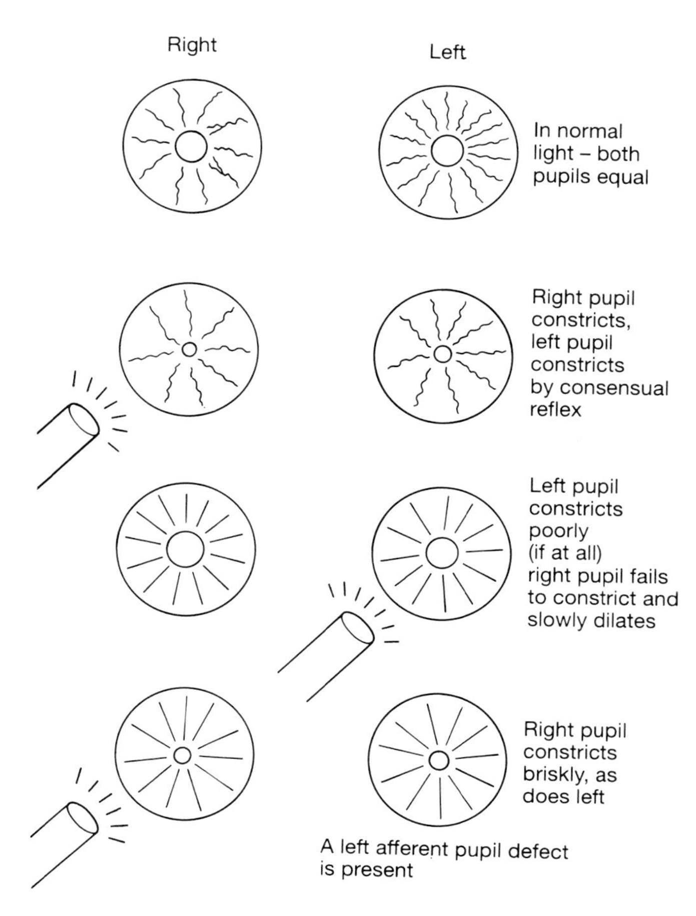

Fig. 2.1 Testing for an afferent pupil defect: the 'swinging flashlight test'.

haemorrhage is small it can be visualized with the direct ophthalmoscope. If there is a large vitreous haemorrhage, which has entered the substance of the gel, then it may not be possible to see any red reflex; in this situation ophthalmoscopy is unhelpful and the examiner has to resort to using an ophthalmic ultrasound to visualize the retina.

Asteroid hyalosis is an interesting but unusual condition in which there are multiple highly refractile particles within the vitreous humour, making it difficult to visualize retinal details. The refractile particles are thought to be due to a particular type of degeneration of the vitreous with formation of calcium soaps. This does not seem to be associated with any particular systemic condition, although the authors' clinical impression is that it does appear to be more common in diabetic patients.

2.4 THE RETINA – NORMAL ANATOMY AND LANDMARKS

Examination of the fundus shows some important landmarks, which can be identified (Fig. 1.5). The optic disc is about 15 mm in diameter and is composed of a central optic cup and a surrounding neural rim, which is usually yellowish-pink in colour. There are usually retinal vessels feeding the optic disc in each quadrant, those on the temporal side arching above and below the macula, the so-called arcade vessels.

The macula itself can be seen about 2 disc diameters away from the temporal side of the optic disc and appears slightly darker than the surrounding retina. The macula is quite large in diameter, being between 3 to 4 disc diameters across, and the central part of the macula is termed the fovea.

On examination the fovea can be distinguished by the presence of the yellow luteal pigment, xanthophyll. This is particularly easy to see in young patients and progressively harder to visualize in older patients. In younger patients the central part of the fovea does have quite a marked reflex and this is from the foveola, which has a pit at the central part. In children and young adults the surface of the retina in this region has a glistening-like quality. This is a normal reflex which is lost in older adults. The central part of the fovea has no retinal vessels feeding it and obtains its nutrition only from the choroid. This part of the fovea is termed the foveal avascular zone and is about 0.5 mm in diameter. This is an important clinical landmark for patients when fluorescein angiography is carried out, as it outlines the central part of the fovea and is an important guide as to where laser photocoagulation burns should be applied. Generally laser treatment is not applied within this area.

2.4.1 The fundus

Fundus examination may show, at 3 and 9 o'clock positions, a yellowish streak passing back from the front of the eye towards the posterior pole and this is the site of the long ciliary nerve and blood vessels. Similar streaks can sometimes be seen near the 6 and 9 o'clock positions in the fundus and these represent the position of the short ciliary nerves and blood vessels. The practical importance of these landmarks is that they are helpful in orientating oneself when examining the peripheral retina, but they are also quite sensitive when treated directly with laser and because of this they are sometimes avoided when using laser.

The appearance of the normal fundus will vary depending on the underlying amount of pigmentation within the body. In negroes and darkly pigmented races the fundus usually does have a darker appearance than in Caucasians and there may often be a ring of pigmentation around the optic disc. In fair skinned patients, particularly with blue eyes and blond hair, the deficiency of underlying retinal pigmentation means that the choroidal vessels can often be visualized very readily through the retina. These choroidal vessels appear as quite large reddish-brown lines, which are much larger than the overlying retinal vessels and arranged in a much more haphazardous fashion. This appearance is a variation of normal and reflects the underlying amount of pigmentation within the eye.

2.5 HAEMORRHAGES IN THE FUNDUS

A common and important physical sign on fundus examination is the presence of haemorrhage. The appearance and character of haemorrhage and its site give an important guide as to its likely source and the level at which it is occurring. Fundal haemorrhages usually occur at four levels (Fig. 2.2).

1. Pre-retinal haemorrhages (Fig. 2.2a) occur between the surface of the retina and the hyaloid face of the vitreous gel. They are sometimes called subhyaloid haemorrhages as a result of this and they have a characteristic appearance, which is very similar to a fluid level. The upper border of the haemorrhage often assumes the position of a horizontal line, but this can be disturbed depending on the posture of the patient. If pre-retinal haemorrhages are large they can break through the inner limiting membrane and into the vitreous humour causing a vitreous haemorrhage.
2. Nerve fibre layer haemorrhages (Fig. 2.2b) are haemorrhages from vessels in the inner retina which tend to infiltrate between the axons of the nerve fibre there and assume a characteristic flame-shape. These haemorrhages are superficial but located within the retina and have their rather feathery appearance because of the presence of the nerve fibres within this layer. Such haemorrhages are often seen in association with systemic hypertension, but also occur in a wide variety of other systemic and ophthalmic conditions.
3. Intra-retinal haemorrhages or dot and blot haemorrhages (Fig. 2.2c) are small haemorrhages originating from deeper capillaries within the retina and are located within the compact inner nuclear and outer plexiform layers of the retina. Because of these constraints the haemorrhages are always very small. In diabetic retinopathy it is often difficult to differentiate between dot haemorrhages and micro-aneurysms, but a useful guide to this is that micro-aneurysms often appear to have sharper borders to them on direct ophthalmoscopy. They can, of course, be readily distinguished during fluorescein angiography.
4. Subretinal haemorrhages (Fig. 2.2d) originate from the choroidal circulation and can become quite large, often lifting the overlying retina upwards. The hallmark of subretinal haemorrhages is that the retinal vessels appear normal overlying them and the haemorrhages themselves are rather darker than normal. Subretinal haemorrhages can arise from subretinal neovascular membranes (networks of vessels), which arise from the choroidal circulation and through deficiencies in Bruch's membrane to lift up the overlying retinal pigment epithelium.

2.6 EXUDATION

Hard exudates are seen in a variety of important retino-vascular conditions:

- diabetes mellitus
- systemic hypertension
- retinal vein occlusion
- retinal telangiectasia
- Coats' disease
- familial exudative vitreoretinopathy
- subretinal neovascular membranes
- retinal capillary angiomata

They have a yellow waxy appearance with sharply defined borders and represent the residue of oedema, which has leaked into the retina from abnormal retinal vessels (Fig. 2.3). Retinal exudates tend to accumulate in the outer plexiform layer, where the tissue is most lax. Exudates which derive from vessels in the macular area are located between the radially arranged fibres of Henle's layer and assume a characteristic stellate pattern or macular star. Where exudates are located further away from the fovea they tend to assume a ringlike or circinate conformation around the site of leakage, such as from a retinal micro-aneurysm or a diseased capillary leakage.

If a large amount of exudate is seen at the macula, it should not be assumed that the site of leakage is wholly at the macula. The so-called 'exaggerated macular response' can occur in conditions where there is enormous peripheral retinal vascular abnormality and as a result of this response, fluid and exudate precipitate out at the macula and are seen as a large macular star and accumulation of lipid. Such an exaggerated macular response is seen typically in conditions such as Coats' disease, familial exudative vitreoretinopathy, Von Hippel-Lindau disease and in some retinal vascular occlusions. This is a reminder that a careful examination of the entire retina is always important when abnormalities are seen at the macula. A particular type of exudation that is seen within the retina is so-called candle wax exudates, which occur along retinal vessels in sarcoidosis. In this situation it is usually accompanied by a papillitis.

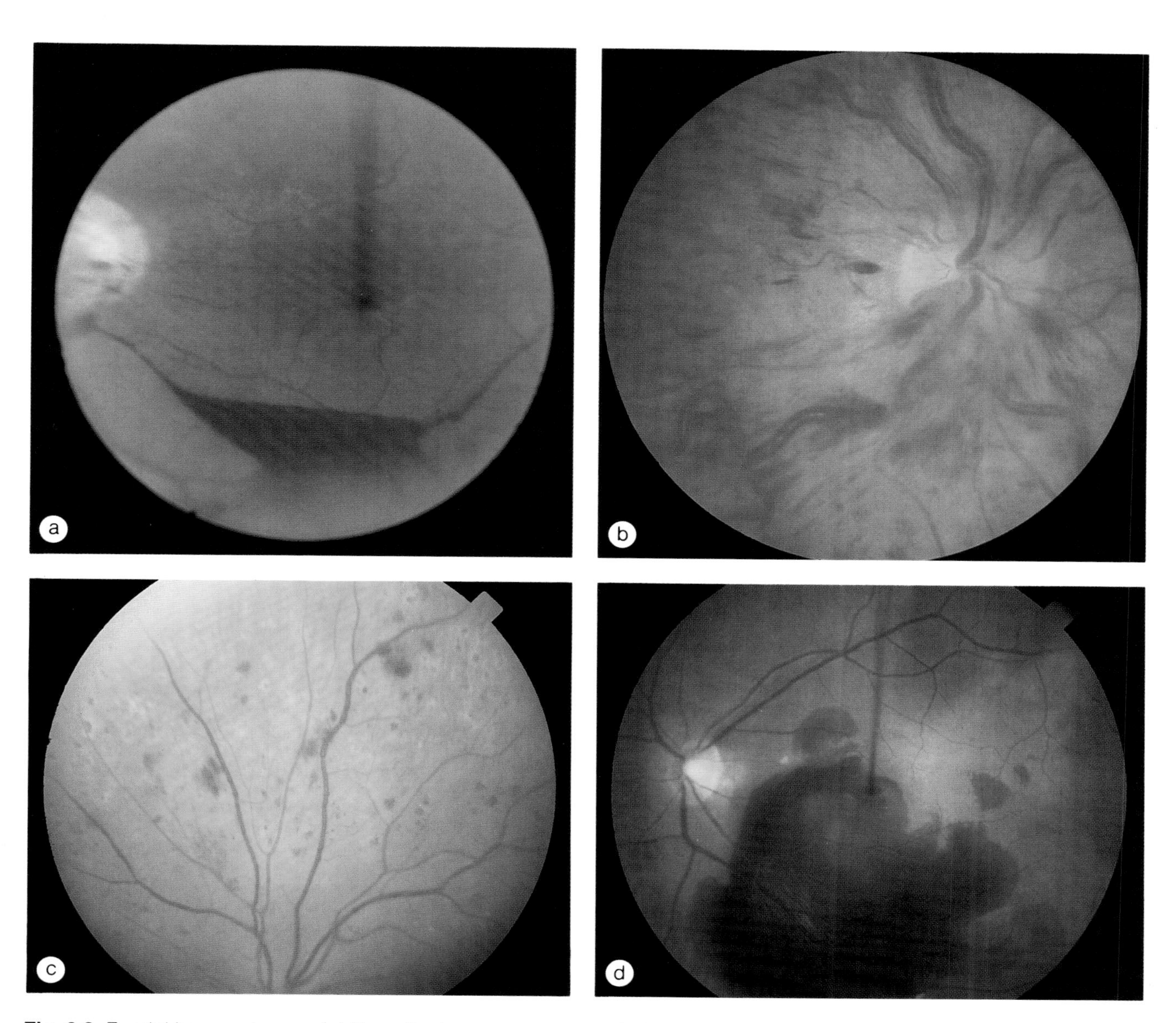

Fig. 2.2 Fundal haemorrhages. (a) Pre-retinal haemorrhage from bleeding of optic disc new vessels in diabetic patient. (b) Multiple nerve fibre haemorrhages in central retinal vein occlusion. (c) Small and large intraretinal haemorrhages in a diabetic patient. (d) Large subretinal haemorrhages in a case of age-related macular degeneration.

2.7 COTTON WOOL SPOTS

Cotton wool spots are discrete lesions found in the nerve fibre layer of the retina, which appear to have a characteristic fluffy white opacification and are a feature of several different types of vascular retinopathies (Fig. 2.4). They are basically a sign of focal ischaemia of the retina. Pathological interpretation of this physical sign is that they represent swelling of the nerve fibre layer and disruption of normal axoplasmic flow, within the nerve fibre layers, as seen in conditions in which focal ischaemia occurs:

- Hypertension
- Diabetic retinopathy (pre-proliferative)
- Retinal vascular occlusion
- Collagen vascular disorders
- Acute ischaemic optic neuropathy
- Leukaemia
- Radiation retinopathy
- Trauma
- Septicaemia
- Dysproteinaemia
- Severe anaemia
- Ocular ischaemic syndrome
- Cardiac vascular disease

In diabetic patients the presence of multiple cotton wool spots implies that the retinopathy has reached an ischaemic stage and this is one of the characteristics of pre-proliferative retinopathy. Following central retinal vein occlusion, the presence of multiple cotton wool spots again implies that the retinopathy is ischaemic and this has the important prognostic significance of a higher chance of neovascular glaucoma developing later. This is usually an indication to carry out prophylactic panretinal photocoagulation.

2.8 MACULAR OEDEMA

Oedema at the macula can assume a characteristic appearance, which is called cystoid macular oedema. Clinically this appears as though there are multiple petals around the macula: these represent cysts full of extracellular fluid. The fluid is thought to arise from the peri-foveal capillaries and these cause cystic spaces to occur within the Henle's nerve fibre layer in the superficial part of the retina. Cystoid macular degeneration may occur due to a variety of reasons:

- Diabetic retinopathy
- Uveitis, retinal vasculitis
- Pars planitis
- Retinal vein occlusion (central/branch)
- Subretinal neovascular membrane
- Retinal dystrophy (retinis pigmentosa)
- Retinal detachment surgery
- Aphakia (especially intracapsular surgery)
- Drug related

Almost always visual acuity is compromised and if the oedema is present for any length of time, the prospect of full visual recurrence is lessened.

Diffuse macular oedema can occur in diabetic patients, when there is a generalized leakage of extra-cellular fluid from multiple perimacular capillaries and micro-aneurysms. Macular oedema is notoriously difficult to assess by direct ophthalmo-

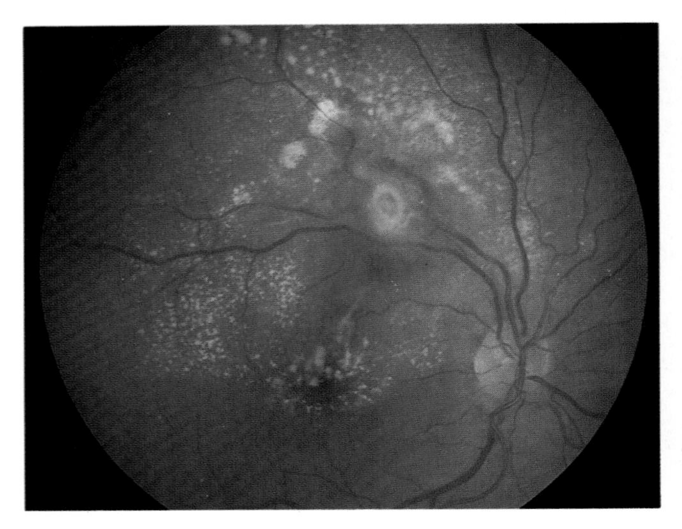

Fig. 2.3 Hard exudates from retinal arteriolar macroaneurysms.

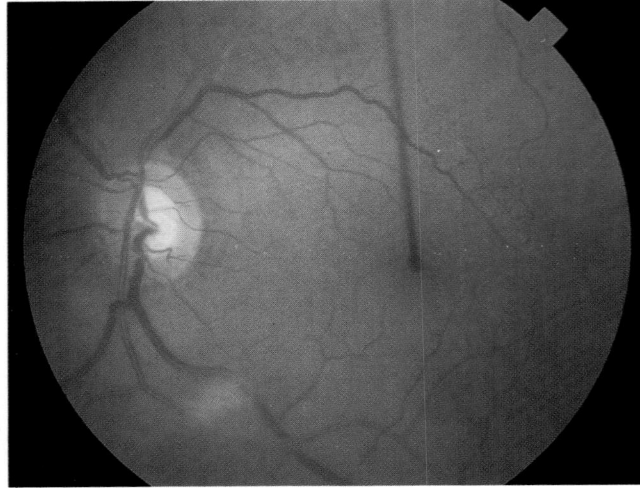

Fig. 2.4 Cotton-wool spot in fundus.

scopy alone and some form of stereoscopic examination is necessary to measure and judge the amount of oedema that is present in the retina. In fluorescein angiography such oedema is seen as leakage of fluorescein in later phases of the angiogram (Fig. 2.5).

2.9 THE RETINAL VESSELS

The appearance of the retinal vessels on fundus examination is quite characteristic with the four quadrants of the fundus each containing and being supplied by a major pair of retinal vessels, comprising a retinal artery and vein (Fig. 2.6). In a normal fundus the retinal arterioles appear a lighter colour than the veins and the veins are somewhat larger than the arteriole at any corresponding point in a ratio of 3:2. Whether the retinal arteries are in fact arterioles is a somewhat arbitrary distinction. Some authors have based their classification of these vessels on their size, the absence of a continuous internal elastic lamina and the number of smooth muscle cells in cross-section of the wall. The distinction as to whether the larger vessels are small arteries or in fact arterioles is probably not helpful, but the important thing is that as the pre-capillary arteriole is reached the amount of muscle present in the vessel wall becomes small and the capillaries themselves are distinguished from terminal arterioles by being entirely devoid of smooth muscle.

The normal retinal arteriole and vein have transparent walls, but with ageing and in other pathological processes these walls can lose their transparen-

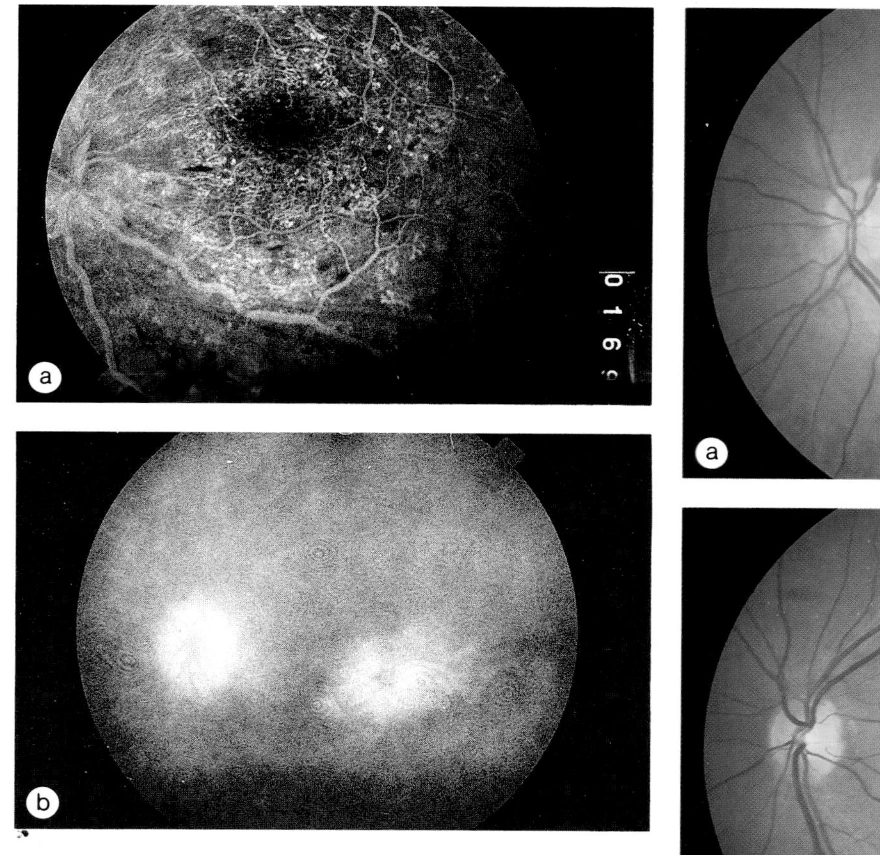

Fig. 2.5 Fluorescein angiogram in a case of macular oedema in a young diabetic patient. (a) Early phase. (b) Late phase showing cystoid macular oedema.

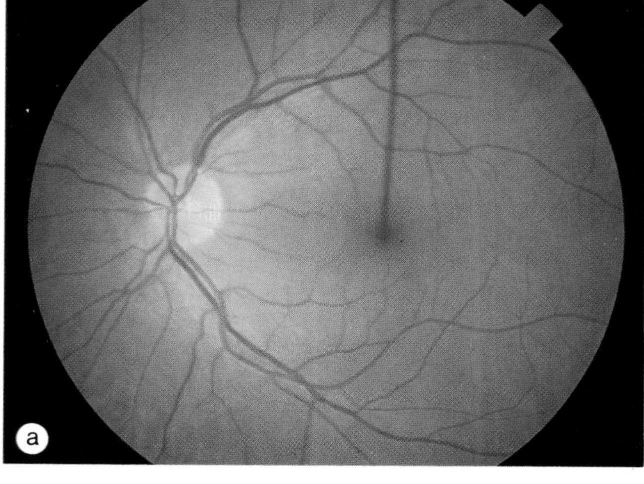

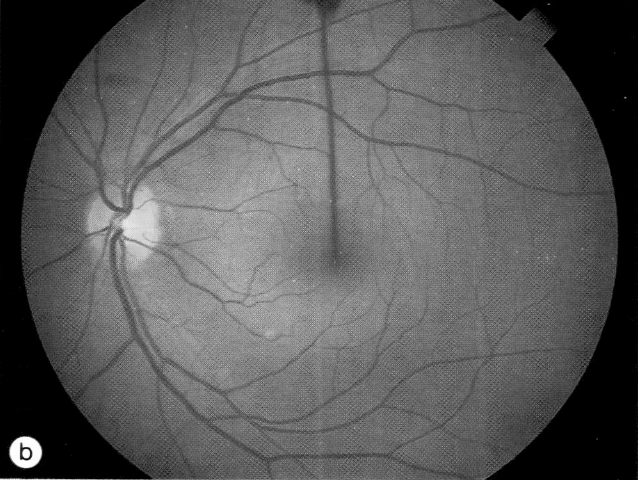

Fig. 2.6 Normal fundus appearance with fixation marker. (a) and (b) are different patients.

cy and become visible. This is seen in arteriolarsclerosis (Fig. 2.7) which may, or may not, be related to essential hypertension.

Arteriovenous crossing changes, the so-called Salus sign, occur at the crossing points of retinal arterioles and attendant vein, where the vein is deviated by the wall of the arteriole. This is thought to occur because the vein and the arteriole are in a common sheath at the point of their crossing. Arteriovenous crossing changes are an indication of atherosclerotic disease in the retinal arterioles, rather than a sign of systemic hypertension. In fact the most relevant sign of hypertension in the fundus is probably focal arteriolar narrowing and this seems to directly represent the amount of hypertensive damage that has been caused to the vessels.

Changes in the retinal veins are commonly seen in retinal vascular and other diseases:

1. Enlarged, tortuous veins – hyperviscosity syndromes, chronic obstructive airways disease, diabetes mellitus.
2. Venous beading and loops – diabetes mellitus, retinal vascular occlusion.
3. Exudative venous leakage – diabetes mellitus, retinal vascular occlusion.
4. Narrowed veins – retinal vein occlusion, retinal arterial occlusion.
5. Sheathing of retinal veins – (periphlebitis) sarcoidosis, multiple sclerosis, retinal vascular occlusion.

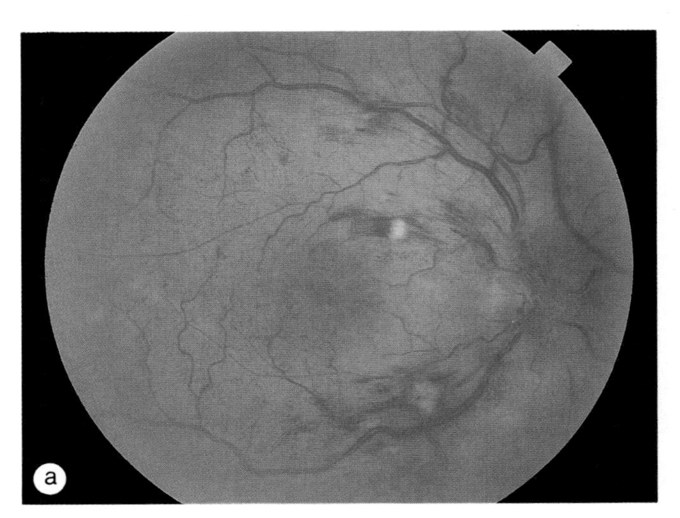

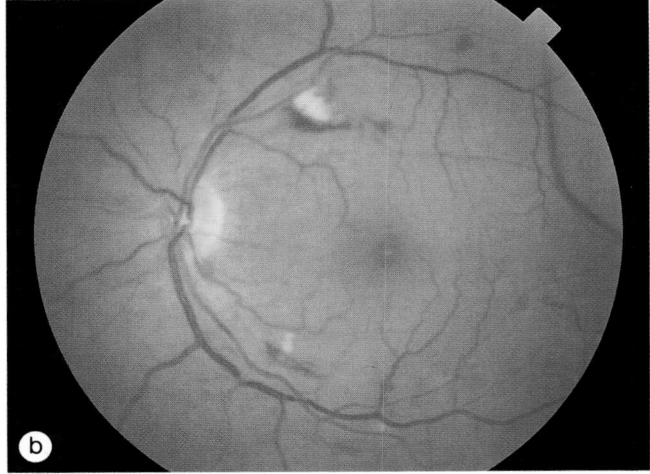

Fig. 2.7 Hypertensive retinopathy (accelerated hypertension). (a) right, (b) left eye.

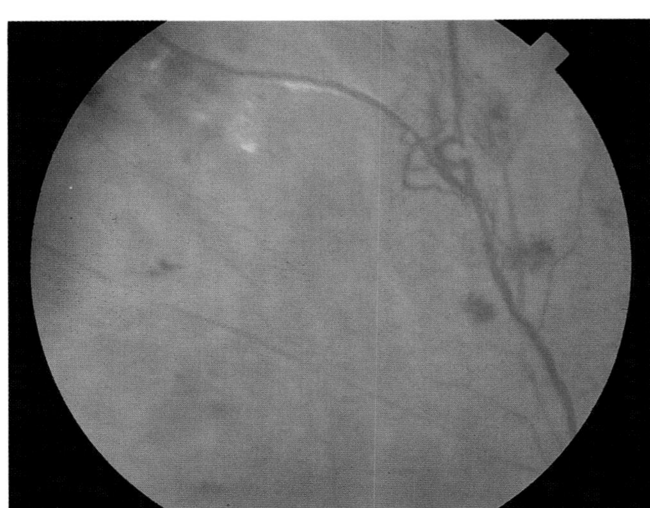

Fig. 2.8 Beading and loops of retinal veins in a diabetic patient.

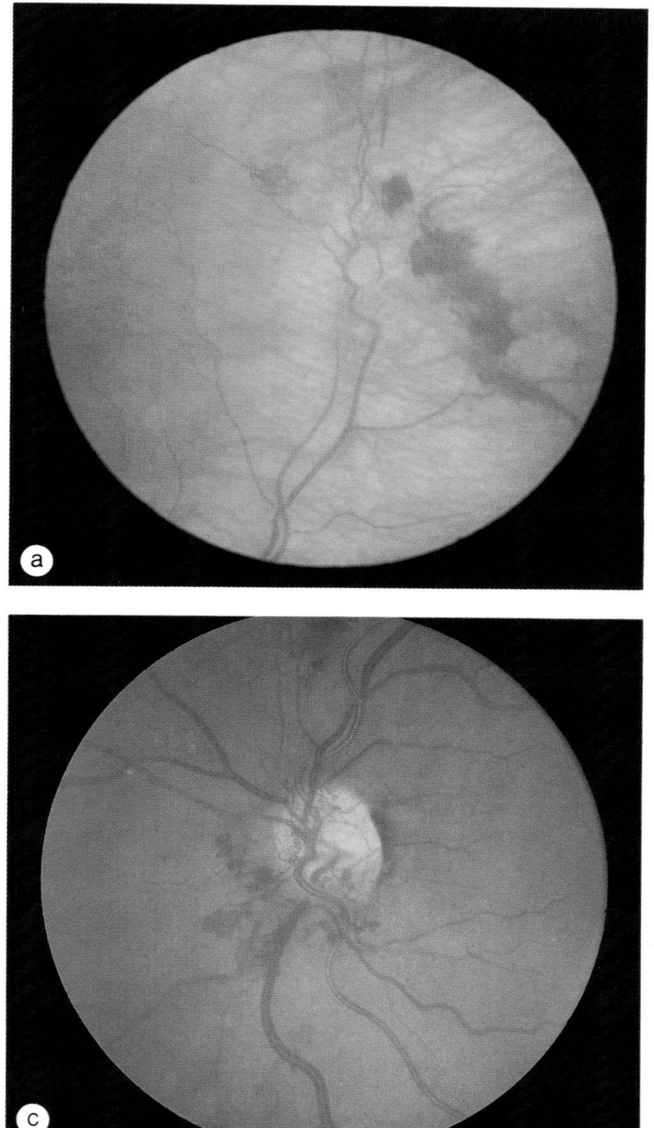

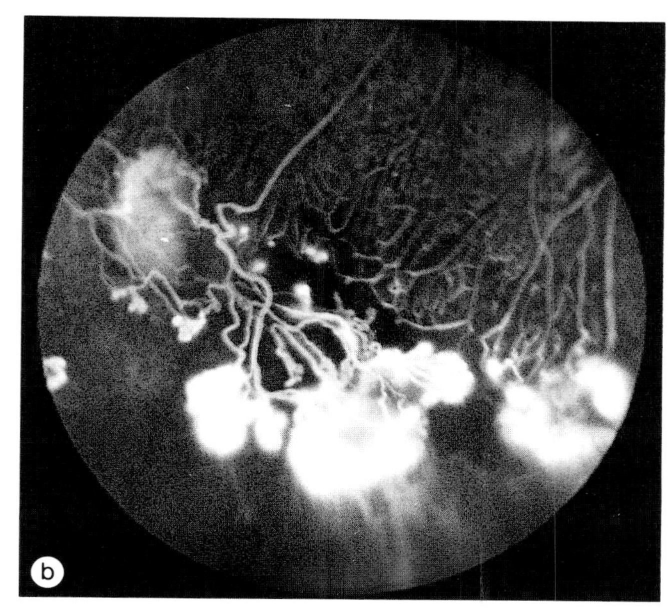

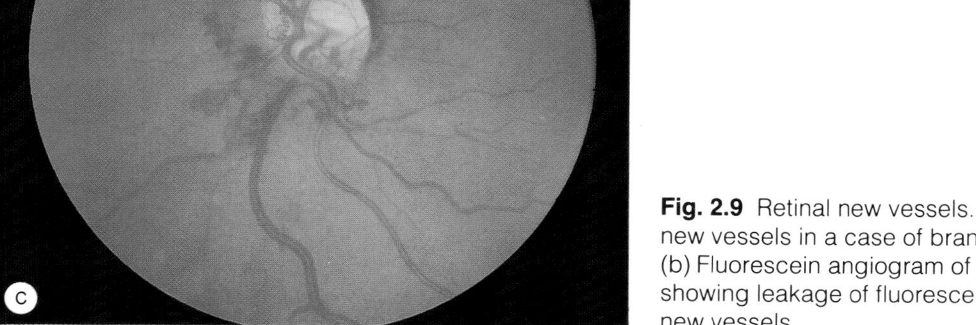

Fig. 2.9 Retinal new vessels. (a) Peripheral bleeding retinal new vessels in a case of branch retinal vein occlusion. (b) Fluorescein angiogram of peripheral new vessels showing leakage of fluorescein in late phase. (c) Optic disc new vessels.

Increased retinal vein tortuosity and diameter occur in conditions in which there is hyperviscosity of the blood. The appearance in these cases is quite characteristic with the veins often looking extremely full and being much larger in comparison to the retinal arterioles which they are paired with. Increased retinal vein size is often a very early sign of diabetic retinopathy, but in pre-proliferative diabetic retinopathy the retinal veins often assume quite bizarre forms with venous beading and venous loops occurring on the veins. The exact cause of these rather unusual signs is unknown but it has been postulated that this may be a type of abortive, neovascular proliferation. These signs are shown in Fig. 2.8.

Retinal new vessels, which occur in diabetic retinopathy or following retinal vascular occlusive disease, have a characteristic appearance, being much smaller than their corresponding retinal veins, and often arising in lacy networks or fans from the vessels (Fig. 2.9). In diabetic retinopathy common sites of such retinal new vessels are from the optic disc, the retinal arcade vessels above and below the macula, in the watershed areas temporal to the macula and on the nasal side of the optic disc.

2.10 AGE-RELATED MACULAR DEGENERATION

Age-related macular degeneration is a common finding in elderly patients and is the commonest cause of visual loss in those aged 65 years and over. Frequently the earliest clinical manifestation of age-related macular degeneration is the presence of retinal drusen (Fig. 2.10a) and these are sometimes quite commonly confused with retinal exudates. Retinal drusen normally occur at the macula and have the appearance of being small, yellowish dots mainly at the posterior pole. Drusen can appear to be 'hard' in which case they have firm borders and are relatively small and this should be compared with so-called 'soft' drusen, which have more indistinct edges and are larger, frequently becoming confluent. Some drusen which have been present for a long time become calcified and these have a very glistening appearance. Normally, with age-related macular degeneration retinal drusen are bilateral and symmetrical in their distribution throughout the retina and this helps to distinguish them from retinal exudates, which often arise in a relatively haphazard fashion around retinal vascular abnormalities. Retinal exudates tend to look harder and waxier than drusen.

Age-related macular degeneration can be divided into two types. In the dry or atrophic type of degenerative change there is atrophy and pigmentary change within the retinal pigment epithelium, giving rise to multiple areas of thinning and degeneration within the central retina. Generally this is associated with a gradual, slowly progressive loss of central vision. This is in contrast to the other type of age-related macular degeneration, the exudative, or neovascular type. This occurs when a small retinal meshwork of blood vessels grows through defects in Bruch's membrane and causes a haemorrhagic detachment of the retinal pigment epithelium and sensory neuroretina to occur (Fig. 2.10b). This usually goes on to form a so-called disciform response in which there is a round shaped area of disturbance in the central macula, which is gradually replaced by a central scar and resulting loss of central vision. This type of macular degeneration often develops very quickly with the cardinal feature being sudden onset of distortion of vision, implying that the retina has been elevated and the photoreceptors disturbed. This type of macular degeneration is in some cases amenable to direct laser treatment when the subretinal network of vessels can be sealed off directly. Unfortunately this seems only to be possible in those cases which are caught at an early stage.

2.11 ANGIOID STREAKS

Angioid streaks have an unusual appearance in the fundus (Fig. 2.11) and are so-called because of their

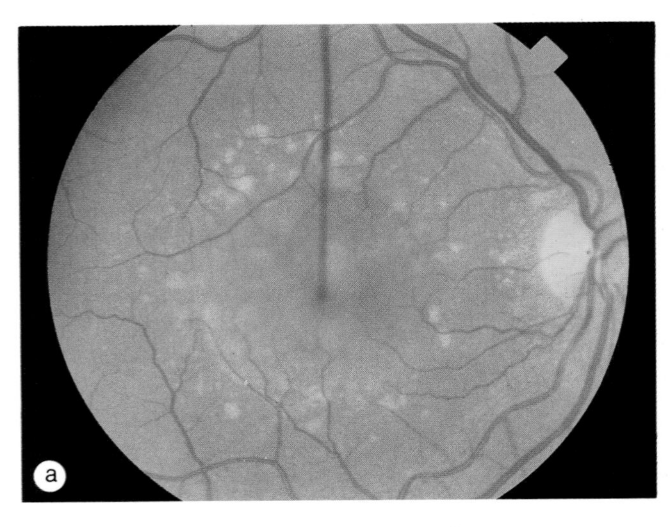

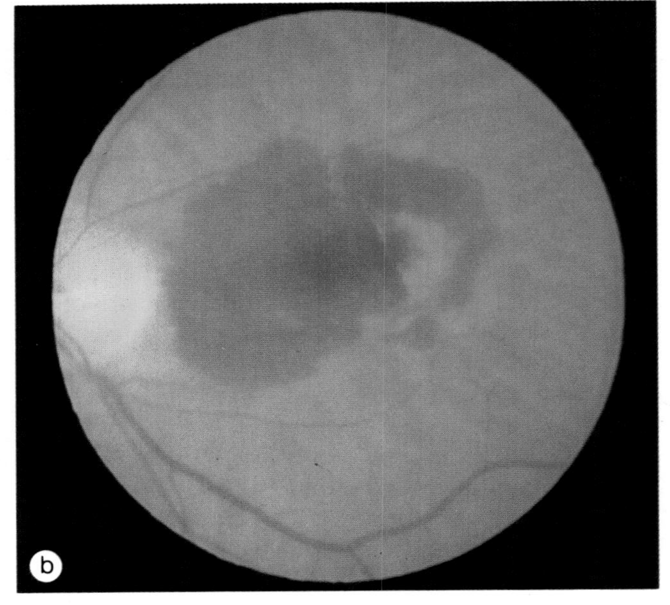

Fig. 2.10 Age-related macular degeneration. (a) Retinal drusen in a case of dry, age-related macular degeneration. (b) Sub-retinal macular haemorrhage in a case with sub-retinal neovascular membrane.

similarity to branching blood vessels. They are caused by separations in Bruch's membrane, which is the underlying basement membrane under the retina. The streaks are a dark brown/orange colour and they radiate out in an irregular fashion from the optic disc. Angioid streaks are associated with a number of systemic conditions:

- Pseudoxanthasma mastium
- Paget's disease of bone
- Ehler's–Danlos syndrome
- Haemoglobinopathies

The cause of the angioid streaks is thought to be degenerative changes within Bruch's membrane. They are associated with the development of the ingrowth of subretinal neovascular networks from the choroidal circulation, under the retina, forming a disciform response. Prompt detection and treatment of these neovascular networks with laser photocoagulation, can preserve central vision if they are referred at an early stage.

Angioid streaks are often associated with secondary changes within the retina such as pigmentary retinal mottling, the so-called peau d'orange appearance, peripapillary chorioretinal atrophy and occasionally optic nerve head drusen. Angioid streaks have a characteristic appearance and once seen in a patient are never forgotten.

2.12 CHOROIDAL AND RETINAL FOLDS

Choroidal folds occur in a number of conditions:

- Proptosis (dysthyroid eye disease, pseudotumour)
- Orbital tumour
- High hypermetropia
- Hypotomy of the eye
- Ocular inflammation (uveitis, scleritis)

They appear as parallel and horizontal folds and are most prominently seen at the posterior pole. Fluorescein angiography can be used to confirm the appearance, with the folds appearing as horizontal, hyper- and hypofluorescent streaks, with the troughs of the folds appearing darker than the crests.

They should be distinguished from retinal folds, which are usually caused by contraction of a chorioidoretinal or fibroglial scar. Retinal folds occur in vascular retinopathies following retinal detachment surgery or occasionally heavy photocoagulation scars. Epiretinal membrane formation, on the surface of the retina, can result in surface wrinkling of the retina, which takes the appearance of wrinkled cellophane, so-called 'cellophane retinopathy'. In some cases if the vision has been threatened by this process, the epiretinal membrane can be removed by vitreoretinal surgery.

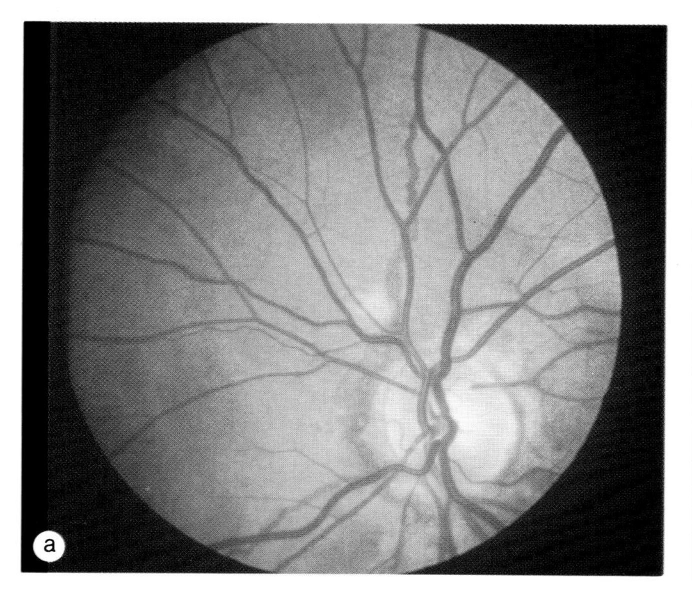

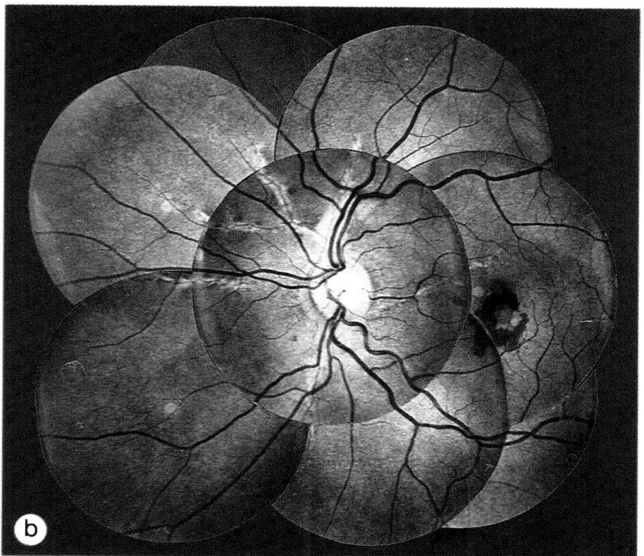

Fig. 2.11 (a) Characteristic appearance of angioid streaks. (b) Composite red-free fundus photograph of angioid streaks with sub-retinal haemorrhage at macula. (Courtesy of the British Journal of Ophthalmology.)

3 *Specific ophthalmological investigations*

Clinical Retinopathies. Paul M. Dodson, Jonathan M. Gibson and Erna E. Kritzinger.
Published in 1995 by Chapman & Hall, London. ISBN 0 412 35930 8

3.1 TESTS OF VISION

3.1.1 Visual acuity tests

Testing the visual acuity of the patient with retinopathy is of obvious importance, but in a busy clinic in hospital or general practice it is easily missed out. Visual acuity testing measures the form vision sense of the eye, which is made up of the resolving power of the eye (the minimum separable stimulus) and the perceptual power of the visual system to recognize the nature of the stimulus (the minimum recognizable stimulus).

The vision of each eye should be checked separately and for this it is helpful to use an opaque occluder or card to cover each eye in turn. It is customary to measure the distance visual acuity at 6 metres with a Snellen test chart (Fig. 3.1), but reduced charts are available which can be used at 3 metres. If the patient normally wears spectacles for distance, these should be worn for the test.

The visual acuity is measured as the last complete line on the chart which the patient reads without making a mistake and it is recorded as an expression of the line of letters which can be discerned at a particular distance. If only the top letter can be read, this is recorded as 6/60, where 6 is the distance from the test chart in metres and 60 equals the distance at which the letter which was read subtends an angle of 5° at the nodal point of the eye. A 'normal' level of vision is 6/6 although many patients are able to see 6/5 or 6/4.

(a) THE PINHOLE TEST

A useful addition to the test is to use a pinhole for the patient to look through. If the patient has poor vision which improves with the pinhole, it means that there is an uncorrected refractive error present. It is particularly useful for those patients who have forgotten their spectacles and have uncorrected poor vision. If the vision does not improve with the pinhole, it usually means that there is an ocular cause for this.

(b) NEAR VISUAL ACUITY

Near vision is measured with reading spectacles if normally worn, for each eye separately and binocularly. The result is expressed in 'N' numbers referring to the print size of the test type. N48 for instance is the largest type, whilst N4.5 is the smallest. An alternative test makes use of 'J' types.

In some conditions distance and near vision are affected disproportionately, and this is why it is important to test at both near and distance. In macular disorders, for example, and in posterior subcapsular cataract, the near vision may be quite severely compromised whilst the distance vision is relatively normal. In other types of cataract near vision may be preserved whilst distance vision has deteriorated significantly.

Contrast sensitivity testing is an additional test of visual function, which can provide information about the patient's ability to see large, low-contrast objects which tests of visual acuity do not. Contrast sensitivity tests will most likely remain an adjunct rather than a replacement for testing visual acuity for clinical purposes.

3.1.2 Visual field testing

Testing the visual field is an important and essential part of the ophthalmic examination, as it tests the integrity of the visual pathway from the retina to the visual cortex. In assessing patients with retinopathy however, perimetry has a limited role to play in routine clinical management. Automated perimetry (Fig. 3.2) has been used as a means of comparing functional and structural changes in the retina but its use is not widespread.

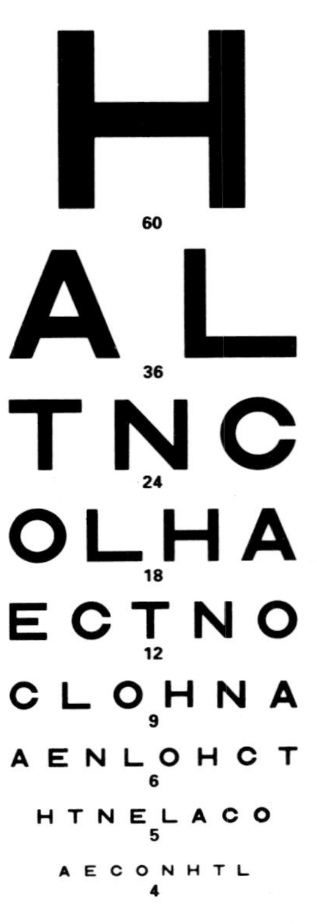

Fig. 3.1 Snellen test chart.

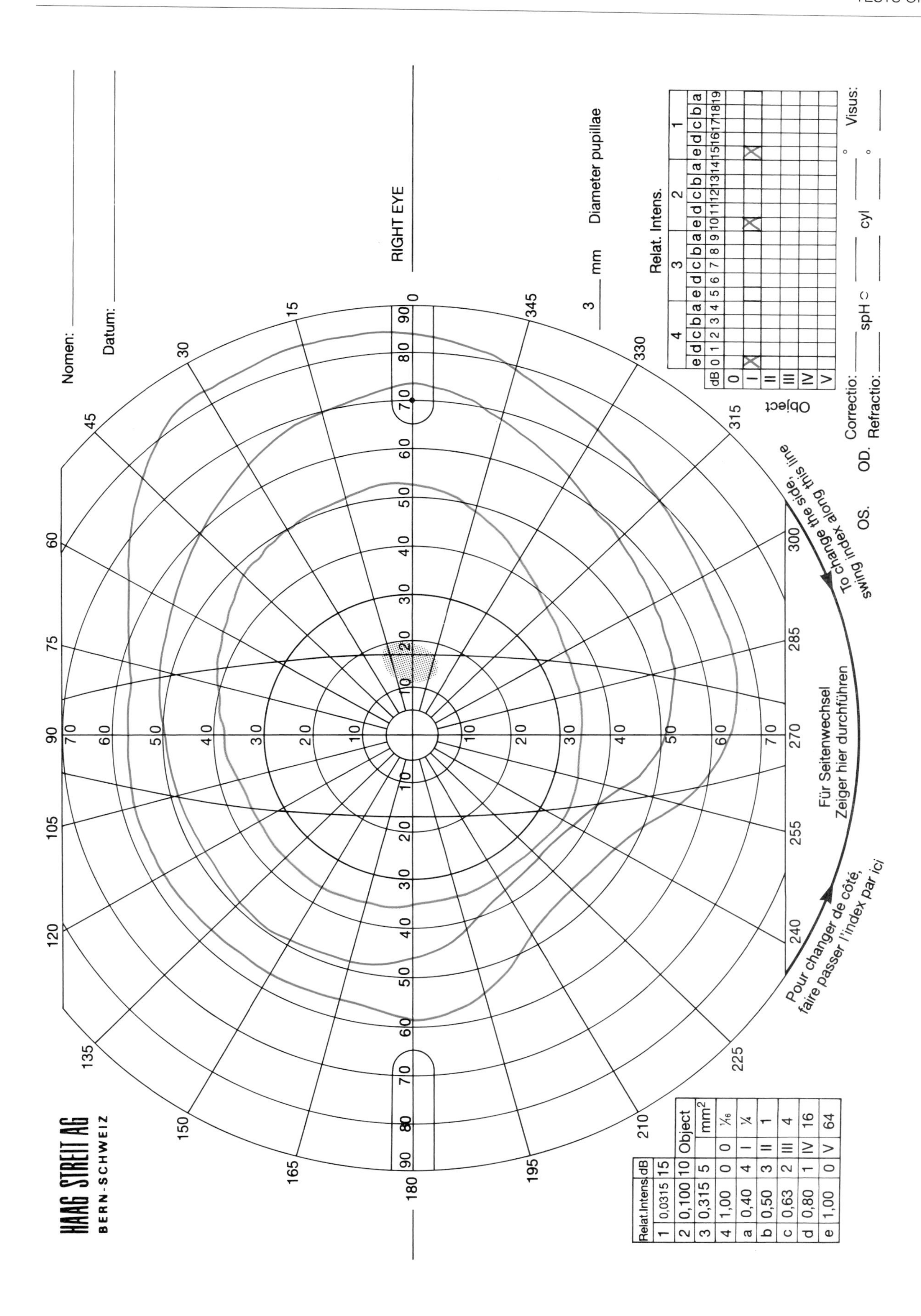

Fig. 3.2 Normal Goldmann visual field. Right eye.

Name ______________________ Age ______________________ Date ____/____/____

85	1	2	3	4	5	6	7	8	9	10	11	12	13	14	15	16	17	18	19	20	21
22	23	24	25	26	27	28	29	30	31	32	33	34	35	36	37	38	39	40	41	42	
43	44	45	46	47	48	49	50	51	52	53	54	55	56	57	58	59	60	61	62	63	
64	65	66	67	68	69	70	71	72	73	74	75	76	77	78	79	80	81	82	83	84	

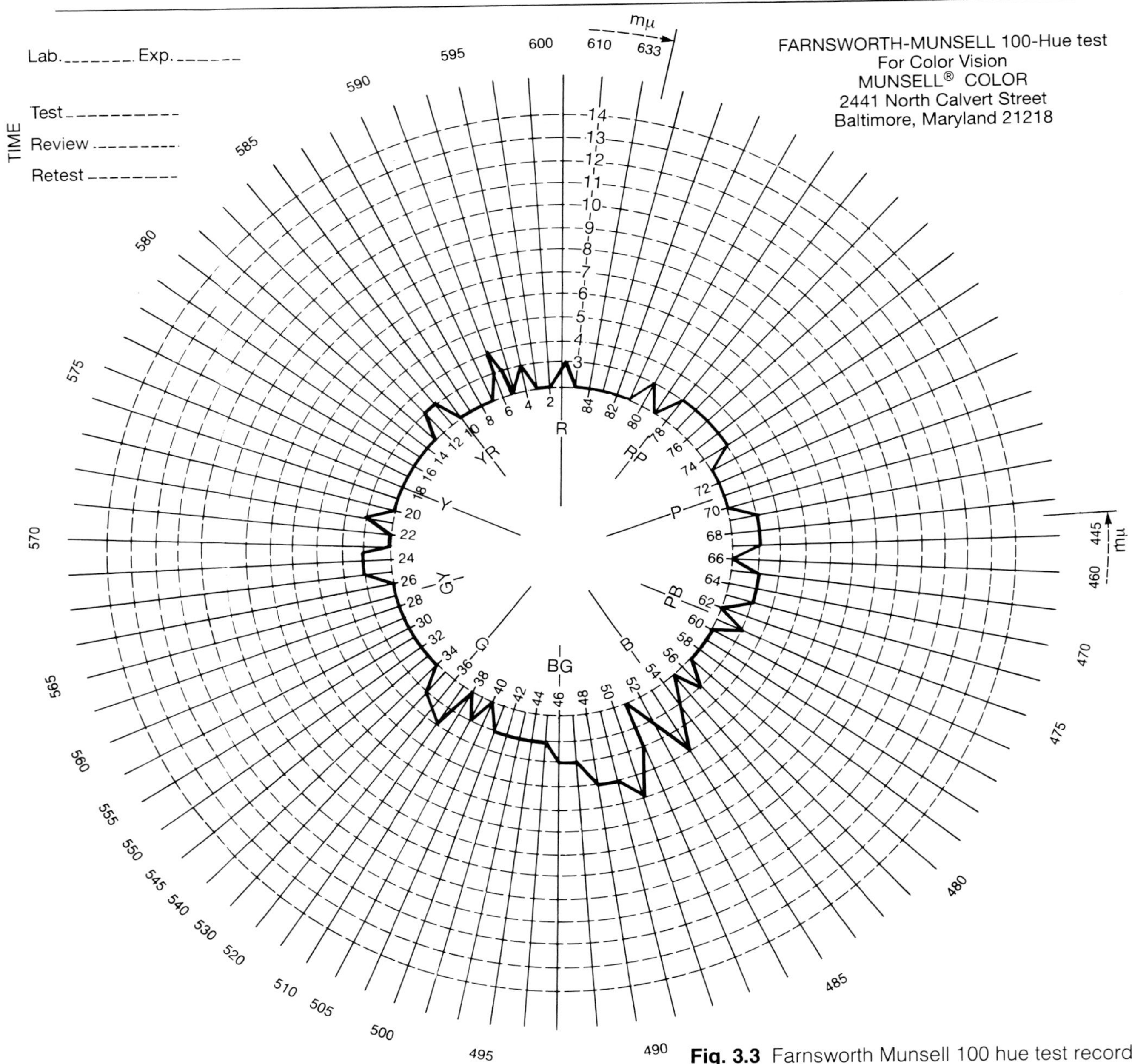

Fig. 3.3 Farnsworth Munsell 100 hue test recording. (a) Normal. TES = 63. (b) Tritanopic (blue-yellow axis) defect. TES = 452 (cf. normal <100).

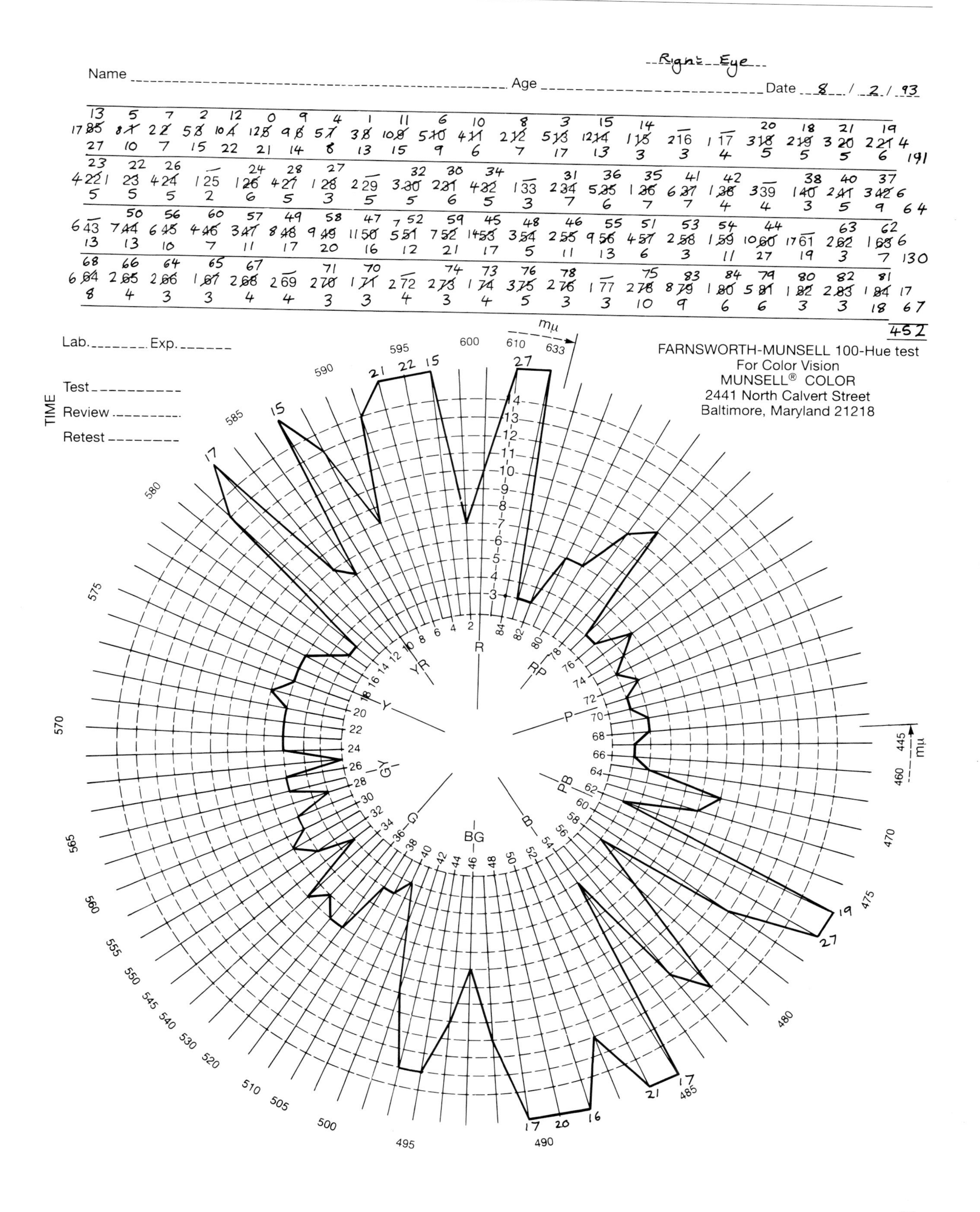
Right Eye
Name
Age
Date 8 / 2 / 93
452
Lab. Exp.
TIME
Test
Review
Retest
FARNSWORTH-MUNSELL 100-Hue test
For Color Vision
MUNSELL® COLOR
2441 North Calvert Street
Baltimore, Maryland 21218
mμ
R
YR
Y
GY
G
BG
B
PB
P
RP

3.1.3 Colour vision

Congenital colour vision defects affect both eyes in the same manner and are usually stationary. Acquired defects may be secondary to retinal or optic nerve disease, are not present at birth and usually change over a period of time.

The most well known colour vision test is the Ishihara test, which consists of a series of coloured plates composed of small coloured dots. The test is easy to carry out but will only detect in the red–green axis. The City University test is a similar but more useful test in that it will also detect abnormalities in the blue–yellow axis. It is in a book form and is easy to perform.

The gold standard test is the Farnsworth Munsell 100 hue test (Fig. 3.3), which uses coloured caps that have to be arranged in a particular order corresponding to their colour. Despite its name the test actually comprises 85 coloured caps divided between four boxes, each with fixed reference caps. The coloured caps are of equal brightness and colour saturation and the test, which is quite time-consuming, is designed to be undertaken in daylight or its artificial equivalent.

The test is scored by means of a special chart which shows the distribution of the errors and the axis of the colour defect. The Farnsworth Munsell D–15 test is an abbreviated version of the 100 hue test and is therefore very useful clinically, especially in patients with poor visual acuity.

In retinal disease colour vision abnormalities have been reported in a variety of different conditions. An important cause of acquired retinal disease that may cause colour vision defects is dabetic retinopathy in which blue–yellow discrimination is affected before red–green.

Abnormalities in colour vision can be detected in some patients before retinopathy is visible, but whether it can be used in screening for diabetic retinopathy is far from clear. A practical aspect of this is that some diabetic patients may have difficulties performing home monitoring of their diabetes if they have colour vision abnormalities. Argon laser photocoagulation causes considerable deterioration in overall colour discrimination for patients, particularly for blue–yellow. In the United Kingdom attention has recently turned to the effect such lasers may have on the colour vision of ophthalmologists.

3.2 TESTS OF MACULAR FUNCTION

The macula lutea is the site of central, fine discriminatory vision and also of colour vision. The important symptom of macular disease is an abnormality of central vision. This may take the form of a positive scotoma (a blind spot), metamorphopsia (distortion of vision), micropsia (diminution of image size) and macropsia (increase in image size). Since most of the cones of the retina are situated within the macula, abnormalities of colour vision also occur (dyschromotopsia).

Clinically the easiest test of macular function is the test of visual acuity, but there are other tests that are available which can yield more information.

3.2.1 Amsler chart

This test, which is named after the ophthalmologist who first described it, is a very useful test for diagnosis of and for following the course of macular disorders. It consists of a squared chart 10 cm × 10 cm in size, with a central black fixation spot (Fig. 3.4). The patient is asked to look at the central spot with each eye in turn, with reading spectacles if they are normally worn. The patient is asked to note any distortion of the squares, any wavy lines, blurred areas or blank spots in the grid, and it is helpful to mark these down on the grid.

The test is in effect a static perimetry test of the central part of the visual field. There are several modifications of the test in the test booklet and recently several authors have described how the test can be made more sensitive and quantified.

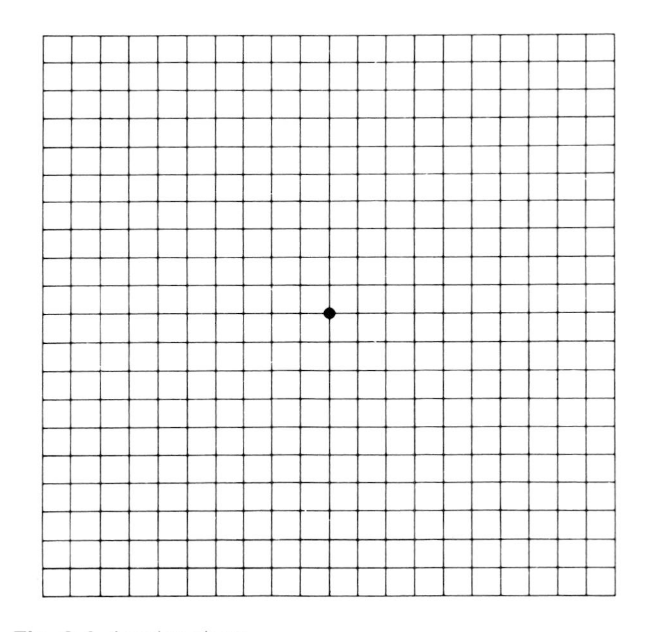

Fig. 3.4 Amsler chart.

3.2.2 Macular photostress test

This test is useful in confirming macular disease when fundus examination is inconclusive. It is particularly useful in differentiating between macular and optic nerve disease. For the test the best corrected visual acuity is measured. The patient is then asked to look at a very bright light from a pen torch or ophthalmoscope, held about 2–3 cm from the eye being tested, for a fixed period of time, normally 10 seconds. The time taken for the patient to read any three letters of the pre-test acuity line is measured and is the photostress recovery time.

The recovery time is dependent on the integrity of the retinal pigment epithelium and photoreceptor layers. It is measured for each eye in turn and then compared. For conditions affecting the macula, such as cystoid macular oedema or central serous retinopathy, the time will be very prolonged. It is extremely useful in distinguishing macular disease from optic nerve disorders, such as optic neuritis, because it will be normal in these. If used under standardized conditions it can be useful in following chronic disease such as diabetic maculopathy.

3.2.3 Maddox rod test

This is a very simple test which uses the Maddox rod, a red-coloured trial lens composed of a series of cylindrical lenses. This has the effect of converting a point source of white light, such as a pen torch, into a bright red line. It is used mainly in assessment of ocular motility, but is also a quick and easy way of screening for macular disorders, such as diabetic maculopathy.

The patient is asked to look through the Maddox rod with the other eye closed, at a pen torch. Normally the subject would be expected to see a red line but if macular disease is present causing a relative scotoma, the line will appear to have a gap in the middle.

3.3 OPHTHALMOSCOPY

The invention of the direct ophthalmoscope has been attributed to Von Helmholtz in 1851, although some authorities also note the ideas proposed by Babbage in 1847. The use of the ophthalmoscope marked the beginning of a new era in ophthalmology because for the first time the structures in the posterior segment of the eye could be visualized during life, and it led to an explosion of interest and information. Today ophthalmoscopy remains a crucial part of the general medical examination of patients and for the assessment of retinopathy it is of obvious importance.

The direct ophthalmoscope, which is the familiar hand-held instrument, is easy to use with practice but it is useful to have a plan of action when examining the fundus. Fundus examination is made much easier with adequate pupillary dilatation and this can be achieved with tropicamide 1.0% or 0.5%, which is a short-acting mydriatic, acting within a few minutes. Phenylephrine 10% drops are a useful adjunct for diabetic patients where the pupils may not dilate very readily.

It is difficult to underestimate the value of using mydriatic eyedrops for ophthalmoscopy, because it is virtually impossible for even the most experienced ophthalmoscopist to examine the fundus properly without the pupils being dilated.

3.3.1 How to use the ophthalmoscope

The direct ophthalmoscope provides an erect, magnified view of the fundus, usually of about ×15 magnification. The observer's right eye should be used in examination of the patient's right eye, with the ophthalmoscope held in the right hand. It is convenient, and looks professional, if the left hand is placed on the patient's forehead, to steady the patient and help retract the upper eyelid if required. The process is reversed for the left eye, which is examined with the observer's left eye, with the ophthalmoscope held in the left hand.

By convention it is customary to start the examination by holding the ophthalmoscope about 18 inches from the patient to observe the red reflex and detect any opacities in the media of the eye, the cornea, anterior chamber lens and vitreous, which show up as dark areas against the red reflex. This is made easier by rotating a plus (convex) lens into the view on the ophthalmoscope. After the media have been inspected, the ophthalmoscope is brought close to the patient's eye, and the fundus can be examined. It may be helpful to follow a routine when examining the fundus:

1. Find any retinal vessel and follow it towards the optic disc. The peculiar branching pattern of the retinal vessels will point like arrows towards the optic disc.
2. The optic disc, which is the anterior part of the optic nerve, should be examined carefully. It is important to look at the margin, the optic cup and the colour, (cricket enthusiasts may remember it as MCC).

3. Examine the macula and fovea. This is most easily achieved by asking the patient to look directly at the ophthalmoscope light. It can only be properly visualized if the pupil is dilated, as otherwise the pupil will constrict very strongly.
4. Follow the retinal vessels out from the optic discs in all four quadrants and compare the calibre of the arterioles and the veins (normal ratio 2:3) and the arteriovenous crossings.
5. Examine the more peripheral retina.

Most ophthalmoscopes have various auxiliary items on them to facilitate examination and it is wise to be familiar with these.

1. The green light, or more properly red-free filter, is useful to examine retinal blood vessels. As retinal vessels and haemorrhages show up as black, it is particularly helpful in examining patients with vascular retinopathies such as diabetic retinopathy. The red-free filter also shows up the retinal nerve fibre layer, which appears as a very fine layer of slits, on either side of the arcade vessels.
2. The small aperture beam of light is sometimes helpful to examine through the undilated pupil, or to examine the macula.
3. Some ophthalmoscopes provide a slit-beam which allows it to be used like a hand held slit-lamp to examine the anterior segment.
4. A pattern target like a cross or series of concentric circles is sometimes provided and this can be projected on to the fundus to assess fixation. It can also be used to assess whether the retina is elevated, although the binocular indirect ophthalmoscope is much better for this purpose (see below).

Most modern ophthalmoscopes have very bright halogen bulbs and rechargeable batteries, ensuring that a bright beam is always available. There is nothing more awkward than to try and carry out a fundus examination with an ophthalmoscope that has dud batteries!

3.3.2 Binocular indirect ophthalmoscope

This instrument is difficult to use for the occasional user as unlike the direct ophthalmoscope it has a definite learning curve to its use. Its main advantage is that it provides a less magnified, wider view of the fundus and since both of the observer's eyes are used it is stereoscopic, allowing depth perception. It is used in conjunction with a hand-held condensing lens, usually a 20 dioptre lens, which gives about 3× magnification.

The wider stereoscopic view allows large and elevated lesions such as retinal detachments and tumours to be examined. The peripheral retina can be examined by means of a scleral indenter, and this is the basis for the assessment and treatment of retinal detachments.

3.3.3 Slit lamp biomicroscopy

The slit lamp can only be used to examine the fundus if some form of auxiliary lens is added to the optical system to allow visualization. The Hruby lens is a high minus (concave) lens of about −57 dioptres, which can be attached to the slit-lamp and gives a virtual, erect image of the fundus. It is however difficult to use. Alternatively small hand-held convex lenses of +60, +78 and +90 dioptres are now very popular. They are easier to use than the Hruby lens, produce a real and inverted image of the fundus, and are particularly good for providing a magnified, stereoscopic view of the posterior pole of the eye, for detailed examination of the macula and optic disc.

3.4 FUNDUS PHOTOGRAPHY AND FLUORESCEIN ANGIOGRAPHY

3.4.1 Fundus photography

The fundus is readily photographed provided the optical media are clear. Modern fundus cameras offer a choice between a wide field view of 50–60 degrees, and a narrower, more magnified view of 30–35 degrees. The latter is particularly suitable for the macula.

Colour fundus photographs (Fig. 2.6) are an excellent means of documenting pathology and for following the changes in the character of a lesion over a period of time. For clinical trials, fundus photography provides an 'objective' means of recording lesions and most grading systems are now based on photography. For this purpose colour slide film is essential although for routine clinical management polaroid print film is very convenient, and can be affixed in the case notes. Special red-free retinal photography is useful for assessing blood vessels and the nerve fibre layer.

The non-mydriatic fundus camera has been advocated by some authors as a means of screening for diabetic retinopathy. The camera uses infrared light to visualize the fundus and because of this pupillary dilatation is in most cases not essential to get a picture of the fundus. Photographs of diabetic patients can be assessed by an experienced practitioner, and appropriate cases referred to an ophthalmologist for laser treatment in good time. Unfortunately the quality of image may not be good enough in some cases to identify abnormalities and it does not show peripheral retinal new vessels, which are a common site of haemorrhage. At present it is undergoing evaluation in several centres and its role in screening for diabetic retinopathy is being defined.

3.4.2 Fluorescein angiography

Fundus fluorescein angiography (FFA) (Fig. 3.5) is a dynamic means of assessing the retinal and choroidal circulations. It measures the integrity of the inner blood retinal barrier, the retinal vessels, and the outer blood retinal barrier, the retinal pigment epithelium. The original description by Alvis and Novotny has passed into medical folklore, because their paper was initially rejected by the larger, better known ophthalmic journals.

Nowadays it is considered an essential investigation which is routinely performed in virtually all eye departments. Usually 35 mm black and white film is used to record the angiogram, but polaroid film, video recording and digitization systems are all available. For a full description of the technique and uses of fluorescein angiography, the reader is referred to one of the many excellent texts on the subject (see bibliography).

3.5 ELECTROPHYSIOLOGICAL TESTS

The electroretinogram (ERG) and the electrooculogram (EOG) are functional tests of the retina which often are helpful in the assessment and recognition of fundus abnormalities. The visual evoked response or potential (VER or VEP) is a measure of the function of the visual pathway as a whole, but as it is not particularly useful for assessing retinal disorders, it will not be described.

It is important to have a working knowledge of the basics of the ERG and EOG, so that an idea of their limitations and uses can be gained, which is of importance when ordering or interpreting these tests.

3.5.1 The electroretinogram (ERG)

The ERG (Fig. 3.6) represents the combined electrical activity of different cells within the retina. The recording is performed using a corneal contact lens electrode placed in the eye using local anaesthesia, a ground electrode placed on the earlobe and a reference electrode on the forehead. Recently gold foil or fine cotton wick electrodes have been used instead of the contact lens electrode.

The patient is tested under photopic (light-adapted) and scotopic (dark-adapted) conditions and is exposed to a single or multiple bright flash of light, the test taking about 30–60 minutes in total. The responses are recorded and passed through a

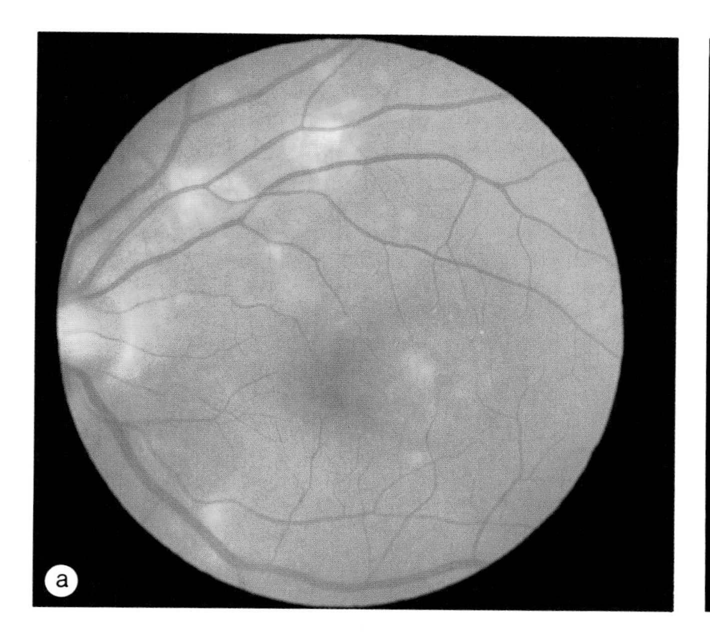

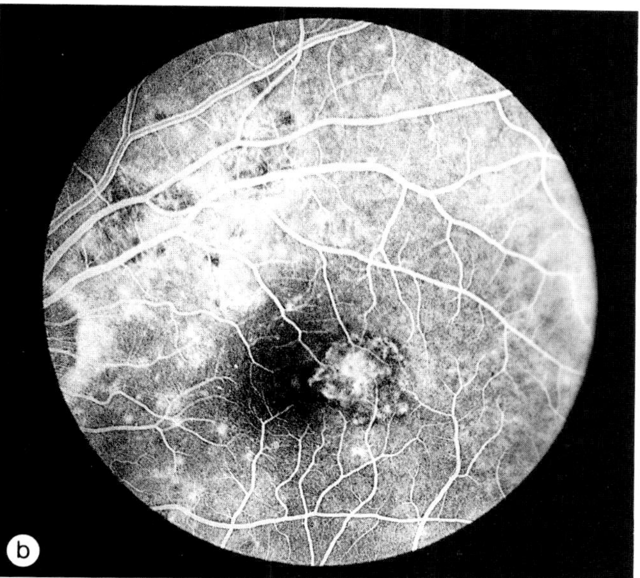

Fig. 3.5 Fundus photograph (a) and Fluorescein angiogram (b) in a case of presumed ocular histoplasmosis.

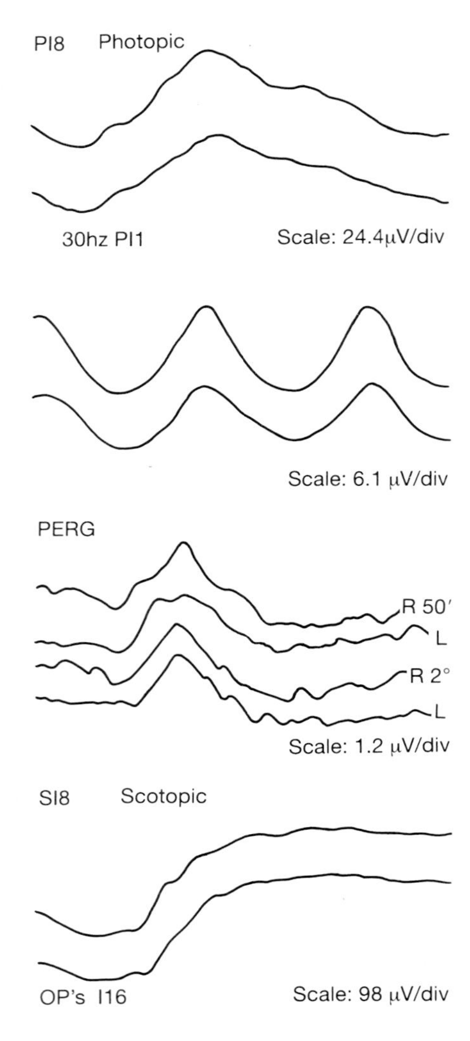

Fig. 3.6 Normal ERG.

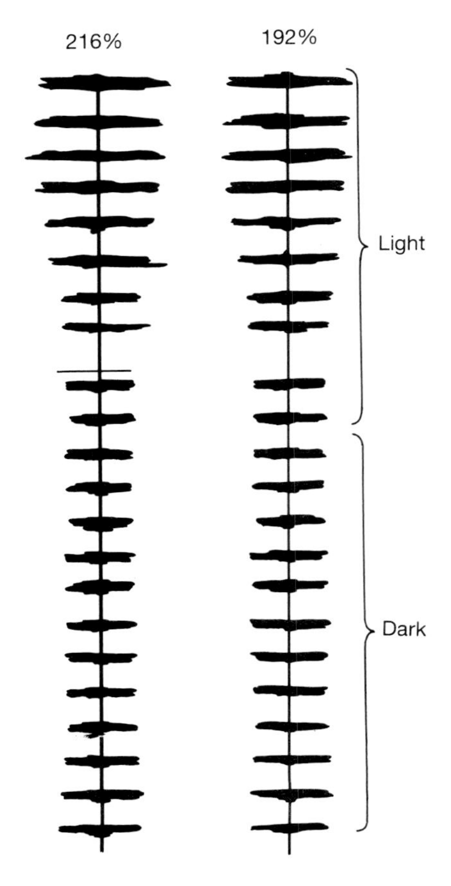

Fig. 3.7 Normal EOG.

differential amplifier and display system and are averaged to filter out the inevitable background noise.

It is customary to divide the normal trace into the 'a' wave, which is an initial negative deflection thought to arise from the photoreceptors, the 'b' wave which is the subsequent positive component which is normally greater in amplitude and probably arises from the Muller cells and bipolar layer of the inner retina and finally the prolonged positive component, the 'c' wave, which probably arises from the retinal pigment epithelial cells.

Abnormalities of the ERG can occur in both time (delay in components) and in the amplitude of the waveform. The ERG is a mass response of the retina and generally disease processes involving less than 15% of the retina cannot be detected by the ERG. In localized macular disease the ERG therefore remains normal and because the ganglion cells do not contribute to the ERG, it is also normal in optic atrophy.

The pattern ERG (PERG) measures a retinal response to a pattern stimulus, and is thought to arise in the ganglion cell layer. It has been used to investigate patients with glaucoma and distinguish them from ocular hypertensives, and also to predict which patients with central retinal vein occlusion might develop neovascular glaucoma subsequently.

3.5.2 Electro-oculogram (EOG)

The EOG (Fig. 3.7) is a measure of the resting potential between the cornea and the back of the eye. To record the EOG, electrodes are placed on the skin at the medial and lateral canthus of each eye and the patient is asked to look at fixed targets, moving the eye from side to side.

The EOG is recorded in the photopic and scotopic states of adaptation. It is measured as the ratio of the maximum level of the light peak to the minimum level of the dark trough. A normal value is 1.85 (185%) or greater, and the EOG is abnormal in conditions which primarily affect the retinal pigment epithelium and photoreceptors.

3.6 DIAGNOSTIC ULTRASOUND

Ultrasound is an acoustic wave which by definition has a frequency greater than 20 kHz (20 000 cycles per second). Clinical ophthalmic ultrasound machines comprise a probe that emits an ultrasound wave and then detects and processes the returning echoes. The basis of all the systems is the piezoelectric effect; this is the physical property of certain substances, such as quartz crystals, which enable them to transduce acoustic energy into electrical energy. Ophthalmic ultrasound is divided into the A-scan and B-scan. The A-scan is a one-dimensional display in which echoes are represented by vertical spikes along a baseline, the amplitude of the spike depending on the acoustic properties of the structure reflecting the ultrasound waves. The B-scan (Fig. 3.8) is useful in producing an overall picture of the nature of the intraocular structures and lesions. The uses of ophthalmic ultrasound are summarized below.

1. Examination of the retina and vitreous when ophthalmoscopy is impossible.
2. Assessment of intraocular lesions.
3. Investigation of ophthalmic trauma.
4. Detection of intraocular foreign bodies.
5. Biometry of the eye prior to cataract/implant surgery.

Ultrasound is particularly useful in assessing the state of the retina when the media are not clear enough to allow fundus examination. An important example is when there is a vitreous haemorrhage, where it is important to check that the retina is flat and not detached. For intraocular masses it allows the dimensions, thickness and acoustic nature of the lesion to be measured. This is of great importance for ocular tumours where ultrasound is very useful in documenting the growth of lesions with time and in the diagnosis of such lesions.

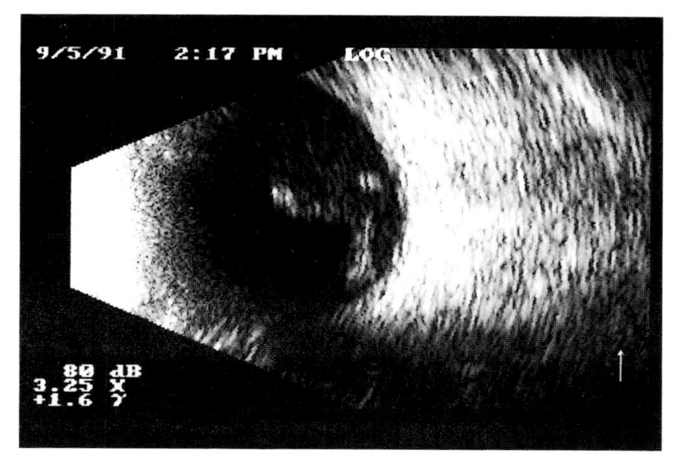

Fig. 3.8 Ultrasound scan of the normal eye.

3.7 SPECIAL TESTS OF RESEARCH INTEREST

3.7.1 Entoptic phenomena

Entoptic phenomena are visual images that arise from optical phenomena within the eye. The most familiar example of this is the Purkinje effect, the visualization of the retinal blood vessels when a small, bright light source is moved from side to side against the eye. The 'blue field phenomenon' or 'flying corpuscular test' has been used to study the blood flow in the retinal circulation. The observer looks at a bright uniform field of blue light and can see the corpuscles moving through the perifoveal capillaries. This has been used to study the blood flow in the retina in diabetic patients but because it is essentially a subjective test it is difficult to accurately quantify.

3.7.2 Vitreous fluorophotometry

This technique is a method of measuring the integrity of the various components of the blood retinal barrier. In the test an intravenous injection of fluorescein dye is given to the patient and following this the fluorescence arising within the vitreous is measured. It is possible to measure the concentration of fluorescein at different sites within the eye and in this manner create a profile of the ocular fluorescence.

The test has been used extensively in diabetic patients as a means of detecting blood retinal barrier breakdown before overt retinopathy is present. As an 'objective' test it has also been used to evaluate the role of drugs which might modify the onset of diabetic retinopathy. Unfortunately the great expense of current machines makes it unlikely that these techniques will gain widespread use.

3.7.3 Scanning laser ophthalmoscope

The scanning laser ophthalmoscope (SLO) is a new and exciting means of assessing the fundus. It works on the principle of scanning the fundus with a focused laser beam and forming an image which is presented in 'real time' on a television monitor. Different lasers can be used as the illumination source and the principal advantage of these is that the laser is more efficient than normal white light, hence lower power settings can be used. With the red HeNe (helium–neon) laser, the fundus can be visualized without the pupils needing to be dilated.

The blue argon laser can also be used to perform fundus fluorescein angiography in which a much lower dose of fluorescein dye needs to be used compared to conventional angiography. Indocyanine green dye (ICG) is a technique that allows better visualization of the choroidal circulation and choroidal neovascularization.

The depth of focus and quality of image with the SLO is far greater than a conventional fundus camera and as such it can detect and record very subtle fundal changes. In addition by using the laser to project targets directly onto the retina, fundus perimetry and scotometry can be performed. The SLO seems to have great potential as a new means of assessing the posterior segment of the eye, but it is at present expensive.

3.7.4 Laser Doppler velocimetry

This research technique permits quantitative evaluation of blood flow within the retinal vessels. It uses an argon laser beam and the Doppler effect to measure flow within the major retinal vessels and has been used to investigate autoregulation of the retinal circulation in normal and diabetic patients.

3.7.5 Computerized tomography

Computerized tomography (CT), in common with other X-ray procedures, shows bony structures, such as the orbit, with the greatest detail. The soft tissues of the globe of the eye do not show up very well, with poor contrast. Calcified lesions that can be easily confirmed by CT are osseous choristoma of the choroid, optic disc drusen and calcification that occurs in certain tumours, such as retinoblastoma. Apart from these, CT scanning for lesions in the globe of the eye is not particularly helpful.

Magnetic resonance imaging (MRI) on the other hand is particularly useful for showing malignant melanomas, and may prove to be an important investigation in the differentiation of intraocular tumours. However, for the moment MRI is considered a useful adjunct in diagnosis of intraocular pathology, rather than an essential procedure.

FURTHER READING

Bek, T. and Lund Andersen, H. (1990) Accurate superimposition of perimetry data onto fundus photographs. *Acta Ophthalmol.*, **68**, 11–18.

Berkow, J.W., Orth, D.H. and Kelley, J.S. (1991) *Fluorescein Angiography, Technique and Interpretation*. Ophthalmology monographs 5: American Academy of Ophthalmology.

Coleman, J.T., Lizzi, F.L. and Jack, R.L. (1977) *Ultrasonography of the Eye and Orbit*. Lea and Febiger, Philadelphia.

Cunha-Vaz, J.G., Mota, C.C., Leite, E.C. *et al.* (1985) Effect of sulindac on the permeability of the blood retinal barrier in early diabetic retinopathy. *Arch. Ophthalmol.*, **103**, 1307–11.

Fishman, G.A. and Sokol, S. (1990) *Electrophysiological Testing in Disorders of the Retina, Optic Nerve and Visual Pathway*. Ophthalmology monographs 2: American Academy of Ophthalmology.

Grunwald, J.E., Riva, C.E., Brucker, A.J., *et al.* (1984) Altered retinal vascular response to 100% oxygen breathing in diabetes mellitus. *Ophthalmol.*, **91**, 1447–52.

Justice, J. Jr. (ed.) (1982) *Ophthalmic Photography*. Boston: Little, Brown and Co.

Loehl, M. and Riva, C.E. (1978) Macular circulation and the flying corpuscles phenomenon. *Ophthalmol.* **85**, 911–7.

Mainster, M.A., Timberlake, G.T., Webb, R.H. and Hughes, G.W. (1982) Scanning laser ophthalmoloscopy. *Ophthalmol.*, **89**, 852.

Maurice, D.M. (1963) A new objective fluorophotometer. *Exp. Eye Res.*, **2**, 33–8.

Nanjiani, M. (1991) *Fluorescein angiography: technique, interpretation and application*, Oxford University Press, Oxford.

Novotny, H.R. and Alivs, D.L. (1961) A method of photographing fluorescence in circulating blood in the human retina. *Circulation*, **24**, 82–6.

Ossoinig, K.C. (1979) Standardised echography: basic principles, clinical applications, and results. *Int. Ophthalmol. Clin.*, **19**, 127–210.

Rabb, M.F., Burton, T.L., Schatz, H. and Yannuzi, L.A. (1978) Fluorescein angiography of the fundus: a schematic approach to interpretation. *Surg. Ophthalmol.*, **22**, 387–403.

Riva, C.E. and Feke, G.T. (1981) Laser Doppler velocimetry in the measurement of retinal blood flow, in *The Biomedical Laser Technology and Clinical Applications* (ed. L. Goldman), Springer-Verlag, New York, pp. 135–61.

Timberlake, G.T., Mainster, M.A., Webb, R.H., Hughes, G.W. and Trempe, C.L. (1982) Retinal localisation of scotomata by scanning laser ophthalmoscope. *Invest. Ophthalmol. Vis.*, **22**, 91.

Webb, R.H., Hughes, G.W. and Pomerantzeff, O. (1980) Flying spot TV ophthalmoscope. *Appl. Opt.*, **19**, 299.

Wiegan, W., de Keizer, R.J.W. and Guthoff, R. (1991) Diagnostic imaging of the eye and orbit by magnetic resonance and x-ray computed tomography (update), in *New Frontiers in Ophthalmology* (ed. Khoo Chang Yew), *Excerpta Medica*, Amsterdam, pp. 210–5.

4 *Retinopathy and diabetes*

Clinical Retinopathies. Paul M. Dodson, Jonathan M. Gibson and Erna E. Kritzinger.
Published in 1995 by Chapman & Hall, London. ISBN 0 412 35930 8

4.1 INTRODUCTION

Microangiopathy is a disorder of the small blood vessels specific to diabetes and is clinically apparent in the eye as retinopathy as well as in other organs such as the kidneys and nerves. Diabetic retinopathy is the most common cause of blindness in the working population of the Western world and also a significant cause of blindness in the elderly. Amongst diabetics the overall prevalence of retinopathy is approximately 26%, and is responsible for approximately 400 new cases of blindness per year. It is most common in Type I diabetes as a large proportion of Type I diabetics will develop retinopathic changes with increased duration of the disease. However, in clinical practice many Type II diabetics are seen with diabetic retinopathy; this reflects the fact that Type II diabetes is far more common than Type I.

4.2 AETIOLOGY OF MICROVASCULAR DISEASE

The pathogenesis of microangiopathy is still poorly understood. The major susceptibility factors for its development are duration of diabetes and may relate also to the degree of metabolic glucose control. However, neither of these factors really explain the mechanisms of development of retinopathy. In clinical studies the major factors relating to the development of diabetic retinopathy are:

1. duration of diabetes;
2. type of diabetes (more common in Type I diabetes than Type II);
3. systemic hypertension;
4. diabetic control – particularly control in the early years of diabetes;
5. presence of macro- or micro-albuminuria;
6. pregnancy;
7. smoking (controversial).

Pathogenesis of microvascular disease probably reflects many factors. These include:

1. functional abnormalities within the microcirculation;
2. consequences of enhanced glucose metabolism via different pathways;
3. genetic susceptibility;
4. hypertension;
5. haemostatic abnormalities with
   (a) increased platelet aggregation
   (b) increased Factor 8 (VIII)
   (c) increased fibrinogen
   (d) decreased fibrinolysis
   (e) an imbalance between thromboxane and prostacyclin in favour of thromboxane;
6. non-enzymatic glycosylation with formation of a Schiff base, e.g. with collagen;
7. increase in a polyol pathway with accumulation of sorbitol;
8. increased free radical activity.

A summary of the various possible interactions producing capillary basement thickening, endothelial cell damage and tissue ischaemia, which are all involved in microangiopathy, is shown in Fig. 4.1. Hyperglycaemia itself may be involved in the excessive accumulation of basement membrane collagen seen in microangiopathy. It also stimulates the intracellular polyol pathway. This pathway will lead

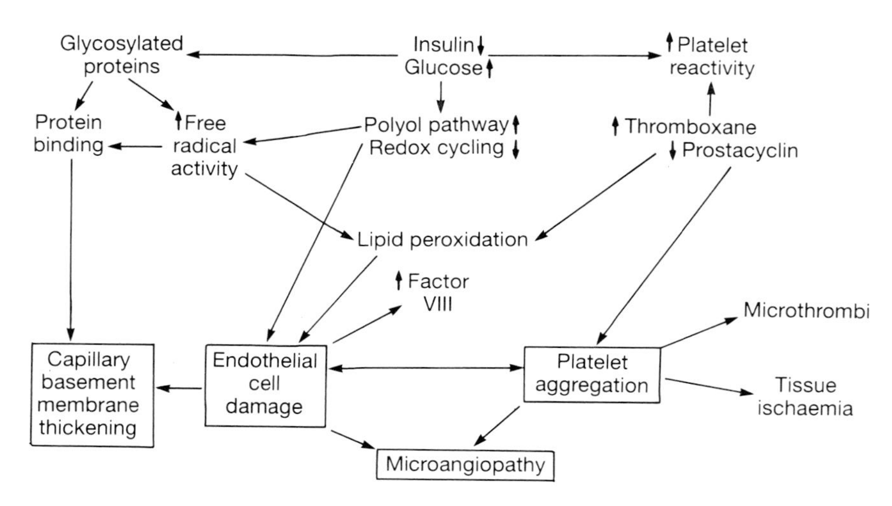

Fig. 4.1 Possible pathways involved in the pathogenesis of diabetic microangiography.

to excessive utilization of the energy source NADPH. This results in reduced levels of antioxidants which are required to scavenge free radicals. Free radicals are violently reactive chemical species produced during metabolism which contain an unpaired electron in their structure. These are powerful oxidants which cause lipid peroxidation as well as protein denaturation and aggregation. The potential consequences of these metabolic processes include capillary endothelial cell damage and dysfunction as well as the abnormalities of increased platelet aggregation and release of platelet factors, thromboxane and factor VIII. This sequence culminates in capillary basement membrane abnormalities, protein leakage, microthrombus formation and tissue ischaemia which are all features of diabetic retinopathy.

4.2.1 Mechanisms of retinal damage

Endothelial cell damage appears to be a major feature leading to the changes of diabetic retinopathy. This will result in leakage giving rise to exudates, and haemorrhage into the retina. Specific changes occur within the pericytes lining the capillaries which result in the formation of microaneurysms. The pericyte appears to have a key role in the maintenance of normal endothelial cell structure. Pericyte degeneration is an early histological feature of cell changes as shown in Fig. 4.2. Although leakage is a prominent part in the evolution of diabetic retinopathy (Table 4.1), microthrombi leading to progressive ischaemia with capillary closure and the formation of cotton wool spots (retinal infarcts), are ominous features.

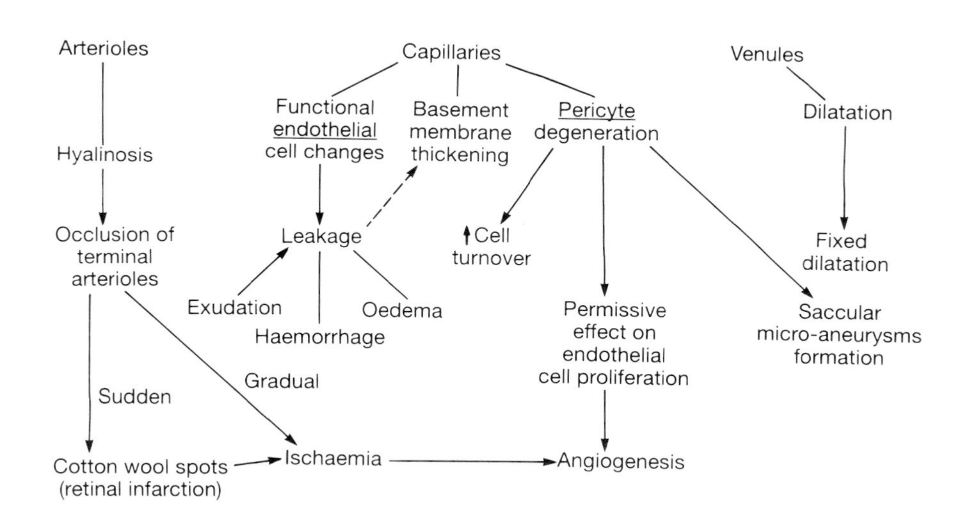

Fig. 4.2 Changes that may occur in the genesis of diabetic retinopathy.

Table 4.1 Microvascular haemodynamics in the retina in relationship to diabetic control

Increased capillary permeability	Glycosylation relation?
Over-perfusion and capillary hypertension	Probably glycaemic control related
Under perfusion	Relates to vascular limitation and vasodilatation
Loss of autoregulation	Relates to intraoccular pressure and systemic blood pressure

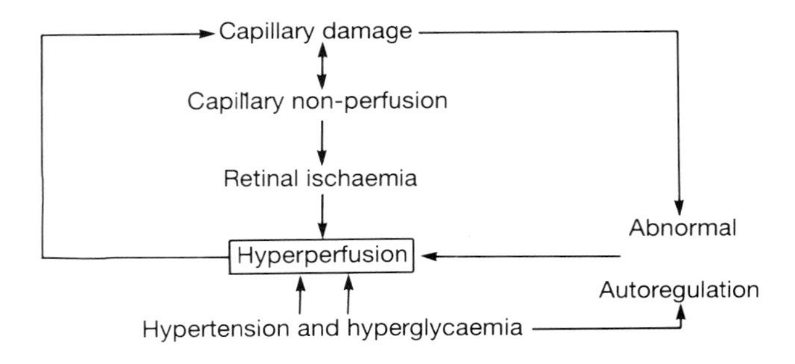

Fig. 4.3 Scheme of haemodynamic changes in the evolution of diabetic retinopathy.

It is thought that retinal ischaemia produces stimulation of the production of angiogenic growth factors, some of which have now been identified. Possible angiogenic growth factors are:

- basic fibroblastic GF (b-FGF);
- transforming GF-beta (TGF-b);
- platelet derived GF (PDGF);
- insulin-like growth factor (IGF-I);
- epidermal GF (EGF);
- growth hormone (GH);
- angiotensins 1–3;
- endothelin-1.

Other changes are observed in the retina with special techniques. For example, retinal blood flow may be increased in volume in the large veins of the retina, as well as disruption of retinal vascular autoregulation. If there is formation of microthrombi in the capillaries, there may be a reduction in linear flow. A summary of changes that may occur is shown in Fig. 4.3.

4.3 CLASSIFICATION OF RETINAL CHANGES IN DIABETES

The major classifications of diabetic retinopathy are:

1. background retinopathy
2. maculopathy
3. pre-proliferative retinopathy
4. proliferative retinopathy

4.3.1 Background retinopathy

The early changes of micro-aneurysm formation, small retinal haemorrhages and the formation of exudation (from leakage) is determined as the background form (Fig. 4.4). Providing these changes do not affect the fovea, the patient will remain asymptomatic. Background changes are very common particularly with long duration of Type I diabetes. They may equally be seen in Type II diabetics and may be a feature at presentation. This suggests that diabetes has been present for a considerable length of time before diagnosis.

4.3.2 Maculopathy

Retinopathic changes due to diabetes in the macular region (circular area of 2 disc diameters from the fovea) are always significant. Diabetic maculopathy is the commonest cause of blindness due to retinopathy in diabetes. Three forms of macular disease may occur. The most common is the exudative form characterized by yellow waxy deposits thickly formed in a flattened star or ring shape (circinate pattern) which may surround the macula or be distributed throughout the posterior pole of the fundus (Fig. 4.5). Other changes characteristic of diabetic maculopathy, namely retinal oedema or capillary fallout and ischaemia, are difficult to assess accurately with the ophthalmoscope.

The second form is ischaemic maculopathy due to capillary closure. Detection of this is not possible with the ophthalmoscope unless there are other changes suggestive of ischaemia (e.g. cotton wool spots). The usual method of detection is using a fundus fluorescein angiogram on which the ischaemic areas can then be identified (Fig. 4.6). Retinal oedema owing to leakage may also be

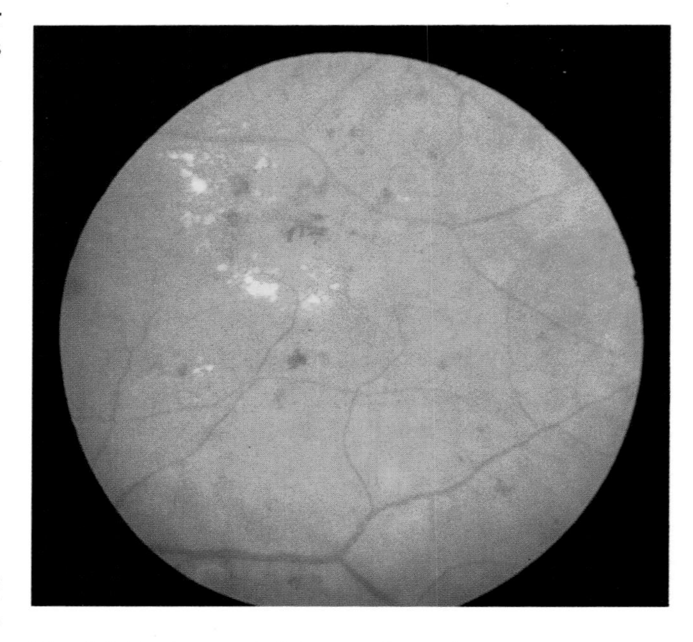

Fig. 4.4 Background diabetic retinopathy.

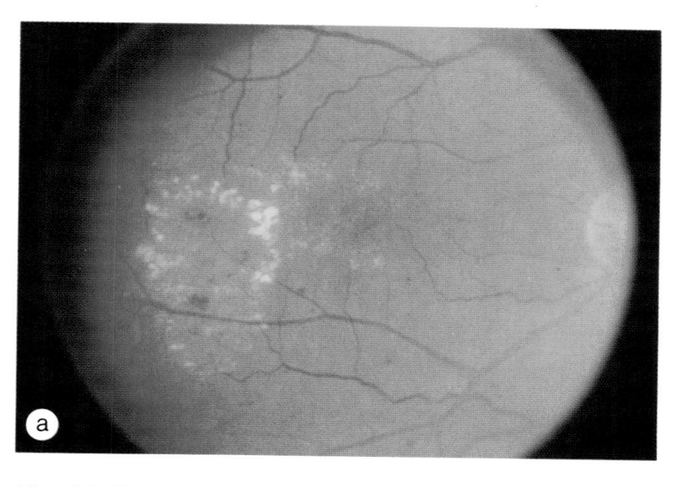
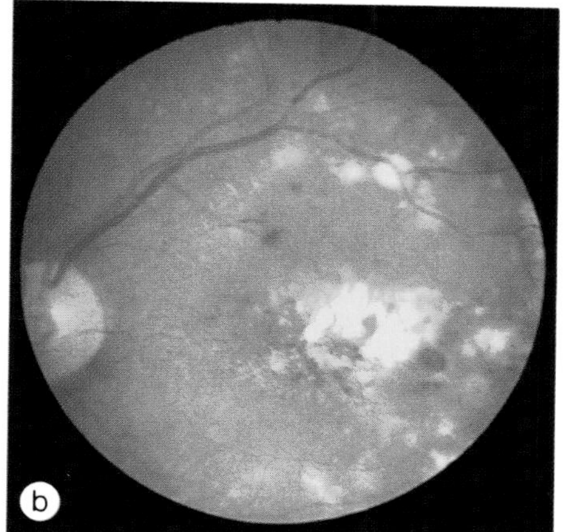

Fig. 4.5 Examples of maculopathy (a) early, and (b) late.

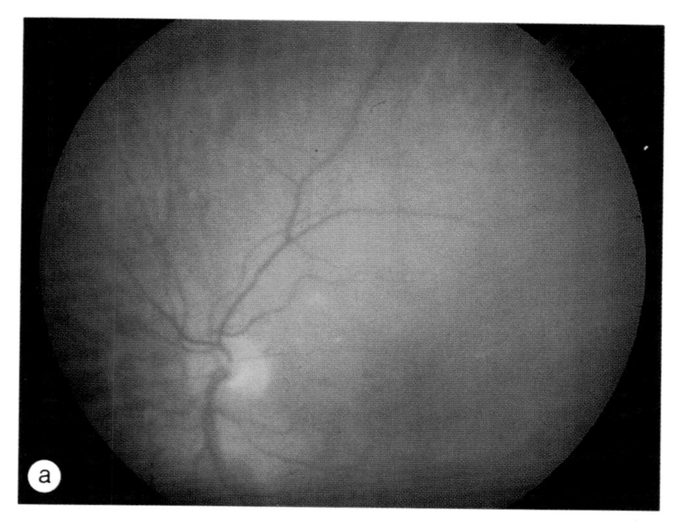
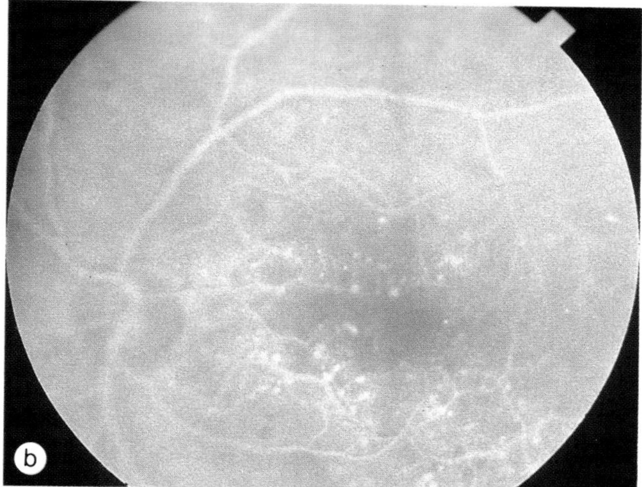

Fig. 4.6 (a) Ischaemic maculopathy – left fundus. (b) Fluorescein angiogram of same eye in mid-venous phase, showing areas of capillary closure around left macula.

detected by slit lamp or biomicroscopy, which will show up the areas of retinal thickening. The third form of diabetic maculopathy is described as a cystoid (Fig. 4.7). This is due to extensive accumulation of fluid in the retina. All three forms may give rise to serious compromise in vision.

4.3.3 Pre-proliferative retinopathy

It has been suggested that certain retinal changes ascribe risk of development of the next stage, the proliferative (new vessel formation) stage of diabetic retinopathy. The changes observed in the retina reflect retinal ischaemia (Fig. 4.8). This may be due to localized retinal infarction or, as seen on a fluorescein angiogram, may reflect capillary closure and ischaemic areas. The main changes associated with pre-proliferative diabetic retinopathy are:

1. cotton wool spots;
2. venous abnormalities – tortuosity, beading, venous reduplication;
3. arteriolar abnormalities;
4. intra-retinal microvascular abnormalities (IRMA), which consist of dilated retinal capillaries.

The risk of developing proliferative retinopathy is approximately 50% over 2 years if these features are

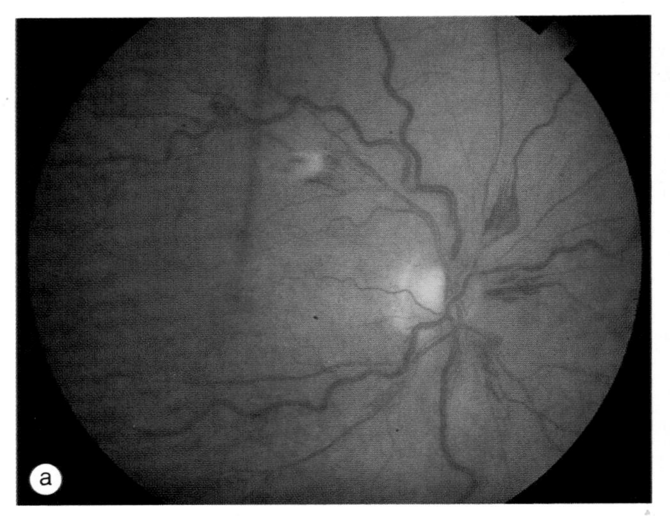

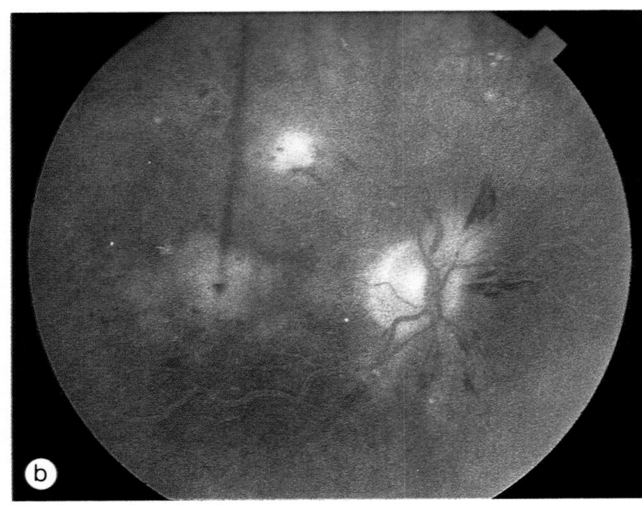

Fig. 4.7 (a) Cystoid macula odema in a diabetic patient's right eye. Cotton wool spots and nerve fibre haemorrhages are evident. (b) Late phase fluorescein angiogram of the same eye, showing cystoid macula oedema.

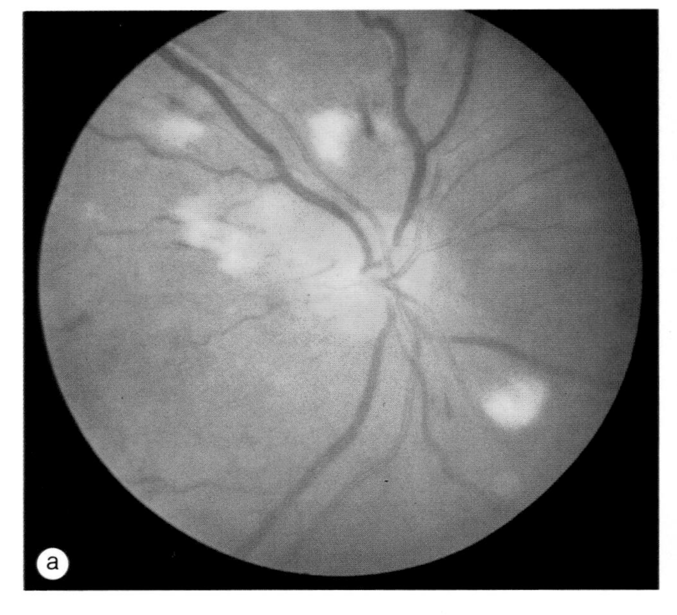

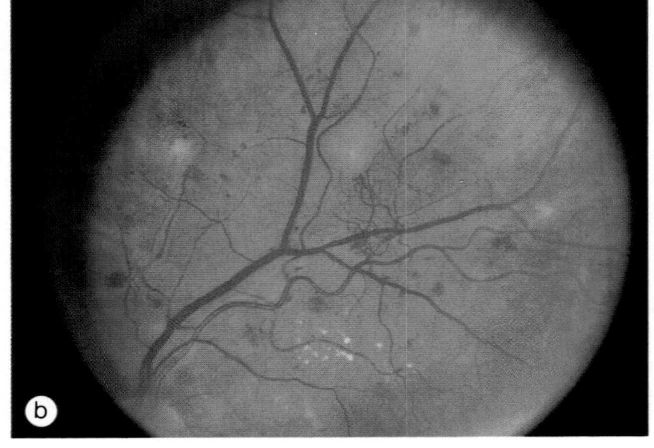

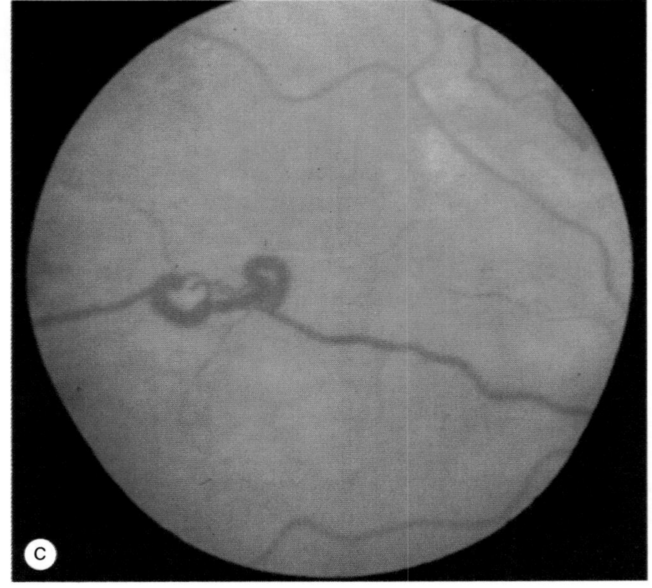

Fig. 4.8 (a) Pre-proliferative diabetic retinopathy. (b) Intraretinal vascular abnormalities. (c) Venous reduplication.

present. The exact degree of pre-proliferative changes with regard to risk of neovascularization needs to be further studied. However, recent research has suggested that at least three cotton wool spots are required to give significant risk of proliferative diabetic retinopathy.

4.3.4 Proliferative diabetic retinopathy

In this stage of diabetic retinopathy, severe retinal ischaemia leads to new vessel formation on the optic disc, the retina or the iris (Figs 4.9–4.11). It is thought that these vessels develop in response to production of angiogenic factors released by the ischaemic retina (Section 4.3). The short and long term consequences of new vessel formation are serious. Affected patients have a high risk of suffering severe visual loss within 2 years. The new vessels form fine, fan-like networks that grow in the vitreo-retinal interface and they are usually asymptomatic until they rupture, leading to the serious complication of vitreous haemorrhage (Fig. 4.12). Initially, haemorrhage into the vitreous may cause the patient to complain of seeing floaters in the vision (variously described as tadpoles, spiders or cobwebs). Large haemorrhages which enter into the gel of the vitreous may cause profound visual loss, and because the vitreous is relatively inert, these haemorrhages may take a long period to clear. Recurrent haemorrhages may be associated with vitreo-retinal traction and in advanced severe cases, fibrous tissue may develop causing a traction retinal detachment (Fig. 4.13). An advanced form of proliferative diabetic retinopathy includes new vessel formation on the iris, termed iris neovascularization (Fig. 4.9). This may lead to glaucoma and carries a poor visual prognosis.

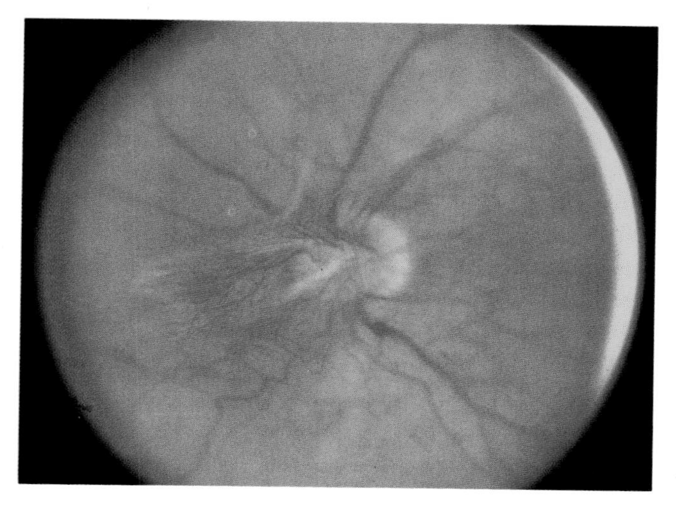

Fig. 4.9 Optic disc new vessels.

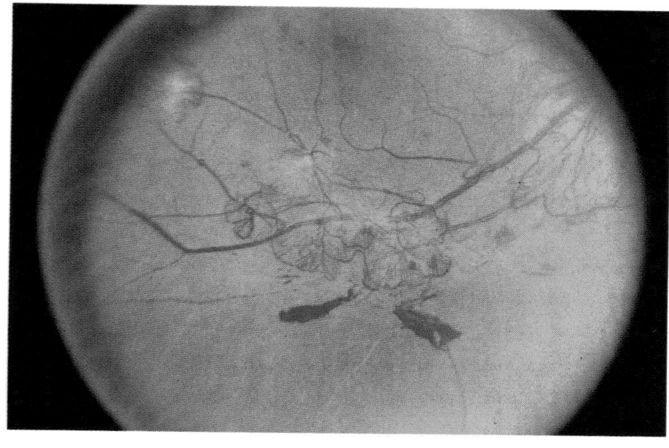

Fig. 4.10 Retinal new vessels.

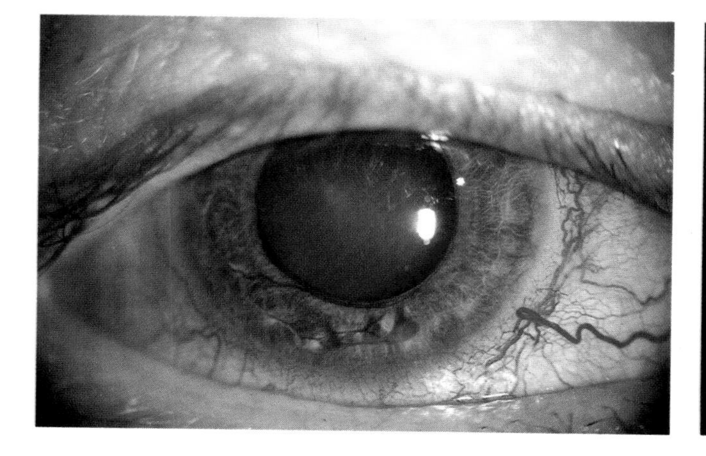

Fig. 4.11 Iris new vessels.

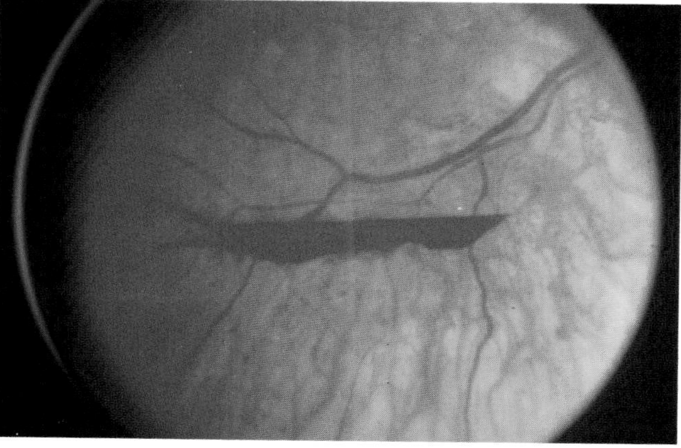

Fig. 4.12 Vitreous haemorrhage from new vessels.

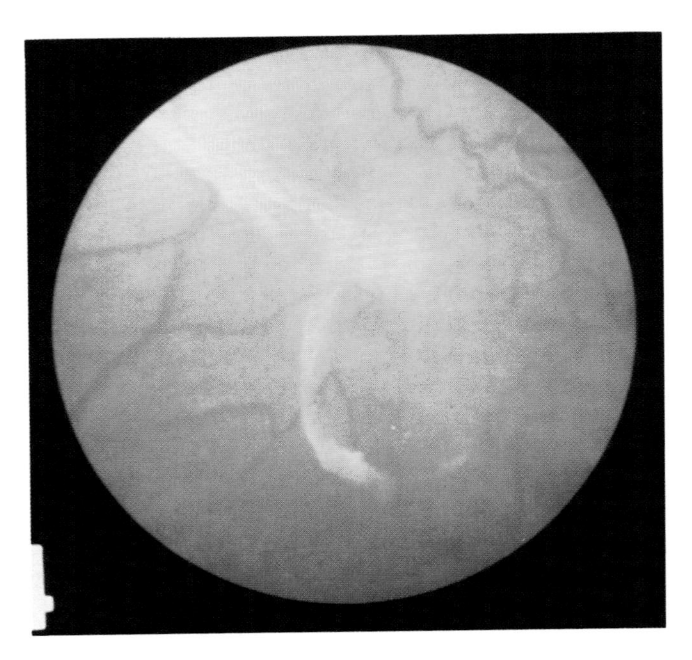

Fig. 4.13 Fibrous tissue formation.

4.3.5 Other features associated with diabetic retinopathy

Cataract, opacification of the lens, occurs more commonly and at an earlier age in diabetic patients than non-diabetics. Cataract is important in diabetics because not only will it affect the vision, but it may also be sufficiently bad to prevent adequate fundus examination to be performed and to prevent laser treatment of the retina. In that situation prompt cataract extraction and lens implantation is important. Cataract surgery in diabetic patients has a small, but significantly higher association with complications and YAG laser capsulotomy is more often required due to posterior capsule opacification.

There is good evidence now that pre-existing retinopathy may advance rapidly following cataract surgery and these patients should be kept under close observation following operation.

Isolated cranial nerve palsies occur in diabetic patients, including those affecting III, IV and VI cranial nerves, which cause diplopia. Third nerve palsies occur relatively commonly in diabetic patients, but caution should be taken before ascribing third nerve palsy to diabetics alone, without excluding other, potentially more serious causes. Retinovascular disease and glaucoma are also associated with diabetes and are discussed in section 4.7.

4.4 MANAGEMENT OF DIABETIC RETINOPATHY: OPHTHALMOLOGICAL MANAGEMENT

Multicentre controlled clinical trials have shown that appropriate retinal laser photocoagulation gives the best chance of preserving vision patients with diabetic retinopathy. The Diabetic Retinopathy Study (DRS) was a randomized, prospective multicentre clinical trial of 1758 patients designed to answer the following questions:

1. Is panretinal photocoagulation or direct treatment of retinal neovascularization effective for preventing severe visual loss in diabetic retinopathy?
2. What is the efficacy of argon compared to xenon photocoagulation?

The results of the DRS showed that photocoagulation reduced the risk of severe visual loss by at least 50% and that argon laser treatment had less harmful effects on vision than xenon photocoagulation.

4.4.1 Management of proliferative retinopathy

Information from the Diabetic Retinopathy Study (DRS) and the Early Treatment for Diabetic Retinopathy Study (ETDRS) have established the role of laser photocoagulation in proliferative retinopathy. Immediate panretinal photocoagulation is indicated for eyes with any of the DRS high-risk characteristics:

1. Disc new vessels which are at least 1/4 to 1/2 disc area in extent.
2. Disc new vessels associated with pre-retinal or vitreous haemorrhage.
3. Peripheral new vessels, which are at least 1/2 disc area in extent and associated with pre-retinal or vitreous haemorrhage.

In current clinical practice, aggressive panretinal photocoagulation is applied if any disc new vessels are detected. Peripheral retinal new vessels (NVE) are usually treated initially by scatter laser photocoagulation and following that by direct coagulation of the new vessels, if this is feasible.

4.4.2 Laser photocoagulation techniques

Panretinal, scatter laser photocoagulation is the standard treatment technique for proliferative retinopathy. The technique involves applying 2000, 500 micron laser spots in a scattered pattern over the

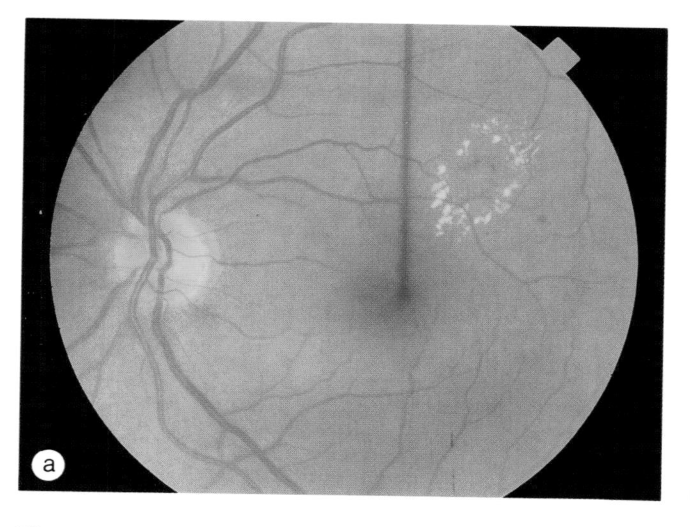

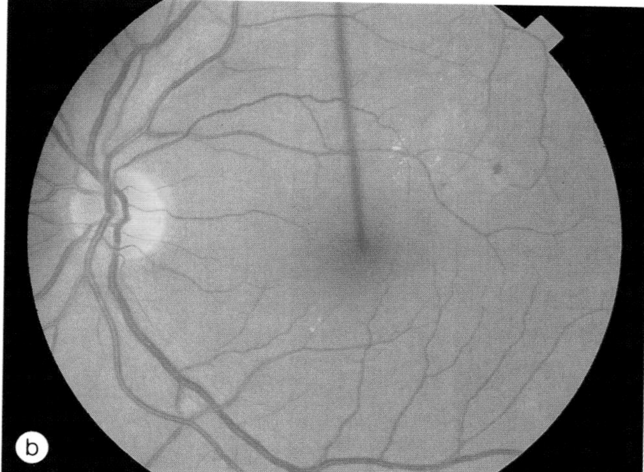

Fig. 4.14 Maculopathy exudative (a) before, and (b) after focal laser.

retina, avoiding the optic disc and retinal vessels, and keeping out of the central macular area of the retina (Fig. 4.14). In practice this is commonly applied within the argon green wavelengths, over two sessions of about half an hour each. The treatment is not usually very uncomfortable for the patient, and reassurance and a relaxed manner are usually all that is required. Occasionally young diabetic patients, particularly men, may find the treatment painful and in these cases local anaesthesia by retrobulbar or peribulbar injections is helpful. Scatter laser photocoagulation should be completed over a short period as there is some evidence that this is much more effective than prolonging the treatment over several weeks. Our practice is to give the treatment in two sessions about 1–2 weeks apart.

In patients with aggressive proliferative diabetic retinopathy, considerably more treatment than the 'standard' 2000 burns may be required before complete regression of new vessels is accomplished. In this situation it is probably better to risk overtreatment of the patient rather than risk the serious complications of not giving enough laser treatment.

All patients undergoing laser scatter photocoagulation must be warned that they may suffer some constriction of their peripheral visual field and night vision. In practice, with 2000 burns this is usually not a major consideration and most patients are not greatly handicapped by this. However, patients who require a large number of laser burns are significantly at risk of suffering loss of peripheral vision, which may prevent them from holding a driving licence, and may make night vision a problem.

Advanced diabetic eye disease with multiple episodes of vitreous haemorrhage, or traction detachment formation will lead to consideration for vitrectomy surgery. This is a highly skilled and specialized technique performed in major centres and may be associated with excellent results.

4.4.3 Diabetic maculopathy

One of the aims of the Early Treatment Diabetic Retinopathy Study (ETDRS) was to answer the question, does photocoagulation alleviate diabetic macular oedema? The results of the ETDRS showed that photocoagulation was of benefit in preventing visual loss in eyes with clinically significant macular oedema. The following guidelines, as indications for laser photocoagulation, have been drawn up, based on the ETDRS:

1. All leaking lesions 500–3000 microns from the centre of the macula, thought to be causing clinically significant macular oedema, should be treated with focal photocoagulation.
2. Areas of diffuse retinal thickening 500–3000 microns from the macular centre, should be treated with grid laser photocoagulation.
3. Retinal avascular zones (ischaemic areas) 500–3000 microns from the macular centre associated with clinically significant macular oedema, should be treated with grid photocoagulation.

Diabetic maculopathy is the most common cause of loss of vision in diabetic patients with retinopathy, so it is an important problem to recognize

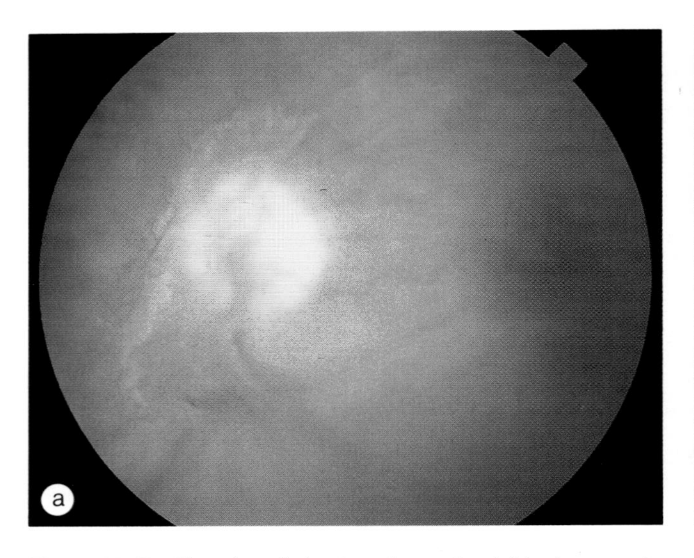

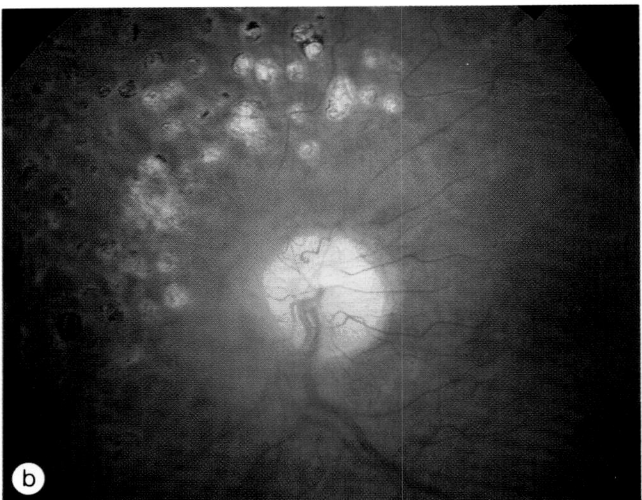

Fig. 4.15 Proliferative diabetic retinopathy (a) before, and (b) after pan-retinal photocoagulation.

and treat (Fig. 4.15). Screening for diabetic maculopathy can be difficult but measuring visual acuity testing and direct ophthalmoscopy with a dilated pupil are important. Special attention should be paid if significant retinal ischaemia is present in the macula region, i.e. ischaemic maculopathy, as laser treatment may be hazardous.

4.4.4 General ophthalmological management

Multicentre controlled clinical trials have shown that appropriate retinal laser photocoagulation gives the best chance of preserving vision in patients with retinopathy. Background retinopathy without involvement of the macula needs review on a 4–6 monthly basis. If any visual symptoms occur, careful visual acuity recording and ophthalmoscopy is appropriate. Any complaint of diminution of visual acuity with blurring of vision or sudden vision loss should be carefully examined. Visual acuity is a very important test and should be recorded, as many patients complain of visual symptoms but have normal visual acuity on testing. It should be noted that alterations in diabetic control, particularly with poorly controlled diabetes, may produce diminution of visual acuity. This will correct once good diabetic control is established. For this reason there should

Table 4.2 When and how to refer patients for ophthalmological review

Background retinopathy	View by diabetic physician no referral necessary
Diabetic maculopathy	Visual acuity normal, referral appropriate by letter – not urgent. Visual acuity abnormal, (≤6/12) urgent referral
Pre-proliferative diabetic retinopathy	These patients should be referred by letter, in view of the risk of developing proliferative diabetic retinopathy; should be seen in ophthalmology clinic
Proliferative diabetic retinopathy	New undetected cases urgent referral by telephone – all patients with proliferative diabetic retinopathy should be managed and treated appropriately in a diabetic ophthalmology clinic

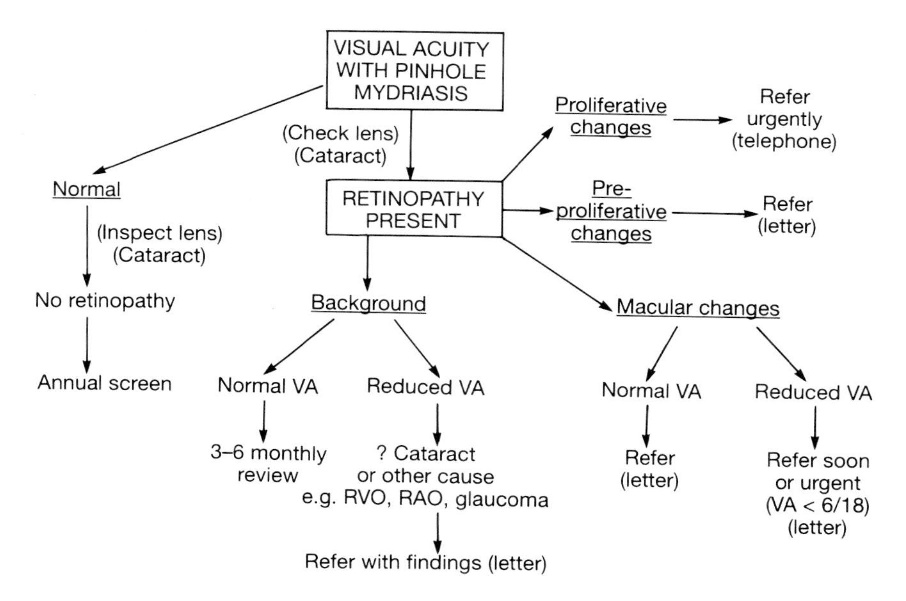

Fig. 4.16 Schematic of management and referral of diabetic patients.

be delay in prescription of new glasses in a patient with poor diabetes control until attention is paid to obtain the optimal glycaemic control. For guidance, the principles of when to refer diabetic patients for ophthalmological review is shown in Table 4.2 and Fig. 4.16.

4.5 MEDICAL MANAGEMENT OF DIABETIC RETINOPATHY

(a) GLYCAEMIC CONTROL

Modern diabetic practice is based around the concept that good diabetic control will prevent the diabetic complications associated with the increased duration of the disease. The weight of evidence relating diabetic complications to poor diabetic control is overwhelming but data proving that improved diabetic control over many years will reduce microvascular complications is now apparent. Two major prospective trials have been set up to answer this.

The UKPDS trial is studying the effects of good diabetic control achieved with differing treatment arms in Type II diabetes, and is due to report its findings in 1994–5. More recently, the Diabetic Control and Complications Trial (DCCT) studying the effects of tight glucose control in Type I diabetic patients, has finished and reported one year early. The key points of the DCCT trial design are:

1. primary and secondary prevention (i.e. with and without retinopathy)
2. 10 years prospective study
3. 1441 Type I diabetic patients studied
4. mean age: 27 years
5. random allocation to:
   (a) *usual regimen*
      (i) once or twice daily insulin injections
      (ii) mean glycosylated haemoglobin (a measure of average blood glucose control over a six-week period) 9%
   (b) *intensive treatment*
      (i) three to four daily insulin injections
      (ii) 'tight control' mean glycosylated haemoglobin 7.2% (NR < 6.05)

Note that the intensive insulin treatment group had a mean glycosylated haemoglobin of 1% above the normal range, and had a three-fold higher prevalence of hypoglycaemia.

The impressive reduction in both primary and secondary prevention of microvascular end points over the nine-year period were:

- diabetic retinopathy reduced by 76%;
- diabetic nephropathy reduced by 35–56%;
- diabetic neuropathy reduced by 60%.

It has been suggested from this trial that good blood glucose control should have a similar effect in Type II diabetic patients, but the results of the UKPDS are eagerly awaited.

From other work, it appears that the level of diabetic control in the early years, particularly with Type I diabetes, is very important.

Once retinopathy is established, should diabetic control be improved? It would be anticipated that if there is a tight relationship between diabetic control and complications, improvement in glycaemic control would be beneficial.

Several small trials in patients with diabetic retinopathy have clearly demonstrated that over the first 18 months of treatment with tight diabetic control, diabetic retinopathy may deteriorate. However, after an 18-month period, patients with tight diabetic control when compared to those maintained on their normal regimens, do indeed have less progression of diabetic retinopathy. The large DCCT trial has subsequently confirmed these findings. It is therefore recommended that patients with established complications should improve diabetic control but this should be done over a period of time not to produce acute dramatic changes in glycaemia.

(b) HYPERTENSION

Importance of hypertension as a risk factor for diabetic retinopathy has recently been realized. Several reports have shown an association of systemic hypertension with exudation, haemorrhage, and other severe forms of diabetic retinopathy. This appears to hold for both diastolic and systolic hypertension. This was well illustrated in a study of Pima Indians in whom over a 5-year period, the incidence of retinal exudation in diabetic subjects with systolic pressure greater than 145 mmHg, was more than twice that of the subjects whose systolic pressure was less than 125 mmHg. In another study one factor protective against retinopathy in patients with Type I diabetes free of retinopathy for 30 years, was lower diastolic blood pressure.

Logically, treatment of systemic hypertension in association with retinopathy should have benefits. For example, with advanced retinopathy there is significant capillary damage and leakage and also disruption of the retinal auto-regulatory system (Fig. 4.3). However, the influence of hypertension on microvascular disease is still not well defined and the value of hypotensive treatment in terms of progression of diabetic retinopathy, is not well studied. Treatment of the complication diabetic nephropathy has been studied in detail and the results are relevant to retinopathy. There is now significant evidence that control of even mild to moderate hypertension diminishes urinary protein excretion (microalbuminuria) and slows the decline in renal function in diabetic nephropaths. Studies of angiotensin converting enzyme drugs have suggested a specific effect of these drugs on the renal microcirculation which may be independent of the effect on systemic blood pressure. A recent large randomized trial of captopril treatment in patients with diabetic nephropathy has demonstrated definite protection in renal function over a median three-year period. This group of drugs is of major interest with regard to retinopathy as one of the possible angiogenic factors which may be involved in the formation of proliferative diabetic retinopathy is angiotensins 1–3. The possibility, therefore, that ACE inhibitors could be of value in preventing development of proliferative retinopathy from the pre-proliferative stage is under current research.

(c) HYPERLIPIDAEMIA

Some studies have previously suggested a relationship between hyperlipidaemia and diabetic retinopathy. This idea was put forward in 1969 in a study of lipid lowering using the agent clofibrate in those patients with marked exudative diabetic maculopathy. This trial did demonstrate significant reduction in retinal exudation but was not associated with any improvement in visual outcome. The latter is not surprising as the patients had advanced disease and even with laser therapy no improvement would have been anticipated. More recent evidence from two centres have suggested that cholesterol lowering in hyperlipidaemic diabetic patients with exudative maculopathy may be of benefit. Trials using the new class of cholesterol lowering agent, the HMG CoA-reductase inhibitors, are awaited.

(d) OTHER TREATMENT

Other agents have been tried which alter other possible pathogenic pathways. For example, aldose reductase inhibitors which prevent the accumulation of sorbitol, have been studied but the results have generally been disappointing. In view of the abnormalities in haemostasis in diabetics, trials of aspirin have been performed. The results are inconclusive and do not show benefit of treatment with this drug. In view of increased free radical activity that might be involved in the pathogenesis of diabetic retinopathy, specific free radical scavenging agents (usually anti-oxidants) could theoretically be of benefit. These would include Vitamin C and E and glutathione.

(e) DIABETIC RETINOPATHY OCCURRING IN PREGNANCY

Diabetic retinopathy may develop or indeed be pre-existing in a diabetic patient who becomes pregnant. Reports have shown that diabetic retinopathy may progress very rapidly with the impairment of vision during pregnancy. The exact mechanisms for this are not entirely clear. Predictive factors for deterioration in retinopathy in pregnancy include the presence of proteinuria and pre-existing changes of retinopathy before pregnancy.

Management of retinopathy during pregnancy is similar to that in the non-pregnant state. However, it is worth noting that retinopathic changes do regress in the post-partum period, and because of this some authors feel that laser treatment need not necessarily be so aggressive. Diabetic retinopathy is also not a contraindication to pregnancy if adequate laser treatment has been given for diabetic maculopathy or proliferative retinopathy previously. In this case, the retinal findings may remain stable for the duration of the pregnancy.

4.6 SCREENING FOR DIABETIC RETINOPATHY

With the modern emphasis on early detection of diabetic retinopathy, methods of reliable screening for early disease has become more imperative. In many countries with suitable numbers of trained ophthalmologists, ideal routine eye screening is performed by this specialist group. In the United Kingdom and other countries, this approach is not feasible owing to the overwhelming number of patients per trained ophthalmologist. Furthermore, organizational changes may also put more emphasis on screening for diabetic retinopathy outside the hospital diabetic clinics into primary health care. The other methods of screening are:

1. fundoscopy – dilated pupil;
2. optometrist screening;
3. non-mydriatic camera;
4. visual acuity with pinhole correction;
5. macular function tests.

The traditional way in hospital diabetic clinics of screening for diabetic retinopathy is using the ophthalmoscope. The current European recommendations are that this should be on at least an annual basis and should be done through a dilated pupil. In patients with established background retinopathy, retinal examination should be performed on a 4–6 monthly basis. Dilatation of the pupil in diabetic clinics (albeit in hospital or primary care) should be the aim for every patient who is having fundoscopy. In clinical practice many centres do not achieve this ideal particularly in view of organizational problems in clinic and the fact that pupil dilatation affects patients' ability to drive home after attendance in out-patients.

Retinal screening, therefore, still occurs through undilated pupils, which may miss peripheral lesions or subtle changes in the macular area and neovascularization. The accuracy of retinal examination with the ophthalmoscope also reflects the degree of specialization and expertise of the doctor examining. An error rate as high as 61% has been observed in some studies in patients with established diabetic retinopathy being screened by junior and senior medical staff. Training in use of the ophthalmoscope and fundoscopy through dilated pupils on an annual basis is vital to the success in terms of screening.

Visual acuity has previously been suggested as a method of screening. As much of diabetic retinopathy is asymptomatic, and the aim of screening is to pick up patients before visual symptoms develop, visual acuity testing will not be adequate. However, visual acuity testing may be an aid as specific changes may be picked up with altered visual acuity; for example a change from 6/6 to 6/9 vision may be highly significant. Equally deterioration in visual acuity with a pinhole correction may suggest underlying macular disease. Other forms of testing may also be helpful in the clinical situation. In particular, the Amsler chart, the Maddox rod and the photostress test are all used in assessment of macular function. Some studies have suggested that these may detect early macular disease even in the presence of normal visual acuity. These tests would not replace fundoscopy but aid in detection of those with significant disease.

Eye tests with optometrists are currently free of charge to diabetic patients in the UK. Optometrists are highly trained in fundoscopy and their role has therefore been assessed with regard to screening for diabetic eye disease. Several studies assessing optometrists versus ophthalmologists and other health professionals involved in diabetic care have shown that they are effective in screening. This is particularly important to patients cared for in a primary care setting.

Considerable assessment has been made of the non-mydriatic fundus camera in screening for diabetic retinopathy. In summary:

1. Used in large studies (>5500 patients).
2. Better performance than untrained internist (especially for maculopathy).

3. Disappointing accuracy: technical problems (sensitivity 35–67%).
4. 37% of new vessels >3 disc diameters from centre and are therefore potentially missed by photography.
5. Useful adjunct to direct ophthalmoscopy: improves sensitivities.

Various studies have shown this to be an effective method for screening but its main drawbacks are the cost of the camera and film and the fact that peripheral retinal new vessels may be missed. It would therefore appear that screening for early diabetic retinopathy can effectively be achieved by examination of a fundus through a dilated pupil by an experienced examiner. This can be performed by an optometrist, particularly if specific training in diabetes has been undertaken. The non-mydriatic camera is also an option buut requires photographic staff as well as medical assessment, and should be used in conjunction with direct ophthalmoscopy.

4.7 OTHER OPHTHALMOLOGICAL COMPLICATIONS

Like hypertension, retinovascular disease is not uncommon in diabetic patients. It is likely that both retinal vein occlusion and retinal artery occlusion (embolic or local occlusion) occur more frequently in diabetics because of the increased prevalence of macrovascular and microvascular disease. The major risk factors associated with non-insulin dependent diabetes are shown in Table 4.3. It is clear that in retinal vein occlusion these complications of either the branch or central form do reflect the other cardiovascular risk factors of hypertension and hyperlipidaemia.

Glaucoma is associated with diabetes, particularly in the chronic open angle variety. This occurs in approximately 1% of a diabetic clinic population. Although the exact etiology of this condition is unclear, several theories have been suggested. These include autonomic neuropathy affecting the pupillary reflexes or vascular disease affecting the aqueous drainage system. Ischaemic optic neuropathy is also associated and may relate to the predeliction of macro- and microvascular disease for the diabetic patient. Uveitis has been identified in association with diabetes but the reason for this association is not clear.

Table 4.3 Major cardiovascular risk factors in non-insulin dependent diabetes (percentages given are approximate and may vary)

	Percentage in clinic population
Smoking	30%
Hypertension	40%
Hyperlipidaemia	40%

4.8 DIAGNOSIS AND MANAGEMENT OF DIABETES MELLITUS

Diabetes mellitus is a syndrome characterized by chronic hyperglycaemia. A high blood glucose level produces an osmotic diuresis, leading to the typical symptoms of:

- polyuria
- nocturia
- weight loss
- weakness (hyperglycaemic lethargy)

In the Western world, most cases of diabetes are non-insulin dependent (Type II) and a minority are insulin dependent (Type I diabetes). The features of these two types of diabetes are shown in Table 4.4.

Diagnosis is usually confirmed by the presence of an elevated random blood glucose (>11 mmol/l) in conjunction with symptoms of diabetes and glycosuria as shown in Fig. 4.17. However, in a minority, the diagnosis cannot be confirmed using these criteria, making the glucose tolerance test essential. The required values to establish or refute the diagnosis are shown in Table 4.5.

All patients with diabetes should be home blood glucose monitoring where possible. The aim of therapy is to abolish diabetic symptoms and to reduce the macrovascular and microvascular complications that are part of the disease process (Table 4.6). Diabetic education is of paramount importance.

4.8.1 Management of diabetes mellitus

(a) TYPE I DIABETES (IDDM OR KETOSIS-PRONE)

Once the diagnosis is established, insulin administration is essential in conjunction with a diabetic diet (see Table 4.7). Patients should be referred urgently to a diabetes centre, where insulin administration, home blood glucose monitoring, education about diabetes, and diabetic diet, can be undertaken. The aim of management is to provide a patient with the information and equipment to become self-caring in order to obtain optimal diabetic control. This is particularly stressed in the early years of diabetes as

Table 4.4 Features of Type I and Type II diabetes mellitus

Type II *NIDDM*	*Type I* *IDDM*
Non-ketosis prone	Ketosis prone
Insulin treatment optional	Insulin treatment mandatory
Insidious onset	Acute
Obese or non-obese	Usually non-obese
Onset usually over 50 years but may occur in young (MODY) and in Asian populations	Typically onset in youth but can be any age

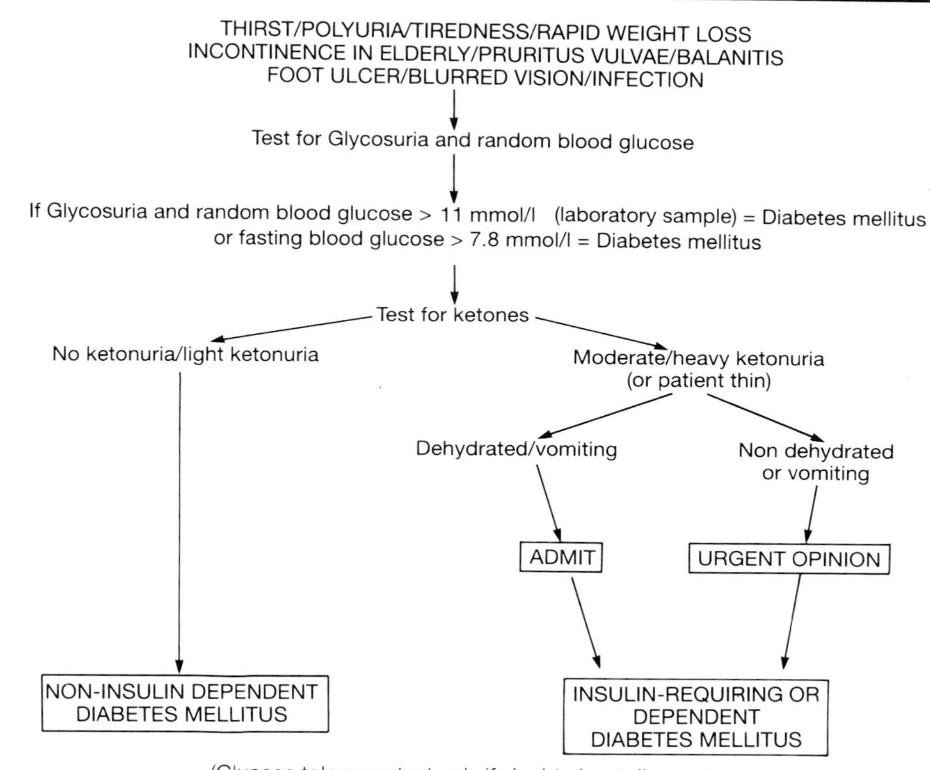

Fig. 4.17 Diagnosis of diabetes mellitus.

Table 4.5 Key glucose values of the glucose tolerance test (75 g glucose load)

	Venous plasma samples (glucose mmol/l)	
	Fasting	*After 2 hours*
Normal	<7.8	<7.8
Impaired glucose tolerance (IGT)	<7.8	7.8–<11.1
Diabetes mellitus	⩾7.8	⩾11.1

(IGT is a category which carries an increased risk of subsequently developing diabetes and also of macrovascular disease)

Table 4.6 Common complications of diabetes mellitus

	Site	Features
Macrovascular	(a) Coronary	Ischaemic heart disease, angina, myocardial infarction
	(b) Peripheral	Ischaemic limbs, intermittent claudication, ulceration, gangrene
	(c) Carotid and cerebral	Stroke (infarction, embolic, haemorrhagic)
Microvascular	(a) Eye	Cranial nerve palsies, cataract, glaucoma, retinopathy
	(b) Kidney (nephropathy)	Micro-albuminuria (30–300 mg/24 hrs, incipient nephropathy) Macro-albuminuria (>300 mg/24 hrs, Albustix +ve, diabetic nephropathy) Renal failure, Nephrotic syndrome
	(c) Nervous system (neuropathy)	Peripheral neuropathy (glove and stocking sensory loss, reduced or absent vibration sense, absent ankle jerks, neuropathic ulcers) Amyotrophy (non-symmetrical muscle wasting, typically quadriceps) Autonomic neuropathy (postural hypotension, diarrhoea, gustatory sweating, bladder atony)
	(d) Skin	Necrobiosis Lipoidica Diabeticorum, Candidal infection common, pyoderma diabeticum
	(e) Joints	Cheiro-arthropathy, frozen shoulder

diabetic control in this period appears to have an influence on subsequent development of microvascular complications. This period is often the most difficult period to obtain control particularly in childhood and during adolescence.

A common insulin regimen will consist of twice daily injections subcutaneously (SC) either of free mixing or fixed mixture insulins (Table 4.7). These are now mostly in the human form, although beef and bovine varieties are still available. Some Type I patients use a regimen of three injections of short acting insulin pre-meals with an isophane injection at bed time. This latter regimen has the advantage of more flexibility, allowing adjustment for individual cases. The results of DCCT trial suggests a target glycosylated haemoglobin level of less than 1% above the normal range.

(b) TYPE II DIABETES (NIDDM OR NON-KETOSIS PRONE)

Following a definite diagnosis of diabetes, the cornerstone of management is diabetic education and dietary advice. Principles of the diabetic diet are to calculate ideal body weight and set total calorie intake. Also to advise:

- high unrefined carbohydrate foods;
- high fibre products;
- avoidance of refined carbohydrate;
- reduce saturated fat;
- increase polyunsaturated and monounsaturated fat;
- alcohol in moderation;
- reduction of salt intake.

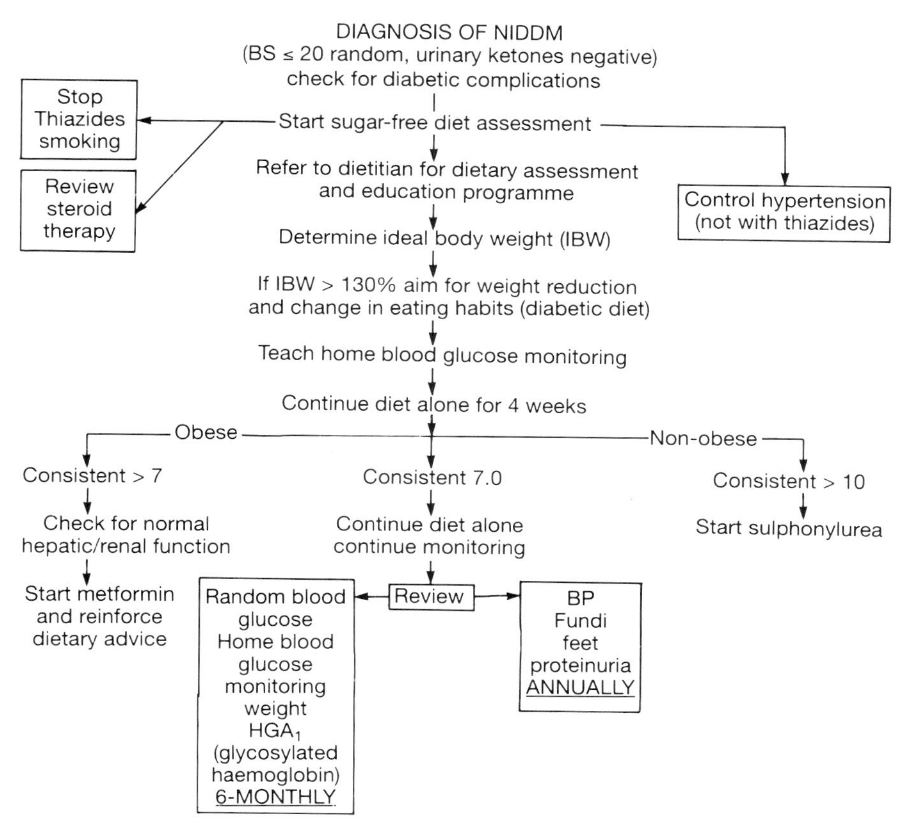

Fig. 4.18 Management of non-insulin dependent diabetes mellitus.

Table 4.7 Types of insulin available in common usage

	Action (h)	*Type*	*Examples*
Short acting	4–6	Soluble	Actrapid, Velosulin, Humulin S
Intermediate acting	12	Isophane	Insulatard, Protophane, Humulin I
		Insulin zinc suspension	Monotard
Long acting	24+	Insulin zinc suspension	Ultratard, Humulin lente and ZN

Fixed mixtures

Ratio (%)			
Short	*Intermediate*	*Humulin range*	*Pen mix range*
10	90	M1	10/90 Penfill
20	80	M2	20/90 Penfill
30	70	M3	Actraphane
40	60	M4	40/60 Penfill
50	50		50/50 Penfill
		Via B-D pen	Via Novopen II

(Mixtard and Initard are 30/70 and 50/50 mixtures respectively.)

Table 4.8 Oral hypoglycaemic therapy in diabetes mellitus

	Biguanides	*Sulphonylureas*
Mechanism of action	↓ Appetite ↓ Intestinal glucose absorption ↑ Muscle glucose uptake	↑ Endogenous insulin secretion ? ↑ Insulin receptor function
Indications	Diet failed in obese type II patient	Diet failed in non-obese
Common drug usage	Metformin 500 mg b.d. or t.d.s.	Tolbutamide (good in elderly) Chlorpropamide (avoid in elderly) Glibenclamide Glipizide Gliclazide Gliquidone (useful if renal failure)

A flow diagram outlining management is shown in Fig. 4.18. Particular emphasis is placed on weight loss in the obese, and encouraging a prudent lifestyle, including reduction of alcohol and cessation of smoking. If the random blood glucose is below 20 mmol (without ketones on urine testing), diet alone should be maintained for one month. If home blood glucose monitoring does not demonstrate good diabetic control (average blood glucose <7.0 mmol/l or glycosylated haemoglobin <7% (normal range <5%)), either a sulphonylurea or biguanide oral hypoglycaemic agent should be commenced, with the biguanide being used as first choice for obese subjects.

Modes of action and examples of each class are shown in Table 4.8. If one class of drug is insufficient to establish optimal diabetic control, a combination may be used. Insulin administration may be needed in this group of patients if inadequate blood glucose control is achieved on maximal oral therapy

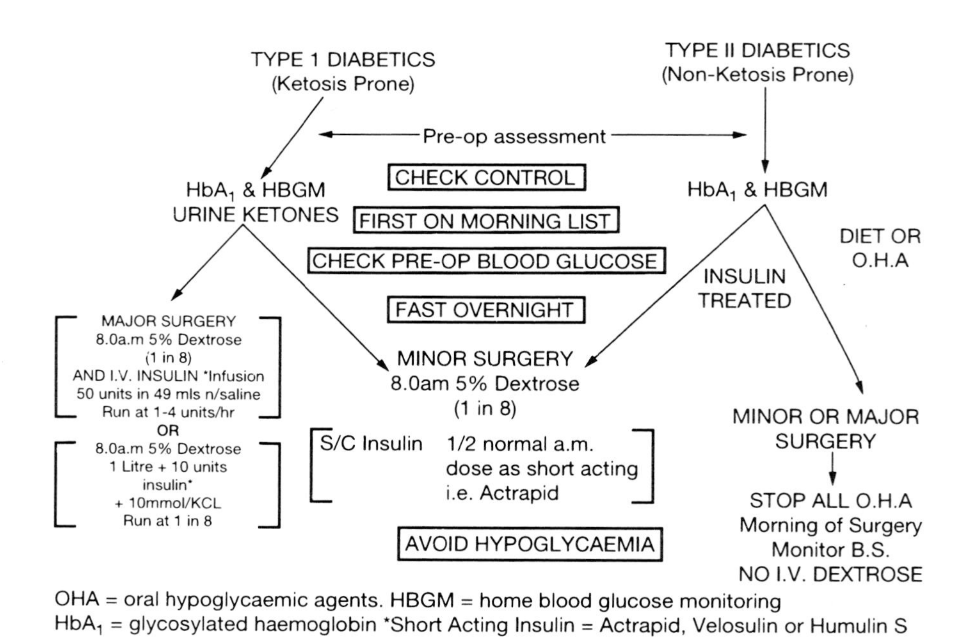

Fig. 4.19 Guidelines of pre-and peri-operative care of diabetic patients undergoing elective surgery.

or a patient is underweight or symptomatic with the presence of urinary ketones. The use of insulin in Type II diabetes management is becoming more common and there is less reluctance amongst such patients to accept insulin, particularly with the advent of new insulin delivery systems, e.g. insulin injection pen devices. This is increasing the number of diabetic patients on insulin treatment undergoing surgical procedures. A schematic to aid perioperative care of diabetic patients is shown in Fig. 4.19.

FURTHER READING

Barnett, A.H. and Dodson, P.M. (1990) *Hypertension and Diabetes*, Science Press, London.

Dodson, P.M. and Barnett, A.H. (1992) *Lipids, Diabetes and Vascular Disease*. Science Press, London.

Dodson, P.M. and Gibson, J.M. (1991) Long term follow-up of and underlying medical conditions in patients with diabetic exudative maculopathy. *Eye*, **5**, 699–703.

Jennings, P.E. and Barnett, A.H. (1988) New approaches to the pathogenesis and treatment of diabetic micro-angiopathy. *Diab. Med.*, **5**, 111–7.

Klein, R., Klein, B.E. and Moss, S.E. *et al.* (1984) The Wisconsin Epidemiologic Study of Diabetic Retinopathy. *Arch. Ophthalmol.*, **102**, 527–32.

Kohner, E.M. (1993) Diabetic retinopathy. *British Medical Journal*, **307**, 1195–9.

Kohner, E.M. and Sullivan, P.M. (1991) Pharmacology of eye care in diabetes, in *Pharmacology of Diabetes*, Vol. 3 (eds Mogensen, C.E. and Standi, E.), W. De Gruyter, Berlin and New York.

Lewis, E.J., Lawrence, G.M., Hunsicker, L.G. *et al.* (1993) The effect of angiotensin-converting enzyme inhibition on diabetic nephropathy. *New Eng. J. of Med.*, **329**, 1456–62.

MacCuish, A.C. (1992) Who should screen for diabetic retinopathy? *Diabetes Rev.*, **1**, 5–8.

Schultz, G.S. and Grant, M.B. (1991) Neovascular growth factors. *Eye*, **5**, 170–80.

The Diabetes Control and Complications Trial Research Group (1993) The effect of intensive treatment of diabetes on the development and progression of long-term complications in insulin-dependent diabetes mellitus. *New Engl. J. Med.*, **329**, 977–1036.

5 *Hypertension*

Clinical Retinopathies. Paul M. Dodson, Jonathan M. Gibson and Erna E. Kritzinger.
Published in 1995 by Chapman & Hall, London. ISBN 0 412 35930 8

5.1 INTRODUCTION AND DEFINITION

The World Health Organization criteria of hypertension are:

- hypertension – above 160/95 mmHg;
- borderline hypertension – 140/90 to 160/95;
- normotension – below 140/90 mmHg.

At least three recordings should be made on separate occasions and cuff correction for obesity (mid upper arm circumference >33 cm) made appropriately.

The definition of arterial hypertension as blood pressure levels above 160/95 mmHg is of practical use but hypertension is best considered to be a state of graded risk. In Westernized societies the height of the blood pressure is an accurate predictor of the subsequent development of heart attacks, strokes, renal failure, heart failure and peripheral vascular disease. The association between blood pressure and risk extends down to 'normal' levels and is quantitative. An alternative definitive of hypertension is to consider it to be that level of blood pressure above which antihypertensive medication has been shown to be of more use than harm. Present knowledge suggests that diastolic blood pressures which are consistently over 100 mmHg are worth reducing because this brings about a large reduction in the risk of hypertension induced stroke and has a modest impact on coronary artery disease.

5.2 OTHER RISK FACTORS

High blood pressure should not be considered a risk factor in isolation, but should be viewed in relation to levels of serum cholesterol, cigarette smoking habits, race, the age of the individual and the family history of vascular diseases including heart attack and stroke. When there is evidence of end organ damage, the prognosis for a given level of blood pressure is substantially worse.

5.3 HYPERTENSION AND THE RETINA

Changes in the retinal vasculature have long been observed in hypertensive individuals and the prognostic significance of such changes has been the source of much interest. The retinal grading systems will now be described, but it is apparent that an updated retinal grading system should be employed and this will be covered towards the end of this section.

Retinal changes were first described in the severe hypertension of Bright's disease shortly after the introduction of the ophthalmoscope but before the widespread use of the sphygmomanometer. Careful documentation of retinal vessel appearances was correlated with renal and cerebrovascular disease and the emergence of essential hypertension as a separate clinical entity brought about interest in retinal vascular changes in hypertension. Changes specific to hypertension alone are still not exactly agreed upon despite a century of observation and investigation. The seminal work of Keith, Wagener and Barker in 1939 in grading hypertension into groups of differing severity and outcome in which retinal features were described, remains in common clinical usage:

Group 1 Mild narrowing or sclerosis of retinal arterioles. No symptoms. Good general health.

Group 2 Moderate to marked sclerosis of the retinal arterioles. Exaggerated arterial light reflex. Venous compression at arteriovenous crossings. Blood pressure higher and more sustained than Group 1. Asymptomatic. Good general health.

Group 3 Retinal oedema, cotton-wool spots and haemorrhages. Sclerosis of retinal arterioles. Blood pressure often high and sustained symptomatic.

Group 4 All the above and optic disc oedema. Cardiac and renal functions may be impaired.

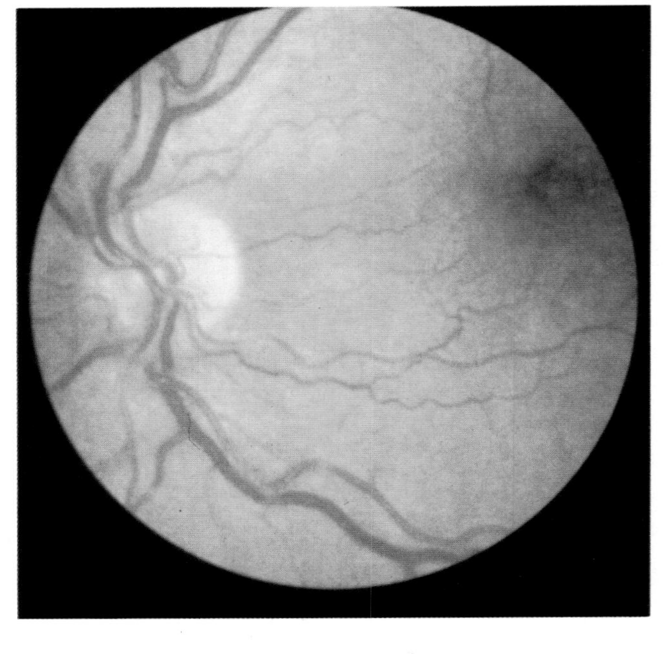

Fig. 5.1 Grade 1 Keith, Wagener, Barker classification.

The strength of the Keith, Wagener and Barker classification was its link between clinical findings and prognosis but its weakness is the fact that the retinal appearance described in Groups 1 and 2 may also be caused by arteriosclerosis and ageing (Figs 5.1 and 5.2).

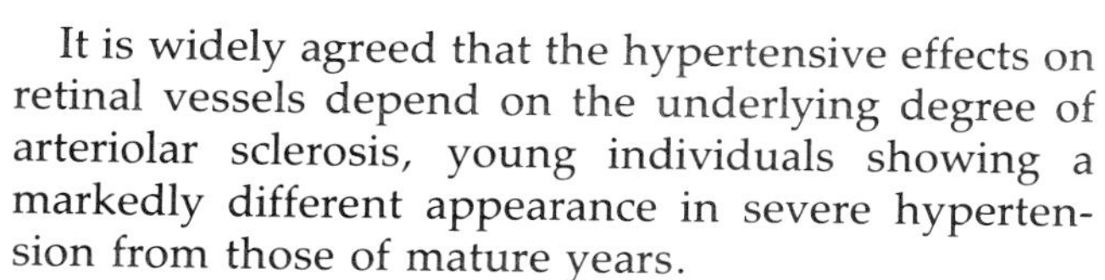

It is widely agreed that the hypertensive effects on retinal vessels depend on the underlying degree of arteriolar sclerosis, young individuals showing a markedly different appearance in severe hypertension from those of mature years.

The first two Keith, Wagener, Barker groups have

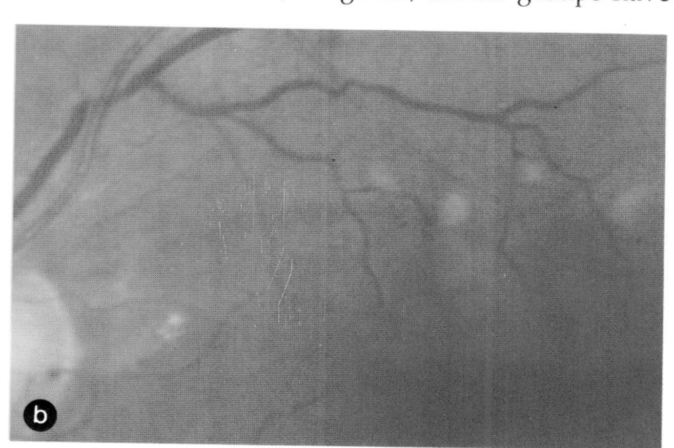

Fig. 5.2 Grade 2 Keith, Wagener, Barker classification. (a) Arteriosclerosis; (b) AV nipping.

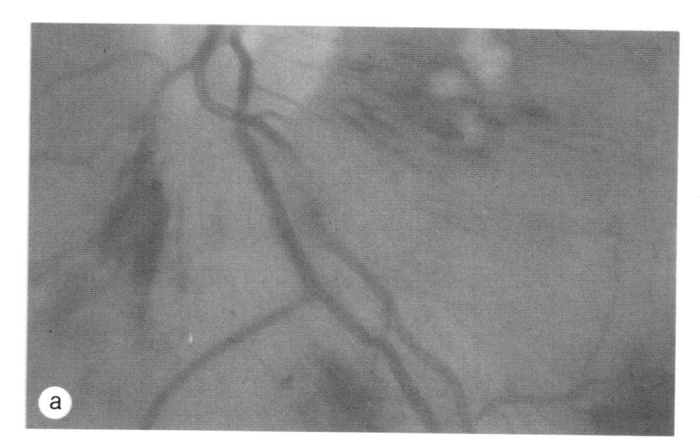

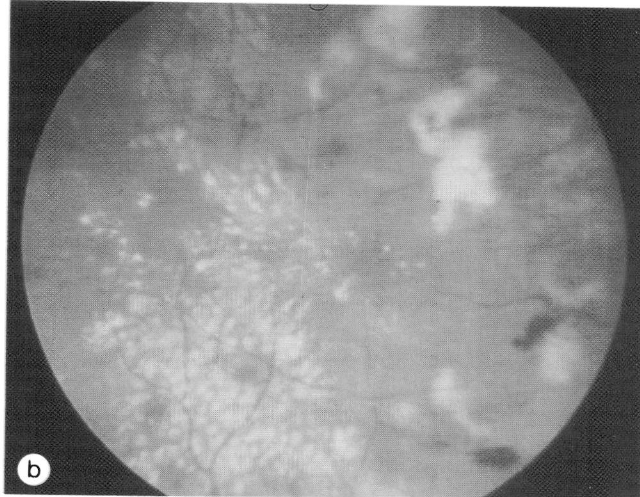

Fig. 5.3 Grade 3 Keith, Wagener, Barker classification. (a) Flame-shaped haemorrhage and cotton wool spots; (b) cotton wool spots, haemorrhage and circinate exudation.

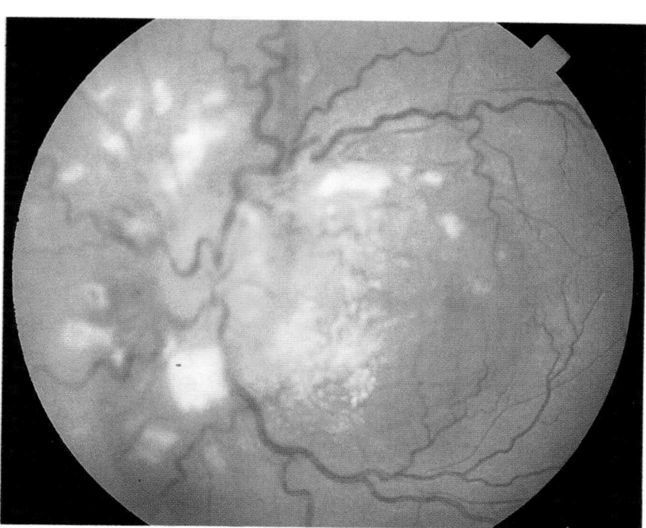

Fig. 5.4 Grade 4 Keith, Wagener, Barker classification.

also been difficult to differentiate clinically. Degrees of light reflectivity from retinal arterioles and the many aspects of arteriovenous crossing appearance can be rather subjective and by no means are all such changes pathological, let alone specific to hypertension.

The third and fourth groups of Keith, Wagener and Barker represent easier grounds for most observers as the presence of haemorrhages, cotton wool spots and papilloedema are much more definite signs (Figs 5.3 and 5.4). The haemorrhages may be flame-shaped and situated at the level of the retinal nerve fibre layer or may be deeper placed and of the dot-and-blot variety. Cotton wool spots are nerve fibre layer infarcts and usually are seen close to the disc and main vessels. Exudates are the result of fluid leakage from terminal arterioles and capillaries, which resorb, leaving behind lipid deposits. If occurring centrally, the exudate may accumulate in Henle's layer (central nerve fibre layer of the retina) and form the so-called macular star (Fig. 5.5).

Keith, Wagener, Barker Group 4 includes the features of papilloedema and is correlated with a poor clinical outcome and prognosis.

The exact cause of the optic nerve head swelling is not known, but raised intracranial pressure, fibrinoid necrosis of small arterioles supplying the optic disc or impeded venous flow may all play a role.

This recognition of a malignant form of essential hypertension pre-dated Keith, Wagener and Barker's 1939 paper. Their Group 4 category, with its very poor prognosis (1% 5-year survival) attracted this term, although some authors have required that proteinuria be added to the diagnostic criteria. Keith, Wagener, Barker's Group 3 has more recently been associated with the term 'accelerated hypertension' (Section 5.4, Table 5.1).

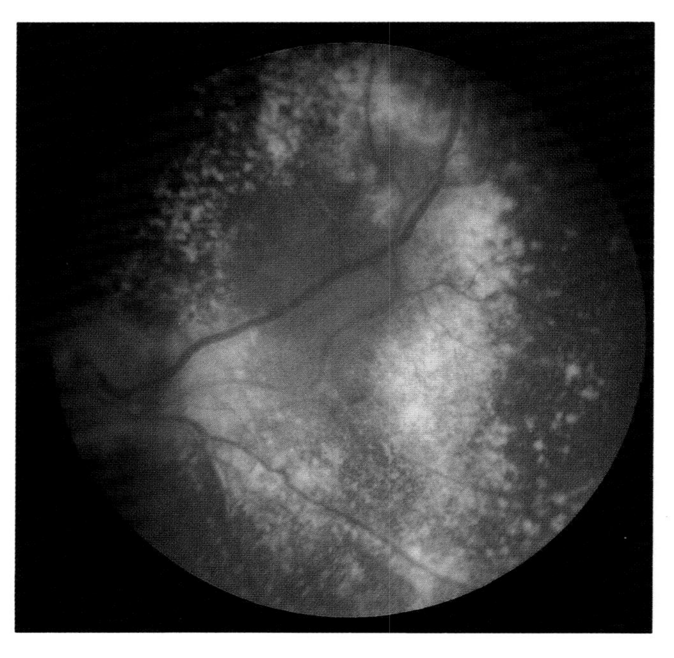

Fig. 5.5 Macular star in hypertension.

More recent studies have found little difference in the present-day survival rates of Groups 3 and 4. Fibrinoid necrosis – once a hallmark of malignant hypertension – has been described without papilloedema, leading many observers to feel that the old groupings are now obsolete. The decline in prevalence of malignant hypertension, in conjunction with the improved prognosis when treated with drugs, and the widespread use of antihypertensive drugs in 'benign' hypertension, have led to a shift in clinical presentation and practice which has now outdated the Keith, Wagener, Barker classification. Since 1939 medicine has, therefore, obscured the natural history of hypertensive disease.

Table 5.1 Suggested revised grading system for hypertensive retinopathy

Grade	*Significance*	*Retinal changes*	*Hypertensive category*
I	Less clinically significant	Generalized arteriolar	Established hypertension
	Non-accelerated	narrowing Focal constriction (NB **not** A-V nipping (nicking))	
II	Highly clinically significant	Haemorrhages Exudation	Retinovascular damage
	Accelerated	Cotton-wool spots ± Optic disc swelling	Accelerated or malignant hypertension

To fulfil Grade II, a lesion of retinovascular damage should be present in both eyes.

Most authors now believe that the grading of hypertension could be simplified into two categories (Table 5.1). Groups 3 and 4, according to Keith, Wagener and Barker should now be considered and classed as accelerated or malignant phase hypertension (Group II), whereas other changes which may or may not be hypertension related, are redefined as Group I.

This latter system has the important advantage of separating out the poor prognostic category relating to features of retinovascular leakage and occlusion associated with hypertension (accelerated or malignant form) as one grade (II). This constrasts with retinal changes of arteriolar sclerosis which may or may not be related to hypertension, and are in any case difficult physical signs in clinical practice. The simple grading system is also practical, and easier to learn, unlike the Keith, Wagener, Barker classification. Why this latter confusing and inappropriate system is still used in worldwide clinical practice and widely taught is not clear. A new simpler clinically relevant grading system has been long overdue.

5.4 ACCELERATED OR MALIGNANT PHASE HYPERTENSION

Sustained hypertension can become accelerated or enter a malignant phase. The presence of papilloedema, or the accompaniment of retinal haemorrhages and exudates defines this condition. The features are:

- Characterized by: arteriolar fibrinoid necrosis;
- Cause: 65% essential in origin;
- Blood pressure: raised (n.b. actual level not defined);
- Fundi: Grade III and IV Keith, Wagener, Barker (or Grade II revised version, Table 5.1);
- Outlook: 10% 1 year survival untreated. Approximately 50% 7-year survival treated.

(Some authors include proteinuria in the definition.)

The blood pressure is often above 200/140. Accelerated hypertension is a significant recent rise in blood pressure levels with evidence of retinal changes with or without papilloedema. Accompanying clinical features are proteinuria, microscopic haematuria, weight loss and renal, cardiac and nervous system malfunction. Usually the histological features of fibrinoid necrosis accompany the syndrome but this is not invariable.

With current treatment, the outlook for accelerated hypertensive patients has greatly improved but the mortality rate is still significant. High levels of blood pressure have been reported in association with fibrinoid necrosis but without retinopathy and this also signifies a bad prognosis.

5.5 CLINICAL AETIOLOGY

In most cases the cause of arterial hypertension is unknown. Over 90% of all cases fall into the group called idiopathic, primary or essential. This figure varies depending on the population studied and the extent of the investigation. Primary renal disease and endocrine disorders are the commoner underlying causes in secondary hypertension.

In accelerated and malignant phase hypertension, underlying causes appear to be commoner than in non-accelerated hypertension. The long term prognosis may vary according to the underlying cause, particularly if a secondary cause is identified. Accelerated hypertension may develop in patients previously in the benign phase, but does also develop *de novo*.

5.6 PRE-ECLAMPSIA

The syndrome of pre-eclampsic toxaemia is not fully understood. It is probable that the prime lesion of pre-eclampsic toxaemia is placental ischaemia related to placental arterial thickening and intravascular thrombosis. This may relate immune complexes with hypertension only as a marker of the underlying disease.

It leads to a rise in blood pressure, development of proteinuria and foetal ischaemia with intrauterine growth retardation and occasionally foetal death. Most women with pre-eclampsia develop fluid retention with leg oedema and facial oedema. Ophthalmoscopy may reveal narrowing of the retinal arterioles (focal or generalized), retinal oedema or, less commonly, retinal haemorrhages. It is likely, therefore, that in pre-eclamptic toxaemia, the high blood pressure is not the main lesion but is merely a marker for the underlying placental disease. Despite the weak association between the height of the blood pressure and the severity of pre-eclampsia, it is usual to reduce blood pressure urgently in such cases. Intramuscular or intravenous hydralazine, labetolol infusions or occasionally oral atenolol, labetolol, hydralazine or nifedipine may prove necessary in order to secure blood pressure control.

If the pregnancy is beyond about 36 weeks gestation and there is severe pre-eclampsia, then the baby should be delivered by emergency lower segment Caesarian section. After Caesarian section, blood pressure commonly returns rapidly to normal range. However, blood pressure may remain elevated up to seven days after delivery and it is usual, therefore, to continue antihypertensive medication in such patients for approximately a week.

During the development of pre-eclampsia, there may be signs of cerebral irritability with headaches, drowsiness and visual disturbance. There may be evidence of intrauterine growth retardation on foetal scanning and the cardiotocograph may reveal transient or prolonged falls in the foetal heart rate, indicative of foetal distress.

5.7 AETIOLOGY OF HYPERTENSION

In the majority (95%) of patients with hypertension, no underlying cause can be found. In the minority (5% or less), there may be an underlying cause found on investigation. The primary and secondary causes of hypertension are:

1. Renal disease
   (a) intrinsic, e.g. glomerulonephritis, pyelonephritis;
   (b) renal artery stenosis;
   (c) chronic renal failure;
   (d) renal tumours;
   (e) polycystic renal disease.
2. Endocrine
   (a) diabetes mellitus;
   (b) phaeochromocytoma;
   (c) primary aldosteronism (Conn's syndrome);
   (d) primary hyperparathyroidism;
   (e) hyperthyroidism;
   (f) Cushing's syndrome, acromegaly;
   (g) oestrogen/progesterone combination therapy.
3. Rarer causes
   (a) coarctation of the aorta;
   (b) Von Recklinghausen's neurofibromatosis.

It is probable that in the accelerated or malignant phase of hypertension, the frequency of underlying renal or adrenal causes of hypertension is greater than in patients without the accelerated phase. Despite this, in the majority of cases of accelerated (or malignant phase) hypertension no underlying cause can be found.

However, many cases present with evidence of renal impairment or failure and it is often not possible to be certain whether there was an underlying renal disease (e.g. glomerulonephritis) causing hypertension. At this late stage, a renal biopsy is rarely performed.

The reason why some patients develop retinal haemorrhages, infarcts, exudates and/or papilloedema for a particular level of blood pressure, whilst others do not, is uncertain. There are some clinical clues. For example, one important finding is that there is a close association between cigarette smoking and accelerated and malignant phase hypertension. By contrast, the prevalence of cigarette smoking amongst people with hypertension without retinopathy is lower than the national average for the general population, i.e. hypertensives are less likely to be cigarette smokers than normotensives. It is possible that cigarette smoking by its effect on platelet aggregation and arterial narrowing increases the tendency towards retinal ischaemia, which in conjunction with a high blood pressure, leads to retinal damage.

It is generally held that accelerated or malignant phase hypertension is particularly associated with high circulating levels of plasma renin. Renin is an enzyme secreted by the kidney which uses the degradation of renin substrate (angiotensinogen) produced by the liver to form the deca-peptide angiotensin 1. Angiotensin 1 is rapidly converted in the lungs to angiotensin 2. This is a powerful pressor agent in its own right and causes stimulation of the adrenal glands, which leads to high plasma levels of aldosterone, together with a rise of plasma sodium and a fall in plasma potassium concentrations. Many patients with accelerated or malignant phase hypertension have mild hypokalaemia at first presentation and this usually improves as the blood pressure is brought under control. It is probable that the high renin levels are partly related to the stimulatory effect of intrarenal arteriolar narrowing with consequent ischaemia in the glomerulus and the juxta-glomerular apparatus.

There are some forms of hypertension where circulating plasma renin levels are typically low. Low renin hypertension is more common in older people and in Afro-Caribbean or black patients. There is no evidence that accelerated or malignant phase hypertension is less common in these groups. Indeed malignant phase hypertension is seen in the elderly although there are only a few case reports.

Plasma renin levels are very low in primary aldosteronism where over-production of aldosterone is autonomous. There is sodium retention and renin release is suppressed. It is generally held that in primary hyperaldosteronism, the malignant phase of hypertension is very rare although occasional reports of the association of malignant phase of hypertension and Conn's syndrome (or primary hyperaldosteronism) have been described. In contrast, there is a strong association between the malignant phase of hypertension and phaeochromocytoma, with 10% of such cases affected. In addition the malignant phase of hypertension does appear to be more common in people with renal artery stenosis, as well as glomerulonephritis, pyelonephritis and other renal conditions. There is also a small number of reports in the literature of malignant hypertension associated with the use of the oral contraceptive pill.

5.8 ASSESSMENT AND MANAGEMENT OF A HYPERTENSIVE PATIENT

A diagnosis of hypertension is made once three abnormal blood pressure recordings have been made, greater than 160 mmHg systolic or 95 mmHg diastolic blood pressure. Accelerated or malignant phase hypertension is defined as hypertension associated with bilateral retinopathy including at least exudation or haemorrhage, as described in the new grading system (Table 5.1). Notice that this definition of accelerated or malignant phase hypertension does not encompass a specific value of diastolic or systolic blood pressure. Particular regard should be paid to measurement of blood pressure as obesity is common. It is important to use the correct sphygmomanometer cuff as measurement of blood pressure using a standard (14 cm) cuff on an obese arm will result in an artificially high recording. If the upper arm circumference is greater than 33 cm, a large (19 cm) cuff should be used.

5.9 CLINICAL ASSESSMENT AND INVESTIGATION

In a newly discovered hypertensive patient, there are a number of important points to consider in the clinical assessment and investigation. Clinical assessment of a new hypertensive should include:

1. age;
2. sex;
3. family history of hypertension;
4. family history of premature cardiovascular disease;
5. smoker or non-smoker;
6. alcohol intake;
7. drug history – e.g. thiazide diuretics, steroids or anti-inflammatory drugs;
8. history of hypertensive complications – such as stroke, myocardial infarction or transient ischaemic attack;
9. cardiovascular disease – e.g. intermittent claudication or angina;
10. previous urinary tract infection or renal disease;
11. history appropriate to secondary causes of hypertension – e.g. endocrine or renal disease.

Contrary to popular belief, hypertension does not have associated symptoms although occasionally headache may be associated with accelerated hypertension. Nocturia may, however, be associated. Following a clinical history, clinical examination should be performed, of which the important features are:

1. degree and type of hypertension, e.g. isolated diastolic, systolic or combined form;
2. correction for obesity with measurement of blood pressure;
3. presence of clinical signs of hypertension, such as displaced apex beat and left ventricular hypertrophy;
4. complications of hypertension, e.g. retinopathy, renal disease, peripheral vascular disease;
5. signs of coexisting hyperlipidaemia;
6. signs of coexisting renal disease (renal artery bruits);
7. signs associated with other endocrinopathies and secondary causes.

Subsequent to this, investigation should be performed as follows:

1. chest radiography for cardiomegaly – coarctation of the aorta with rib notching;
2. ECG, to establish ischaemic heart disease or left ventricular hypertrophy, and left anterior hemiblock;
3. urea, creatinine and electrolytes to establish presence of established renal disease;
4. urine for proteinuria; culture and sensitivity for signs of urinary tract infection;
5. random serum cholesterol and triglyceride estimation to establish concomitant hyperlipidaemia especially hypercholesterolaemia;
6. other endocrine tests may be appropriate, e.g. 24 hour urinary catecholamine or catecholamine metabolite estimation for phaeochromocytoma;
7. random growth hormone for acromegaly; 24 hour urinary free cortisol for Cushing's syndrome;
8. thyroxine for thyrotoxicosis;
9. serum calcium for primary hyperparathyroidism.

In general terms, a practical rule with regard to investigation of hypertensive patients is to investigate those in whom drug treatment is thought necessary. Investigations needed are a urine test, a full blood count, biochemical profile and an ECG. In the majority of patients, however, no abnormalities will be found but most of the abnormalities that are found are important. More detailed investigation should be reserved for those who fulfil the following criteria:

1. below the age of 45;
2. blood pressure resistant to the combination of two drugs;
3. severe hypertension, i.e. diastolic blood pressure 120 mmHg or more;
4. suspicion of a cause or complication of hypertension from clinical assessment or routine investigations;
5. those with retinopathic findings of the grading system of Grade II (Table 5.1).

In general, patients whose blood pressures are very severe or who are resistant to conventional treatment need further specialist investigation. These tests will include a plain X-ray of the abdomen, ultrasound of kidneys, intravenous urography, or renal arteriogram to exclude renal artery stenosis, and CAT scanning of the adrenal gland. Echocardiography is more accurate than the ECG in assessing left ventricular size.

Twenty-four hour urine specimens should be collected on three separate occasions for assessment of catecholamine excretion, urinary protein excretion or 24 hour urinary free cortisol estimation. Renal biopsy may be appropriate to identify a cause of renal impairment particularly if intrinsic renal disease (e.g. glomerulonephritis) is suspected.

When clinical assessment and investigations have been performed and hypertension identified, consideration should then be given to an appropriate line of management.

5.10 MANAGEMENT OF HYPERTENSION

During the 1980s, many large prospective and other studies of the treatment of hypertension were published. As a result of these trials, it is now generally accepted that treating mild or moderate hypertension improves the prognosis of these patients. With accelerated or malignant phase hypertension, the improvement is sufficiently established to justify aggressive treatment. For mild hypertension, despite the differing protocols of the studies, all indicate benefit with treatment. Based on trial evidence, treatment of hypertension is indicated in men and women under 80 years of age who have diastolic blood pressures averaging 100 mmHg or more over a 3–4 month period. There is also a suggestion that patients with diastolic blood pressures of 95–99 mmHg should be actively treated with drugs, but only after careful observation over a period of several months. Two recent studies have looked at drug treatment of systolic hypertension in the elderly. These concluded that treating systolic blood pressure in isolation of greater than 160 mmHg, up to the age of 80 confers significant reduction in cardiovascular end points, and reduction in mortality. The benefit of treatment of hypertension, therefore, in all grades has shown a major impact on the occurrence of stroke, although the effect on myocardial infarction is less clear cut in younger patients. In older patients, the benefit of anti-hypertensive drug therapy on myocardial infarction is impressive in some trials (e.g. STOP and SHEP).

5.10.1 Mild hypertension

The first therapeutic step is usually non-pharmacological (Fig. 5.6). This includes weight reduction, reduction of alcohol intake (if excessive), a diet high in fibre, low in fat and sodium (the diabetic or prudent diet). Patients are encouraged to take more exercise. Obesity is a major problem in hypertensive subjects. There is now clear evidence that weight reduction benefits hypertension as well as improving other cardiovascular risk factors, e.g. hyperlipidaemia and glucose intolerance. The recommendation with regard to alcohol intake is a reduction to less than 2 units of alcohol per day, and with one alcohol free day per week. The recommended intake for males is a maximum of 21 units per week, and 14 units for females (1 unit = 1 glass of wine, 1 measure of spirits, or a half pint of beer). Cessation of smoking in terms of cardiovascular risk is of paramount importance.

Non-pharmacological therapy should be tried in the mild hypertensive for at least 3 months before drug therapy is initiated. Despite the initiation of drug therapy, non-pharmacological measures are still important, particularly with regard to maintaining ideal body weight.

5.10.2 Pharmacological measures

Over the last 20 years, drugs for lowering blood pressure have become more effective and of considerable importance. They now have fewer side-effects. A summary of treatment is shown in Fig. 5.6. Drugs commonly available are:

1. Diuretics
   (a) thiazides
      – bendrofluazide
      – hydrochlorothiazide
   (b) non-thiazides

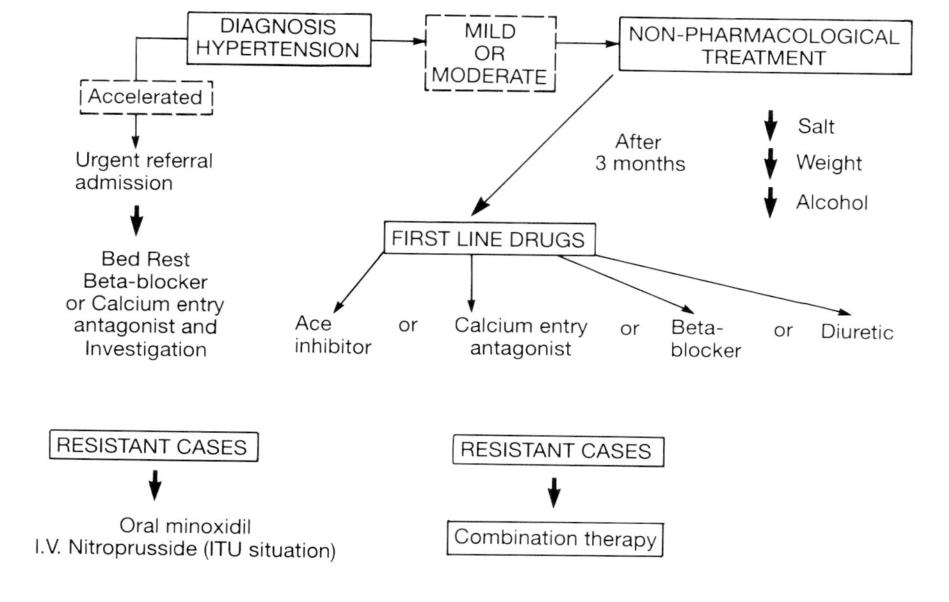

Fig. 5.6 A guide to treatment of a newly diagnosed essential hypertensive.

   - indapamide
   - potassium sparing diuretics
   - loop diuretics
2. Beta-blockers
   - atenolol
   - metoprolol
3. Calcium-entry antagonists
   - nifedipine
   - verapamil
   - amlodipine
   - diltiazem
4. Angiotensin-converting enzyme inhibitors
   - captopril
   - enalapril
   - lisinopril
   - perindopril

Others used are:

5. Alpha-adrenoceptor blockers
   - doxasocin
   - prazosin
6. Peripheral vasodilators
   - hydralazine
   - minoxidil
7. Central acting agents
   - methyldopa

The thiazide diuretics are commonly prescribed but there is increasing concern about potentially harmful metabolic and other side-effects of these drugs. These include impotence, skin rashes, hypokalaemia, hyperuricaemia, deterioration in glucose tolerance, and elevation of plasma cholesterol. Beta-blockers are still widely prescribed and have advantages which are independent of the blood pressure lowering effect. They may reduce the incidence of coronary disease. Preference is given to cardioselective agents which have a greater effect on the cardiac beta-1 receptors. This group of drugs is particularly appropriate for patients with symptomatic ischaemic heart disease or following a myocardial infarction.

The side-effects and contraindications include heart failure, peripheral vascular disease and asthma. Beta-blockers may cause sleep disturbance. They may interfere with insulin secretion, and insulin treated diabetic patients should be warned that the symptoms of hypoglycaemia can be partially masked by beta-blocker therapy. This group of drugs has also been noticed to cause an increase in serum lipids (increase in serum triglycerides with lowering of HDL cholesterol).

The angiotensin converting enzyme inhibitors are a group of drugs which are widely used in first line drug therapy. These drugs block the enzyme that is responsible for conversion of angiotensin 1 to angiotensin 2. They may also act by preventing the breakdown of bradykinin to inactive kinins, which increases circulating levels of this vasodilator hormone. This group of drugs is well tolerated from the point of view of side-effects although chronic cough is recognized as a common symptom and one that is specific to this class of drug. Other problems encountered with ACE inhibitors include hyperkalaemia and skin rashes.

A particular indication for ACE inhibitors is patients who have heart failure associated with hypertension. Patients with these two conditions may do particularly well with an ACE inhibitor with remarkable symptomatic improvement. Caution should be exercised in administration of these agents in combination with diuretic therapy as there may be a first dose hypotensive effect. They may be particularly effective in lowering blood pressure in patients with renal artery stenosis but caution should be exercised in this condition as significant deterioration in renal function may occur. However this is usually reversible when the drug is stopped.

Recent excitement has been generated from research suggesting that this group of agents may prevent or delay progression of diabetic nephropathy. Similarly in patients with scleroderma and accelerated hypertension, recent reports have suggested that ACE inhibitors may reverse or halt the deterioration in renal function.

The calcium entry antagonists are very effective blood pressure lowering agents in all grades of hypertension. Their mode of action is on arteriolar smooth muscle cell with reduction of the concentration of free ionized calcium, thereby causing relaxation of smooth muscle leading to arteriolar vasodilatation. These agents are particularly appropriate in patients with symptomatic ischaemic heart disease, and unlike beta-blockers may be of benefit in patients with peripheral vascular disease. The major side-effects of this group include facial flushing and tingling of the extremities. Headache is not an infrequent symptom particularly with initial doses. A few patients may develop peripheral oedema.

Other agents which are becoming increasingly popular, include the alpha adreno-receptor blockers. Phenoxybenzamine, phentolamine, prazosin and doxasocin are all agents of this group. These should be reserved for patients not responding to beta-blockers, diuretics, calcium antagonists or ACE inhibitors. Major side-effects include a high incidence of failure of ejaculation and the first dose effect of hypotension and collapse. Older agents like the peripheral vasodilators and centrally acting agents (methyldopa) are now rarely used.

5.11 PHARMACOLOGICAL MANAGEMENT OF ACCELERATED OR MALIGNANT PHASE HYPERTENSION

In accelerated or malignant phase hypertension, the blood pressure is usually very high and in the past, physicians have responded by reducing the blood pressure as quickly as possible. This is now realized to be hazardous as cerebral autoregulation is disturbed in accelerated hypertension, so that if the blood pressure is rapidly reduced, cerebral blood flow falls concomitantly. This may lead to cerebral or myocardial infarction. Therefore for this condition, parenteral anti-hypertensive medication should rarely be used. It should only be considered for patients with evidence of hypertensive encephalopathy, in whom there are fluctuating neurological signs or seizures. Under these circumstances an infusion of sodium nitroprusside is the treatment of first choice, but this should be undertaken in an intensive care unit.

In most cases, oral medication is all that is necessary. A single oral dose of atenolol 50 mg or nifedipine (test dose of 5 mg) or oral labetolol have all been employed. These will bring about a steady but controlled reduction of blood pressure over 12 hours. It is best to aim to bring the diastolic blood pressure down to around 110 mmHg at around 24 hours after instituting treatment. Subsequently anti-hypertensive medication should be gradually increased to reduce the diastolic and systolic blood pressure to normal values. Most patients with accelerated or malignant phase hypertension require triple-therapy, with the combination of a beta-blocker, a loop diuretic such as frusemide, and a calcium channel blocker.

In view of the activation of the renin angiotensin system in accelerated hypertension, rapid initial blockade by angiotensin converting enzyme inhibitors may be potentially dangerous and these drugs should not be used as initial therapy. There is also an increased likelihood that patients in this category may have renal artery stenosis, thus the use of ACE inhibitors may cause rapid and dangerous falls in blood pressure and irreversible reduction of renal function.

With regard to prognosis, the survival rate for patients with accelerated or malignant phase hypertension should not be substantially different from those patients without this severity of disease. The prognosis of the patient is more closely related to the accuracy of control of blood pressure rather than the height of the blood pressure at presentation. Most units now report a 5-year survival rate in this condition of around 80%. Patients who have a very poor prognosis are those with renal failure.

FURTHER READING

Ahmed, M.E.K., Walker, J.M., Beevers, D.G. and Beevers, M. (1986) Lack of difference between malignant and accelerated hypertension. *Br. Med. J.*, **292**, 235–7.

Barnett, A.H. and Dodson, P.M. (1990) *Hypertension and Diabetes*, Science Press, London.

Beevers, D.G. and MacGregor, G.A. (1994) *Hypertension in Practice*, Martin Dunitz, London.

Dimmit, S.B., West, J.N.W., Eames, S.M., *et al.* (1989) Usefulness of ophthalmology in mild to moderate hypertension. *Lancet*, **i**, 1103–6.

Eames, S.M., Dodson, P.M. and Gibson, J.M. (1994) Hypertensive retinopathy: Ocular features and grading in the 1990's. *The Journal of Human Hypertension* (in press).

Sever, P., Beevers, G., Bulpitt, C. *et al.* (1993) Management guidelines in essential hypertension: report of the second working party of the British Hypertension Society. *Br. Med. J.*, **306**, 983–7.

Subcommittee of WHO/ISH Mild Hypertension Liaison Committee (1993) Summary of 1993 World Health Organisation/International Society of Hypertension guidelines for management of mild hypertension. *Br. Med. J.*, **307**, 1541–6.

Walsh, J.B. (1982) Hypertension retinopathy – description, classification and prognosis. *Ophthalmology*, **89**, 1127–31.

6 *Retinopathy and hyperlipidaemia*

Clinical Retinopathies. Paul M. Dodson, Jonathan M. Gibson and Erna E. Kritzinger.
Published in 1995 by Chapman & Hall, London. ISBN 0 412 35930 8

6.1 INTRODUCTION

The ophthalmological presentation of the hyperlipidaemias includes xanthelasmata, corneal arcus and lipaemia retinalis. However, the retina and in particular the retinal circulation represents small vessels and therefore has allowed study of the microvasculature. The thrust of lipid research and clinical management is aimed towards prevention and treatment of macrovascular disease (myocardial infarction, stroke, and peripheral vascular disease), whereas less work has been undertaken on the retinal microvasculature. However, there are physical signs and manifestations of the hyperlipidaemias in the retinal circulation. This chapter will concentrate on classification of hyperlipidaemia and its relationship to clinical manifestations in the retinal circulation, as well as management.

6.2 CLASSIFICATIONS OF HYPERLIPIDAEMIAS

Lipids are carried in the blood as soluble particles named lipoproteins. There are five types of particle named, low-density lipoprotein (LDL), very-low-density lipoprotein (VLDL), high-density lipoprotein (HDL), intermediate-density lipoprotein (IDL) and chylomicrons. Each of these particles has different electrophoretic mobility that allowed a classification of the hyperlipidaemias into six types by the World Health Organization study group in 1970.

Tables 6.1 and 6.2 show the outline of this classification although it is helpful to note that the LDL particle is the major cholesterol carrying particle whereas VLDL is the major triglyceride carrying particle. A simpler classification is shown in Table 6.3. In clinical practice Type I hyperlipidaemia (absence of lipoprotein lipase activity) is very rare whereas the most commonly encountered in ophthalmological practice are Types 2A (familial hypercholesterolaemia), 2B, 3 and 4 (combined hypercholesterolaemia and hypertriglyceridaemia). Type 5 hyperlipidaemia is a severe form with very high levels of fasting serum cholesterol and triglyceride and again is rare. This form of hyperlipidaemia is associated with glucose intolerance, alcoholism and pancreatitis.

Attempts have been made to simplify this complex classification and indeed a simpler working form is to classify the hyperlipidaemias into those with isolated hypercholesterolaemia and those with combined hypercholesterolaemia and hypertriglyceridaemia. The former may commonly represent heterozygous familial hypercholesterolaemia whereas the latter may reflect primary familial hyperlipidaemia or may be secondary to other medical conditions:

- diabetes mellitus
- obesity
- renal disease
  - chronic renal failure
  - nephrotic syndrome
- thyroid disease
  - hypothyroidism
  - hyperthyroidism
- liver disease
  - cirrhosis
  - biliary obstruction
- alcohol abuse
- drugs
  - exogenous sex hormones
  - steroids, thiazide diuretics, beta-blocking agents

The lipoproteins are of considerable importance. These have well described relationships, as does serum cholesterol and triglyceride, to the presence of macrovascular disease. These relationships are shown in Table 6.4.

Other ways in which serum lipids and lipoproteins may influence the vasculature include interac-

Table 6.1 Classification of lipoproteins

Lipoprotein group	*Major lipid component*
Chylomicrons	Triglycerides
Very-low-density lipoproteins (VLDL)	Triglycerides
Intermediate-density lipoproteins (IDL)	Cholesterol/Triglycerides
Low-density lipoproteins (LDL)	Cholesterol
High-density lipoproteins (HDL)	Cholesterol

Table 6.2 Classification of the hyperlipidaemias

Type	*Chylomicrons*	*VLDL*	*IDL*	*LDL*
I	++++	N	N	low
IIa	−	N	N	++
IIb	−	++	N, +	++
III	+	+	++	low
IV	−	++	N	N
V	++++	+++	N	low

N = normal
\+ = increased
− = absent
LDL = low-density lipoprotein
VLDL = very-low-density lipoprotein
IDL = intermediate-density lipoprotein

Table 6.3 Simpler three group therapeutic classification of hyperlipidaemias

	Increased concentrations	
	Lipoprotein	*Serum lipid*
I. Hypercholesterolaemia	LDL	Cholesterol
II. Combined (mixed)	LDL + VLDL	Cholesterol and triglyceride
III. Hypertriglyceridaemia	VLDL	Triglyceride

LDL = low-density lipoprotein
VLDL = very-low-density lipoprotein

Table 6.4 Serum lipids and lipoproteins: risk factors for macrovascular disease

Lipid	*Correlation with macrovascular disease*
Total cholesterol	Positive
Total triglyceride	Positive (not independent)
LDL	Positive
HDL	Negative
HDL_2	Negative
Lp (a)	Controversial positive

LDL – low density lipoprotein, HDL – high density lipoprotein, Lp (a) – lipoprotein (a)

tions with platelets. It is known that platelet aggregability is increased in hyperlipidaemia, as has been demonstrated in patients with coronary heart disease and indeed in those with diabetes mellitus. A further lipoprotein has been isolated, called lipoprotein a (Lp(a)). Numerous studies have shown that plasma Lp(a) concentrations above 0.3 g/l (of total Lp(a) mass), which are present in 1 in 5 people, are associated with an increased risk of coronary heart disease and stroke. Lp(a) is produced in the liver and is secreted as very-low-density lipoprotein although the density of most Lp(a) particles falls between the densities of low and high density lipoproteins. Although the function of Lp(a) is not established it appears to have thrombotic and atherogenic properties and along with other risk factors Lp(a) is suggested as a major determinant of macrovascular disease. The relationship of this important particle to microvascular disease will be one of considerable interest.

6.3 RETINAL CHANGES AND HYPERLIPIDAEMIA

The major changes that occur in association with hyperlipidaemia in the retinal vascular circulation are:

- lipaemia retinalis
- retinal infarction
- capillary closure
- vascular leakage
- retinal vein occlusion
- retinal artery occlusion

The majority of patients with hyperlipidaemia have modest elevations in serum cholesterol and/or serum triglycerides.

Lipaemia retinalis occurs only when the serum triglyceride value is above 21 mmol/l. The retinal appearance is that of white arterioles and venules due to excess chylomicrons, giving a creamy colour to the whole retina. An example of this is shown in Fig. 6.1. This finding is always of significance as underlying it will be severe hyperlipidaemia, either Type 3 or Type 5 combined hyperlipidaemias associated with marked rise in hypercholesterolaemia as well as triglycerides. The latter type is associated with pancreatitis, the former specifically with macrovascular disease, particularly peripheral vascular disease.

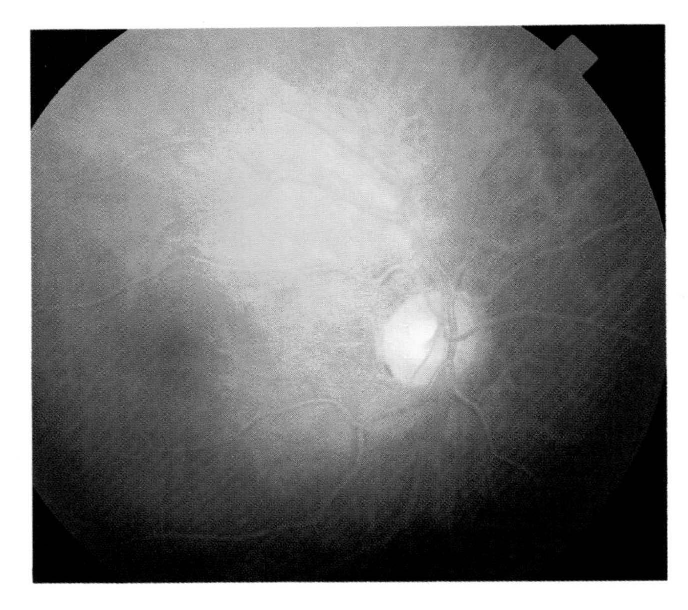

Fig. 6.1 Lipaemia retinalis.

Changes resulting from actual structural vascular damage were initially reported in the 1970s. In particular there were several reports of multiple retinal haemorrhages and intraretinal lipid exudations in patients with severe hyperlipidaemia. Histological examination showed the haemorrhages were in the inner retinal layers and the exudation largely in the outer plexiform layer. A more recent study of 40 hyperlipidaemia patients grouped according to Friedrickson's classification has been made. The patients' details are shown in Table 6.5. The findings on fluorescein angiography demonstrated 32 patients with normal capillary perfusion with no evidence of leakage of fluorescein or capillary closure.

Eight patients were found to have retinal arterial abnormalities and these included:

1. four patients with peripheral vessel closure;
2. two patients with leakage of fluorescein from the peripheral vasculature (Fig. 6.2a);
3. two patients with glucose intolerance and evidence of retinal infarction (Fig. 6.3a).

In this study of patients attending a lipid clinic, just under one-quarter of the patients had retinovascular changes. From this data therefore more changes may indeed be observed in association with the hyperlipidaemia and may be less common than was previously thought.

Interestingly the situation appears different for the retinal micro-circulation compared to large vessels as no abnormalities were found in patients with primary familial isolated hypercholesterolaemia. The only abnormalities were found in patients with combined hypercholesterolaemia and hypertriglyceridaemia. This may suggest that combined hyperlipidaemia is necessary before there is evidence of retinovascular damage.

The relationship between lipoproteins and retinovasculature is most likely different to that of macrovascular disease. In particular HDL cholesterol, which is the cardio-protective lipoprotein, does not appear to be protective with regard to the retinal circulation. In contrast, low HDL cholesterol and its subfractions (HDL 2) levels have been associated with retinal artery and venous occlusion. Studies are awaited as to the relationship of Lp(a) with retinovascular disease.

Table 6.5 The details and groupings of hyperlipidaemic patients studied by fluorescein angiography

	(n)	Mean age (yrs)	Mean serum (mmol/l) Cholesterol	Triglyceride
Familial hypercholesterolaemia				
Type IIa	(6)	48	8.3	2.7
Type III	(8)	56	7	3.5
Type IV	(12)	51	6.8	4
Type V	(13)	51	9.9	12.7

n = number of patients

Definition of hypercholesterolaemia is cholesterol >6.5 mmol/l and hypertriglyceridaemia is triglyceride >2.1 mmol/l.
Abnormalities were found in eight patients on fluorescein angiography.

6.4 RESPONSE TO HYPOLIPIDAEMIC TREATMENT

One report has suggested that there may be regression of retinovascular damage with successful hypolipidaemic therapy. Two examples of this are shown in Figs 6.2b and 6.3b. These changes were achieved in 6 months of normal lipid profiles. Equally it has been shown that with poor control of hyperlipidaemia, the retinovascular disease may deteriorate, in particular with progression of capillary closure.

6.5 OTHER RETINAL VASCULAR ASSOCIATIONS WITH HYPERLIPIDAEMIA

As discussed in other chapters, hyperlipidaemia does associate with other forms of retinovascular damage. In particular retinal vein occlusion, particularly the branch form with hypercholesterolaemia and the central form with hypertriglyceridaemia, has been long established. Retinal artery occlusion in both the central and branch form is associated with hyperlipidaemia in 50% of cases. The relationship with ischaemic optic neuropathy is less clear and has

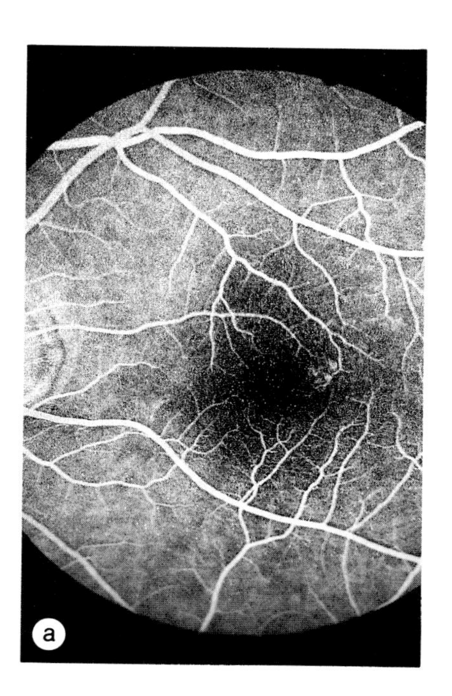

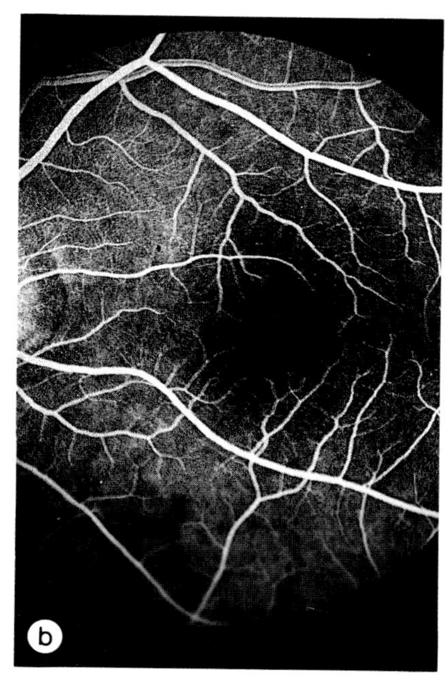

Fig. 6.2 (a) Leakage of fluorescein from peripheral vasculature in type IV hyperlipidaemia; (b) regression of leakage after 6 months treatment.

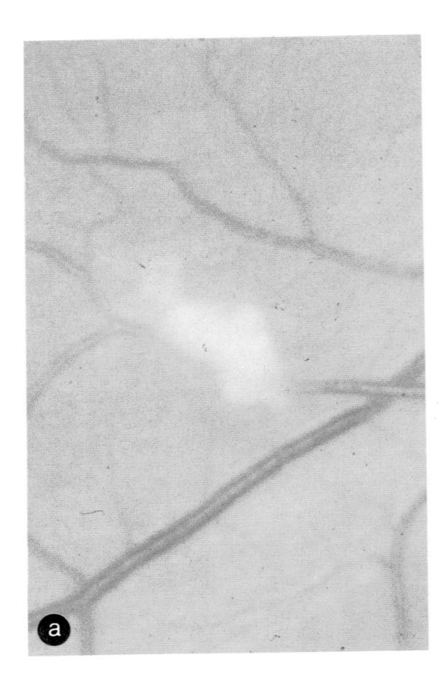

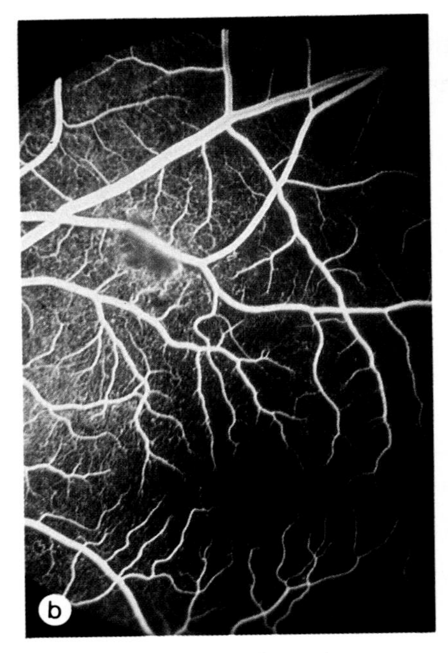

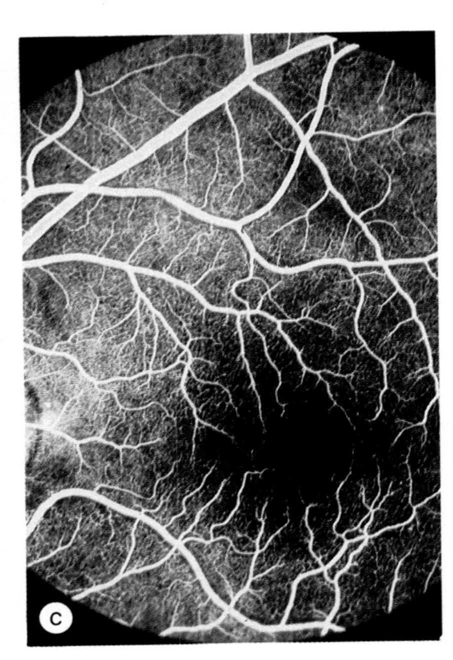

Fig. 6.3 (a) Shows a cotton wool spot; (b) shows fluorescein angiogram demonstrating an area of underlying retinal non-perfusion; (c) re-perfusion of previously non-perfused retina after 6 months hypolipidaemic therapy producing normal lipid profiles.

recently been suggested in a case control study. Rarely, in severe forms of hypercholesterolaemia, cholesterol deposits may be found in the retina giving rise to the 'cholesterol fundus' (Fig. 6.4). Other more controversial associations would include glaucoma and exudative diabetic retinopathy.

6.6 DECISION TO TREAT

In the context of retinovascular changes associated with hyperlipidaemia, there are no long-term prospective large studies showing benefit. However, there are small series showing improvement in retinovascular changes and there does appear to be benefit in terms of reduction of recurrence of retinovascular occlusions in patients who have had treatment with regard to overall cardiovascular risk factors. There are considerable data supporting reduction of coronary heart disease events with treatment of hypercholesterolaemia. Equally patients with retinovascular disease have increased morbidity and mortality from degenerative cardiovascular disease. It would therefore appear logical to treat hyperlipidaemia in the context of retinovascular disease as secondary prevention as is done in secondary prevention of coronary disease.

6.7 MANAGEMENT OF HYPERLIPIDAEMIA

The reasons for treating severe and markedly high lipid levels is to prevent pancreatitis which is associated with high levels of serum triglycerides (>11 mmol/l) by reduction of these to normal levels. However, the reduction of atherosclerosis is a major goal, with reduction of coronary heart disease end points. The majority of lipid lowering trials have focused on males between 30 and 65 years of age. Priorities for lipid lowering suggested by the British Hyperlipidaemia Association are:

1. ischaemic heart disease >5.2 mmol/l (secondary prevention);
2. familial, genetic hyperlipidaemia or multiple risk factors >6.5 mmol/l;
3. asymptomatic hypercholesterolaemic males >6.5 mmol/l;
4. postmenopausal females with hypercholesterolaemia without other risk factors with cholesterol level >7.8 mmol/l.

Table 6.5 shows the significance of serum cholesterol values for clinical practice. The diagnosis of hypercholesterolaemia is confirmed if a fasting serum cholesterol is greater than 6.5 mmol/l. The definition with regard to serum triglyceride levels that are abnormal is more difficult but internationally agreed guidelines suggest that fasting levels greater than 3 mmol/l should be regarded as abnormal. The diagnosis of hyperlipidaemia should not be based on a single estimate. For purposes of screening, a random blood sample for lipid analysis is adequate, and if values of serum cholesterol or triglyceride are abnormal, a repeat fasting sample should be taken.

Once hyperlipidaemia has been identified, the key points to be ascertained in the clinical history are:

- age;
- family history of premature cardiovascular disease;
- smoker or non-smoker;
- alcohol intake;
- drug history – thiazides, beta-blockers, oestrogen preparations;
- presence of macrovascular disease, e.g. angina, myocardial infarctions, stroke, intermittent claudication;
- history appropriate to secondary cause of hyperlipidaemia associated with diabetes mellitus, e.g. hypothyroidism, renal disease.

Important points to consider in clinical examination of a patient with newly diagnosed hyperlipidaemia, are:

- degree of obesity – ideal body weight or body mass index;
- presence of clinical signs of hyperlipidaemia:
  hypercholesterolaemia: arcus senilis, xanthelasma, xanthomata;
  hypertriglyceridaemia: eruptive xanthomata, lipaemia retinalis;
- presence of clinical signs of macrovascular disease:
  presence of bruits – carotid or femoral;
  signs of compromised left ventricular function;
  signs of peripheral vascular disease;
  signs associated with secondary causes;
  signs associated with other cardiovascular risk factors, e.g. hypertension.

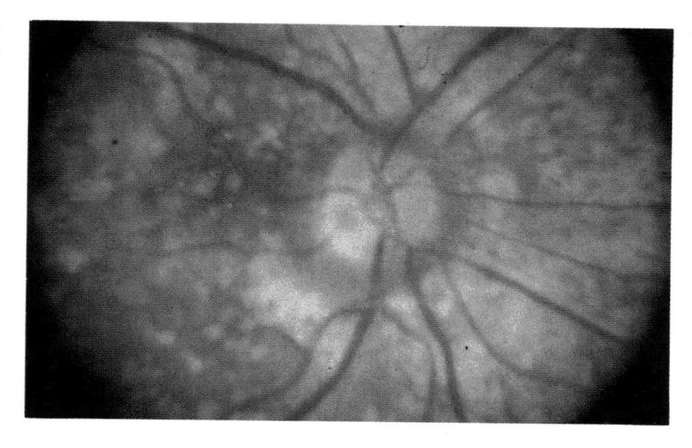

Fig. 6.4 A 'cholesterol fundus'.

Important investigations to be performed are:

- fasting serum cholesterol and triglyceride estimation;
- assessment of HDL-cholesterol concentration;
- assessment of LDL-cholesterol concentration (Friedwald equation);
- lipoprotein electrophoresis (for typing);
- ECG – to establish presence of ischaemic heart disease;
- random or fasting blood sugar – presence of diabetes mellitus;
- serum creatinine – presence of renal disease;
- urine for proteinuria – presence of renal disease;
- liver function tests (glutamyl transferase):
  presence of liver disease;
  alcohol abuse;
- thyroid function tests – free tetraiodothyronine and thyroid stimulating hormone;
- other tests include measurement of:

Table 6.6 Serum cholesterol values

Serum cholesterol concentration	*Significance*
5.2 mmol/l	An ideal serum cholesterol
5.2–6.5 mmol/l	A small but graded increase in coronary heart disease incidence
>6.5 mmol/l Definition of hypercholesterolaemia	Significant increase in coronary heart disease end points

Defined by British Hyperlipidaemia Association, 1993.

apolipoprotein E and C isoforms;
lipoprotein lipase activity (post-heparin);
lipoprotein (a).

Particular emphasis is placed on a history (or family history) of premature cardiovascular disease, and the identification of primary familial hyperlipidaemias (particularly familial hypercholesterolaemia) which may be associated with clinical signs of hyperlipidaemia.

The cornerstone of management is through dietary and lifestyle advice comprising:

- Reduce calorie intake, encourage exercise.
- Reduce weight if subject is obese.
- Reduction of total fat intake to 30% or less of total dietary energy.
- Reduction of saturated fatty acids to less than total dietary energy.
- Encourage intake of monounsaturated (oleic acid) and polyunsaturated (linoleic) fatty acids.
- Reduction of dietary cholesterol to less than 300 mg/day.
- Increase consumption of dietary fibre (vegetables and cereal) and complex carbohydrates.
- Avoidance of alcohol (reduction to at least a maximum of 2 units/day with one alcohol-free day per week).
- Cessation of smoking.

Dietary advice must be given and reinforced in all cases of hyperlipidaemia, until at least three months of dietary treatment have elapsed. Guidelines on the treatment of various lipid levels are listed in Table 6.7. A key factor is to encourage weight loss in the obese subject.

If the response to diet and other measures is inadequate after three to six months, drug therapy should be considered. The indications for drug therapy are shown in Table 6.7. A summary of the lipid lowering drugs is shown in Table 6.8.

In clinical practice, bile sequestrants are often the agent of first choice because of their safety in the treatment of hypercholesterolaemia. However, these agents are commonly poorly tolerated. Fibric acid

Table 6.7 Guidelines for the treatment of various blood lipid levels

Fasting levels (mmol/l)		
Cholesterol	*Triglyceride*	*Management*
<6.5	<3.0	Check for other risk factors Check diet
>6.5	>3.0	Correct obesity Exclude secondary cause Emphasize lipid lowering features of diet Stop drugs exacerbating hyperlipidaemia Check alcohol intake Family history – check lipids of family members
>7.8 Despite good glycaemic control and dietary compliance	>3.0	Consider lipid lowering drug therapy (particularly for males, family history of premature vascular disease, presence of other cardiovascular risk factors)
>10	>10	Consider Type IIb, III or V hyperlipidaemia Exclude diabetes mellitus and alcohol abuse Check history of pancreatitis Dietary and drug therapy appropriate If cholesterol >10 mmol in isolation consider primary familial hypercholesterolaemia Check family history

Table 6.8 A summary of the lipid lowering drugs classified according to their indication for use

Disorder	*Drug group*
Hypercholesterolaemia	Bile acid sequestrants Fibric acid derivatives HMG CoA reductase inhibitors Nicotinic acid derivatives Probucol Guar gum
Combined hyperlipidaemia	Fibric acid derivatives Nicotinic acid derivatives HMG CoA reductase inhibitors
Hypertriglyceridaemia	Fibric acid derivatives Nicotinic acid derivatives Fish oils
Hypercholesterolaemia and renal disease	Fibric acids and/or HMG CoA inhibitors Watch **myositis** and **myopathy**

derivatives and HMG CoA reductase inhibitors are the most popular agents for hypercholesterolaemia treatment.

Special attention is required in the management of severe combined lipaemia of either primary Type III or V forms, or when associated acutely with pancreatitis, alcoholism or diabetic ketoacidosis. Discontinuation of alcohol and normalization of blood glucose with intravenous insulin will lead to rapid reversal of lipaemia. Attention to careful diet and addition of the fibric acid derivatives may be effective therapies in the longer term.

FURTHER READING

Betteridge, D.J., Dodson, P.M., Durrington, P.N., *et al.* (1993) Management of hyperlipidaemia: guidelines of the British Hyperlipidaemia Association. *Postgrad. Med. J.*, **69**, 359–69.

Dodson, P.M. and Barnett, A.H. (1992) *Lipids, Diabetes and Vascular Disease*, Science Press.

European Atherosclerosis Society (1992) European Atherosclerosis Society recommendations: Prevention of coronary heart disease – scientific background and new clinical guidelines. *Nutr. Metab. Cardiovasc. Dis.*, **2**, 113–56.

Feher, M.D. and Richmond, W. (1990) *Lipids and Lipid Disorders*, (Pocket Picture Guides), Gower Medical Publishing, London.

Kurz, G.H., Manoucher, S., Somer, K.K. and Friedman, A.H. (1976) The retina in Type 5 hyperlipoproteinaemia. *Am. J. Ophthalmol.*, **82**(1), 32–43.

Talks, S.J., Chong, N.H.V., Jones, A. *et al.* (1994) Fibrinogen, Cholesterol and smoking as risk factors for non-arteritic anterior ischaemic optic neuropathy. *Eye* (submitted).

Vinger, P.F. and Sachs, B.A. (1980) Ocular manifestations of hyperlipoproteinaemia. *Am. J. Ophthalmol.*, **70**(4), 563–73.

Winder, A.F., Dodson, P.M. and Goulton, D.J. (1980) Ophthalmological complications of hypertriglyceridaemia. *Trans. Ophthalmol. Soc. U.K.*, **100**(1), 119–22.

7 *Retinal artery occlusion*

Clinical Retinopathies. Paul M. Dodson, Jonathan M. Gibson and Erna E. Kritzinger.
Published in 1995 by Chapman & Hall, London. ISBN 0 412 35930 8

7.1 INTRODUCTION

Occlusion in the retinal arterial system is a common cause of visual loss in Britain, particularly in the middle-aged and elderly population. This retinal abnormality is associated with a wide variety of systemic disorders. Atherosclerosis and its risk factors are prominent in the aetiology and influence both investigation and management.

The clinical symptoms and signs of this condition can be divided according to the primary sight of obstruction, i.e. the central retinal artery or the branch retinal artery. It is important to recognize that the branch retinal artery form is commonly due to embolism which relates to disease proximal to the retinal circulation.

7.2 AETIOLOGY AND PATHOLOGY

Atherosclerotic changes are the major causative factor in central retinal artery occlusion. This is usually due to local atherosclerotic disease of the central retinal artery but may rarely occur due to cholesterol emboli. Both central and branch retinal artery occlusion may be a result of inflammatory eye disease but these are rare.

In contrast to the central form, branch retinal artery occlusion is usually caused by embolism; this is an important difference which influences both investigation and management. The most common embolus consists of cholesterol. To reinforce the origin, the chemical composition is similar to atheromatous lesions in the carotid artery. Cholesterol emboli do not persist indefinitely, as they usually fragment. Once emboli have dispersed, areas of vascular sheathing may arise at a previous site of impaction. These represent a giant cell reaction to cholesterol crystals in the arterial wall. Other emboli, which consist of mixed thrombus, calcified fragments, or myxomatous material, are generally of cardiac origin and are rarer than the cholesterol form. Septic emboli found in subacute bacterial endocarditis (termed Roth spots) may cause retinal arterial occlusion.

Atherosclerotic disease also occurs in the posterior ciliary circulation giving rise to ischaemic optic papillopathy. This will be considered in Section 12.3.1.

7.3 CLINICAL FEATURES AND SYMPTOMS

The main objective symptom is painless unilateral reduction in visual acuity. As in retinal vein occlusion, the degree of visual acuity loss varies according to the sight and extent of the occlusion.

Central retinal artery occlusion usually leads to an acute loss of vision corresponding to discontinuity in the circulation of the retina. If a portion of the retina is supplied by a cilio-retinal artery (derived from the choroidal circulation) perception of light or hand movements may be preserved in a small central segment of the visual field. In branch retinal artery occlusion, visual loss may be sudden but may equally be asymptomatic and unnoticed. The visual loss is variable in site and severity. The visual field abnormalities correspond to distribution of retinal oedema and infarction.

Although atheromatous disease is by far the most common cause of retinal artery occlusion, hypertensive small vessel disease may give rise to this syndrome. Equally hydrostatic occlusion due to either high intraocular pressure or low retinal blood pressure may be involved.

Amaurosis fugax may well precede the development of retinal artery occlusion. This is characterized by a typical clinical history. Importantly there are no signs in the retina as this is due to short-lived interruption of the retinal artery blood flow. Spasm of the retinal arterial circulation may also occur. This may be associated with vasoactive drugs, for example the ergot derivatives.

As discussed in Chapter 9, retinal artery and retinal venous occlusion may occur together.

7.4 CLINICAL SIGNS

Retinal artery occlusion is classified into central or branch forms according to the appearance on ophthalmoscopy (Figs 7.1 and 7.2). In central retinal artery occlusion, there is discontinuity in the circulation of the retina or segmentation of the blood column (box-car segmentation) in the veins and, later, there may be attenuation in the retinal arteries, arterioles and veins. Pallor of the retina especially around the macula, due to cloudy swelling of the ganglion cells, is a typical feature, as is a cherry red spot due to swelling and accentuation of the normal fovea. A pink triangular area of retina may be seen lateral to the disc which reflects healthy normal tissue, due to this area being supplied by the ciliary circulation.

Branch retinal artery occlusion is normally demonstrated with evidence of embolic occlusion of a branch of the central retinal artery. This is associated with oedema and infarction of the distal retina. The retina typically is swollen and pale. The presence of emboli may be detected, though this will depend on the duration from the occlusion to the examination. Typically cholesterol emboli are yellow and discrete, whereas the other forms of emboli may be more difficult to detect.

7.5 CLINICAL COURSE

The ocular prognosis of retinal artery occlusion is dependent on the site of the disease. The visual prognosis with central retinal artery occlusion is generally poor. A good visual acuity is often preserved in patients with branch occlusion but it may be severely affected if the macular vessels are involved. Some limited recovery of visual acuity occurs in 20% of patients following central retinal artery occlusion on long-term follow-up.

In contrast to retinal vein occlusion, the prognosis for vision in the contralateral eye is generally good. As discussed later, patients with retinal artery occlusion are at a much higher risk of other serious vascular events than recurrence of retinal artery disease.

7.6 UNDERLYING MEDICAL DISORDERS

The central form of retinal artery occlusion is most commonly found in association with cardiovascular risk factors of macrovascular disease. Hypertension, smoking, hyperlipidaemia and carotid vascular disease are the common underlying medical conditions as shown in Table 7.1. Carotid bruits are found in approximately 10–20% of patients. Hypertension is usually of the essential type and often poorly controlled. The observation of hypertension in 60% of patients with the central form in contrast to the lower prevalence in those with branch arterial occlusion, supports the idea that central occlusion is a consequence of more localized disease. Therefore, potentiation of atheroma in the ophthalmic artery by hypertensive disease might partly account for the differences between central and branch arterial occlusion. However, central occlusion may rarely be caused by embolism.

In some studies hypertension is much less prominent as the underlying medical condition in branch retinal artery occlusion compared to the central form. In our recent studies from Birmingham, there was no major difference between the two forms but a recent series from Moorfields Eye Hospital showed the figures at 25% for branch retinal artery occlusion and 57% for the central arterial occlusive form. Cardiac valvular abnormalities were found in one-third of patients and atheromatous disease of the carotid in 50% of patients with embolic branch retinal artery occlusion.

The types of valvular abnormalities that have been reported in association with branch retinal occlusion are shown in Table 7.2. Aortic stenosis is the

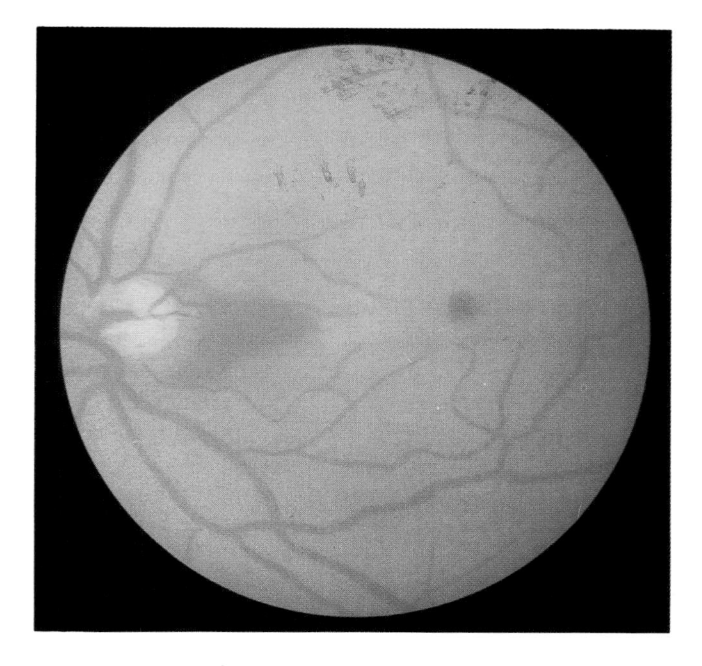

Fig. 7.1 Central retinal artery occlusion.

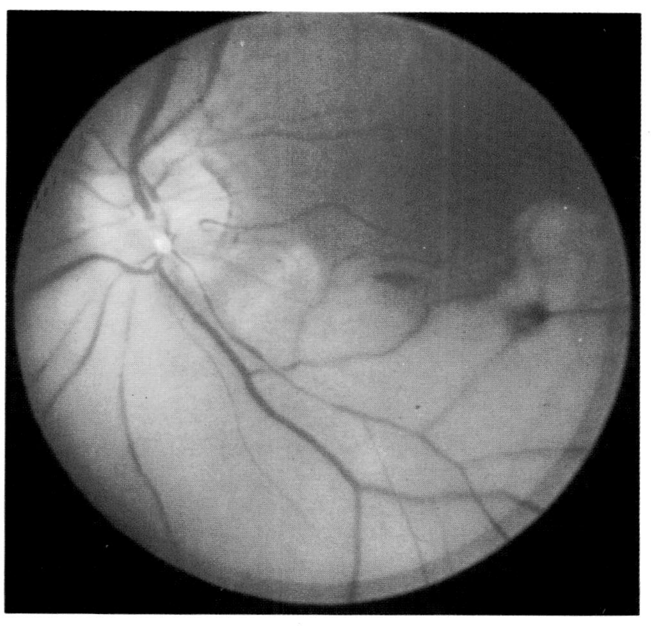

Fig. 7.2 Branch retinal artery occlusion.

Table 7.1 Medical conditions underlying retinal artery occlusion at presentation

	Branch retinal artery occlusion	*Central retinal artery occlusion*
Prevalence of:		
Smoking	60%	43%
Hypertension	59%	66%
Hyperlipidaemia	50%	45%
Diabetes mellitus	7%	5%
Carotid bruits	11%	25%
Previous angina/myocardial infarction	23%	12.5%
Previous TIA/CVA	11%	10.5%
Peripheral vascular disease	9.8%	8.9%
Valvular disease (from echocardiography)	*30%	*15%

n = 120, data from Physicians Clinic, Birmingham and Midland Eye Hospital
*data from Moorfields Eye Hospital

Table 7.2 Common cardiac abnormalities underlying retinal artery occlusion

Cardiac abnormality	*Frequency (%)*
Aortic stenosis	38
Mitral leaflet prolapse	34
Rheumatic mitral valve disease	7
Mitral incompetence	7
Valve prosthesis	7
Patent foramen ovale	7

Table 7.3 Results of carotid angiography in patients with retinal artery occlusion

	Branch RAO (%)	*Central RAO (%)*
Normal circulation	37	33
Internal carotid origin irregular or stenosed	55	39
Frank occlusion	7	28

commonest cardiac abnormality underlying retinal artery occlusion, followed by mitral valve abnormalities. Patients with valve prostheses are also at risk of branch occlusion in spite of the use of anticoagulants and other therapies.

Angiographic studies have been made of the carotid circulation in patients with retinal artery occlusion. Many patients had lesions in the carotid arterial vascular tree as shown in Table 7.3. However, it is important to note that only a minority of these lesions were amenable to surgical intervention.

It would be anticipated that retinal artery occlusion should have a link with vascular disease and stroke. In the series shown in Fig. 7.1, 12 to 23% of patients with retinal artery occlusion had evidence of previous or existing angina or myocardial infarction. Ten percent had previous transient ischaemic attacks or a cerebrovascular accident. Ten percent also had evidence of peripheral vascular disease. These data suggest a strong link between retinal arterial occlusion and other more widespread macrovascular arterial disease.

Retinal arterial occlusions occurring as a result of inflammatory disease are uncommon. However, retinal ischaemic changes may occur in polyarteritis nodosa, systemic lupus erythematosus, syphilis, giant cell arteritis and Takayasu's disease. Other conditions that may present with arterial occlusion are migraine, hyperlipidaemia and diabetes mellitus. The clinical presentation of hyperlipidaemia is mostly of the severe form with combined hypertriglyceridaemia and hypercholesterolaemia (Friedrickson Type 5 hyperlipidaemia).

As with retinal vein occlusion, retinal artery occlusion may occur in young patients taking contraceptive preparations containing oestrogen, and in post-menopausal women on oestrogen replacement therapy. This is particularly the case in post-menopausal females who have existing borderline or mild hypertension.

7.7 MANAGEMENT

7.7.1 Ophthalmic management

(a) INITIAL EXAMINATION AND DIAGNOSIS

Patients presenting with retinal artery occlusion require a full ophthalmological examination. Particular emphasis is placed on the form of occlusion, visual acuity and the appearance of the retina.

It is important to categorize the type of retinal occlusion: central or branch. If of the branch form, it is important to try and characterize the type of embolus visible. The history should include the timing and date of the symptoms of visual loss. Medical examination should include a careful search for abnormalities in the cardiovascular system. Of particular relevance to the central form of the disease are:

1. pulse (for cardiac arrhythmias);
2. blood pressure (presence of hypertension or hypotension);
3. palpation of temporal arteries (any evidence of temporal arteritis?);
4. evidence of other vascular disease (e.g. presence of angina, myocardial infarction, or intermittent claudication. Examination for all peripheral pulses);
5. history of smoking, alcohol intake;
6. history of pre-existing disease (e.g. diabetes mellitus, hyperlipidaemia);
7. family history of premature cardiovascular disease;
8. presence of amaurosis fugax, transient ischaemic attack, cerebrovascular accident.

In addition, if a branch retinal artery occlusion is identified, special emphasis should be paid to examination of the carotid vascular tree. Assessment should include the following:

1. Is the common carotid normal on the side of the occlusion on palpation?
2. The presence of a carotid bruit.
3. Is there a heart murmur (to indicate valvular disease with emboli)?
4. If a carotid bruit is heard, is it transmitted or a genuine bruit?
5. Look for hints of rarer causes of retinal emboli, e.g. subacute bacterial endocarditis.

(b) INITIAL TREATMENT AT THE TIME OF DIAGNOSIS

It is crucial to determine clinically when the retinal arterial obstruction occurred. This can be obtained from the duration of symptoms from the time of onset, which gives guidelines as to the possible approaches to improving retinal arterial flow. Once 24 hours has elapsed since the onset of symptoms, there is no significant treatment, particularly in the central form of the disease, that will have any major influence. In the branch form, vision may not be affected by a small embolus if it lodges in a part of the retinal arterial tree that is not supplying the macula.

There are two approaches that have been used to improve retinal blood flow. The aim of the immediate ocular treatment is to restore the arterial circulation to the retina. There are several reports of restoration of vision where early measures have been undertaken and it is certainly worth attempting to restore the retinal circulation if a patient is seen within 6 hours of suffering a central retinal artery occlusion. Although the retina presumably can only theoretically withstand a short period of retinal circulatory arrest, in practice visual recovery has been reported even after several hours following the retinal artery occlusion.

Ocular massage is sometimes an effective way of dislodging a small retinal embolus and can be carried on by a nurse or attendant whilst the ophthalmologist prepares other measures. Probably the most effective means of restoring the ocular circulation is by suddenly reducing the intraocular pressure, by means of an anterior chamber paracentesis. A small, very sharp needle is introduced at the limbus of the cornea and the needle directed anterior to and parallel with the iris plane so that the lens is not damaged. Using an insulin syringe (with the syringe as a handle) is one method of carrying this out under local anaesthesia and a small amount of aqueous humour can be removed (*Not* by aspirating with the syringe). Acetazolamide given intravenously has been tried but in our experience this is not often successful in lowering the intraocular pressure fast enough. Rebreathing causes vasodilatation in the retinal arterial tree and this combined with ocular massage is a useful manoeuvre to carry out whilst the patient is being transferred to ophthalmologist care. Unfortunately the visual prognosis for most patients is poor following a central retinal artery occlusion because of the initial delay in seeking treatment. However, early paracentesis gives a reasonably good prognosis for the patient and it is our experience that good visual recovery can occur.

The other approach, which is currently undergoing investigation, is with streptokinase or tissue plasminogen activator (tPa). The latter approach is used in patients who present shortly following the onset of visual symptoms, as once 6–8 hours have elapsed then permanent retinal damage will ensue. Therefore it would be anticipated that there would be little benefit after this time period. It is also our experience that intravenous heparin therapy in the acute stages is not of benefit.

7.7.2 Medical management

(a) TREATMENT AND IDENTIFICATION OF UNDERLYING MEDICAL FACTORS

Initial investigations should include a chest x-ray, ECG, full blood count, ESR (plasma viscosity), urea and electrolytes, creatinine, liver function tests, blood glucose and random lipid profile. Management will be appropriate to the underlying condition found. Rare causes may be encountered including myeloproliferative disorders, myeloma, temporal arteritis, systemic lupus erythematosus, polyarteritis nodosa and Takayasu's disease. However, the more common conditions of hypertension, diabetes and hyperlipidaemia will need treatment and are frequently encountered. The management of hypertension is described in Chapter 5. However, a blood pressure recording of systolic greater than 200 mmHg and diastolic greater than 120 mmHg should cause concern and result in urgent treatment of hypertension. Other retinal changes of hypertension should be sought and if exudation or haemorrhage is present, particularly in the unaffected eye, the diagnosis of malignant or accelerated hypertension should be made. Urgent treatment and review by a physician is mandatory in this clinical situation.

Diagnosis of diabetes is made from a typical triad of symptoms (polyuria, polydypsia and weight loss) in combination with the presence of glycosuria. A random blood glucose greater than 11 mmol/l in combination with symptoms is sufficient for the diagnosis. If the random blood glucose is equivocal with the presence of symptoms or glycosuria, a glucose tolerance test is necessary. The majority of patients presenting with central retinal artery occlusion and diabetes will have the Type II or maturity onset form which will require dietary treatment initially, although an oral hypoglycaemic agent may be necessary.

The management of hyperlipidaemia is based on conventional lines. Secondary causes such as diabetes, hypothyroidism and the use of thiazide diuretics must be excluded. Severe hypercholesterolaemia or hypertriglyceridaemia which is resistant to diet and therefore requires drug therapy, is uncommon but may occur. Special attention should be given to patients under the age of 65 with cholesterol values greater than 6.5 mmol/l. A strong family history of premature cardiovascular disease and high serum cholesterol may suggest a heterozygous familial form of hyperlipidaemia and these patients should be assessed by a physician.

In the branch form of retinal arterial occlusion, evidence of carotid artery disease and cardiac abnormalities must be sought. If carotid stenosis is suggested clinically, a decision has to be made as to whether patients will be suitable for more detailed investigations. Although this has been previously debated, patients should be referred for specialist opinions. The results of carotid angiography in both branch and central retinal artery occlusion, published in a recent series, are shown in Table 7.3. A scheme was suggested for the predictive value of clinical features with regard to operability of carotid abnormalities. Three features were highlighted. These are: age over 50 years, carotid bruit present and visible retinal embolus. These three clinical features were of value in predicting a potentially operable carotid lesion on angiography. No operable lesions were found in patients under 50 who did not have either a carotid bruit or the presence of a cholesterol embolus in the retinal circulation.

Medical versus surgical treatment for carotid stenosis is still open to debate. Large prospective trials originally demonstrated that female patients faired no better with carotid surgery than with aspirin treatment on a once daily dose (75 mg or 300 mg daily), but there was some evidence of benefit of carotid surgery in male subjects, particularly those under the age of 65.

However, two recent large international randomized multicentre trials have suggested definite benefit with carotid endarterectomy in patients with severe carotid stenosis (>75%) and recent cerebrovascular symptoms in the carotid artery territory. The benefits of surgery in mild carotid stenosis (30–70% reduction in diameter) remain uncertain. Patients with mild stenosis (<30%) should not be considered for surgical referral. In clinical practice, many centres use the modern noninvasive technique of Doppler imaging. Intra-arterial angiography can be limited to patients with moderate to severe stenosis identified by Doppler studies. Intravenous digital subtraction angiography is an alternative noninvasive screening technique. Following these investigations, referral to a surgeon with an interest in carotid endarterectomy should only be made if there is a history of symptoms or signs attributable to a severe carotid stenosis (≥75%).

Our current medical policy is to use aspirin 300 mg daily, but if there is a significant contraindication to aspirin other antiplatelet agents may be used (e.g. dipyridamole).

If a cardiac cause is found (e.g. mitral stenosis or aortic stenosis) on echocardiogram, it is imperative to assess the patient for the necessity of treatment with warfarin and long-term anticoagulation. Many factors will dictate for or against this approach and a cardiology opinion should be sought.

(b) INITIAL TREATMENT TO IMPROVE ARTERIAL FLOW

As previously mentioned, anterior chamber tap may be performed if the retinal artery occlusion is indeed very acute. Treatment with streptokinase or tissue plasminogen activator may be of benefit but trials are awaited. Infusions of prostacyclin have been used with some anecdotal evidence of benefit. Treatment with aspirin or Persantin is aimed at longer-term management.

(c) PREVENTION OF RECURRENCE

Prevention of recurrence is through general assessment of underlying risk factors. In a recent study of prognosis of patients with retinal artery occlusion, the recurrence rate was reported at 1% over a mean follow-up of 4.2 years.

It would therefore appear that treatment should be aimed at cardiovascular risk factors to improve the prognosis with regard to mortality or morbidity from coronary, carotid and peripheral vascular disease.

(d) PREVENTION OF OTHER ASSOCIATED CARDIOVASCULAR DISEASE

The prognosis of patients with retinal artery occlusion has been poorly studied. An early report suggested that 60% of patients had died within 2–3 years of the retinal arterial event. However, a more precise study in 99 patients showed that the mortality rate was 8% per year, with 7.4% sustaining stroke in the first year and 2.5% per year following. However, the major cause of mortality was accounted for by a coronary event (59% of all deaths). The prognostic factors associated with increased mortality were increasing age, peripheral vascular disease, cardiomegaly and a carotid bruit. Interestingly the risk rate from stroke was only 3%.

With regard to prevention of recurrence and coronary heart disease, it is important to ascertain the cardiovascular risk factors present. This highlights smoking, hypertension, hyperlipidaemia and diabetes mellitus. Cessation of smoking is paramount, as in our recent studies, at least 53% of patients with retinal artery occlusion were regular current smokers.

Treatment of other underlying medical conditions is as previously described. With regard to benefit of this treatment, no such trial has been run specifically looking at retinal infarction. However lowering of myocardial infarction and stroke rate would be expected as large prospective trials of the individual treatment of hypertension or hyperlipidaemia have demonstrated significant reduction in vascular disease end points. There is evidence that aspirin at 75–300 mg daily is of benefit in prevention of stroke. Other factors that might be considered include reduction of stress, adopting the prudent diet (the high fibre, low fat, high unrefined carbohydrate dietary regimen), and reduction of excessive alcohol (i.e. to less than 21 units per week).

FURTHER READING

Brown, M.M. and Humphrey, P.R.D. (1992) Carotid endarterectomy: recommendations for management of transient ischaemic attack and ischaemic stroke. *Br. Med. J.*, **305**, 1071–4.

Dodson, P.M. (1988) Medical aspects of retinal artery occlusion. *Postgrad. Update*, November, 775–80.

Hankey, G.J., Slattery, J.M. and Warlow, C.P. (1991) Prognosis and prognostic factors of retinal infarction: a prospective cohort study. *Br. Med. J.*, **302**, 499–504.

Orme, M. (1988) Aspirin all around. *Br. Med. J.*, **297**, 307–8.

Wilson, L.A., Warlow, C.P. and Ross Russell, R.W. (1979) Cardiovascular disease in patients with retinal arterial occlusion. *Lancet*, **i**, 292–4.

8 *Retinal vein occlusion*

Clinical Retinopathies. Paul M. Dodson, Jonathan M. Gibson and Erna E. Kritzinger.
Published in 1995 by Chapman & Hall, London. ISBN 0 412 35930 8

8.1 INTRODUCTION

Occlusion in the retinal venous system is a common cause of visual loss in Britain, particularly in the middle-aged population. Until the 1970s this condition had been generally regarded as untreatable. However, the successful use of laser photocoagulation for diabetic retinopathy has prompted its application to the ocular complications of retinal vein occlusion. In addition, investigations into the aetiology have suggested possible new approaches to medical management.

The clinical symptoms and signs of this condition can be divided according to the primary site of obstruction, i.e. of the central retinal vein or the branch retinal vein.

8.2 AETIOLOGY AND PATHOLOGY

Conditions known to predispose to retinal vein occlusion include vasculitis, chronic glaucoma and hyperviscosity syndromes (Table 8.1). Many of the associated conditions are rare, and generally the aetiology remains imprecise, although recent research has provided new insights.

Retinal vein occlusion is due to damage of the walls of the venous vasculature. Cell proliferation is the primary histological change in the venous endothelium at the site of occlusion. This appears to be associated with either degeneration of endothelium and secondary intramural thrombus formation or severe phlebosclerosis. The mechanism underlying initial endothelial swelling has not been precisely defined, although clinical findings indicate that it is multifactorial: hypertension, hyperlipidaemia, abnormal platelet function and perhaps increased inflammatory activity have been implicated.

Observations that retinal arterial abnormalities commonly accompany the clinical signs of venous occlusion, and that retinal arterial and venous occlusion may occur in the same patient, gave rise to the concept that retinal arterial disease is responsible for venous occlusion. This was supported by evidence of branch vein occlusion at the site of arteriovenous crossings, as well as established cardiovascular risk factors related to macrovascular arterial disease underlie retinal vein occlusion. It was thought that thickening of the arterial wall caused indentation of the vein at the site of arteriovenous crossings, due to the constraint in a common sheath; this would be responsible for endothelial cell proliferation, resulting in a reduction of venous outflow. However, results of recent animal and human studies have provided contrary evidence, showing that arterial changes follow the experimentally induced venous occlusion rather than preceding it.

Inflammatory processes have been implicated in the aetiology: inflammatory cell infiltration was demonstrated in 48% of histological studies of eyes with retinal vein occlusion. Significantly elevated serum levels of C-reactive protein, immunoglobulin A, as well as increased plasma viscosity and ESR have been reported; the severity of retinal damage following occlusion appears to be positively related to increasing blood viscosity. It is clear that a number of patients with retinovascular occlusion are found on investigation to have classically benign gammopathy, although once occlusion has occurred the designation 'benign' to this form of long-standing immunoglobulin abnormality becomes questionable.

Special mention should be given to the role of thrombosis. Indeed, retinal vein occlusion was previously termed 'retinal vein thrombosis'. Histologically, thrombus formation is probably a secondary event and may be responsible for the resulting total occlusion of the vein. Platelet function has been reported to be abnormal in patients with retinal vein occlusion, even where there is absence of associated medical conditions known to predispose to this abnormality. Abnormal red cell deformity has also been recorded. These are important aspects, as effective anti-platelet and thrombolytic therapies are available which could have considerable therapeutic potential.

8.3 CLINICAL FEATURES

8.3.1 Symptoms

The main objective symptom is a reduction in visual acuity which varies according to the site and extent of the occlusion. In the fully developed central form of retinal vein occlusion visual acuity is considerably reduced, whereas in the branch form the degree of visual loss depends on the extent of oedema and haemorrhage in the macular area. There may also be a visual field defect corresponding to the drainage area of the occluded vein.

Branch vein occlusion may therefore be asymptomatic unless the degree of damage is extensive, resulting in a field defect. Many patients appear to sustain retinal vein occlusion at night, so that visual loss is noticed in the morning.

Visual acuity may be compromised at a later stage by the associated complications of retinal vein occlusion (maculopathy, vitreous haemorrhage from neovascularization and neovascular glaucoma).

There is a well recognized stage of preocclusion which is asymptomatic and reveals retinal abnormalities. This condition may be detected by the optician or during other incidental investigations.

8.3.2 Clinical signs

Retinal vein occlusion is classified into 'central' or 'branch' forms, according to the appearance on ophthalmoscopy (Figs 8.1 and 8.2). In the acute phase, extravasated blood collects in the retina forming deep and superficial haemorrhages.

A blocked central retinal vein leads to a 'battlefield' or 'sunset' fundus appearance. There is dilatation and tortuosity of the retinal veins, extensive oedema of the optic disc and retina, and leakage giving rise to exudation. Oedema and haemorrhages on and around the optic disc often obscure its margin, and in many cases the disc shows a prominence of 1–2 dioptres (papilloedematous appearance). Cotton wool spots are mainly seen around the optic

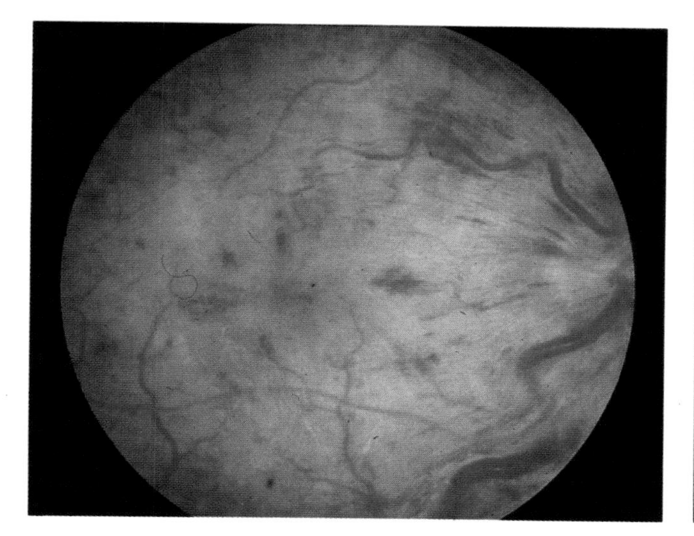

Fig. 8.1 Central retinal vein occlusion.

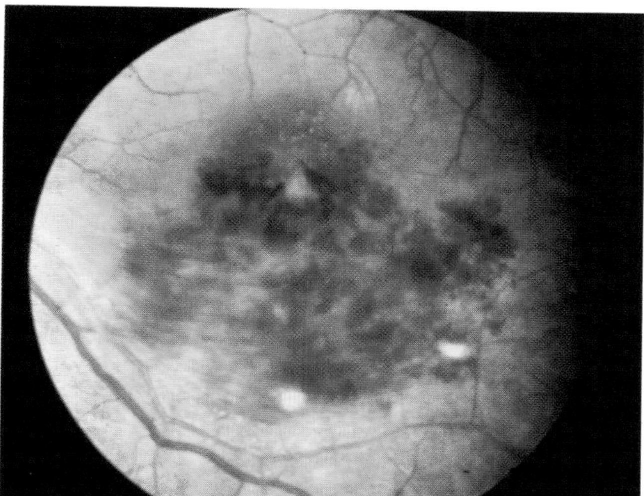

Fig. 8.2 Branch retinal vein occlusion.

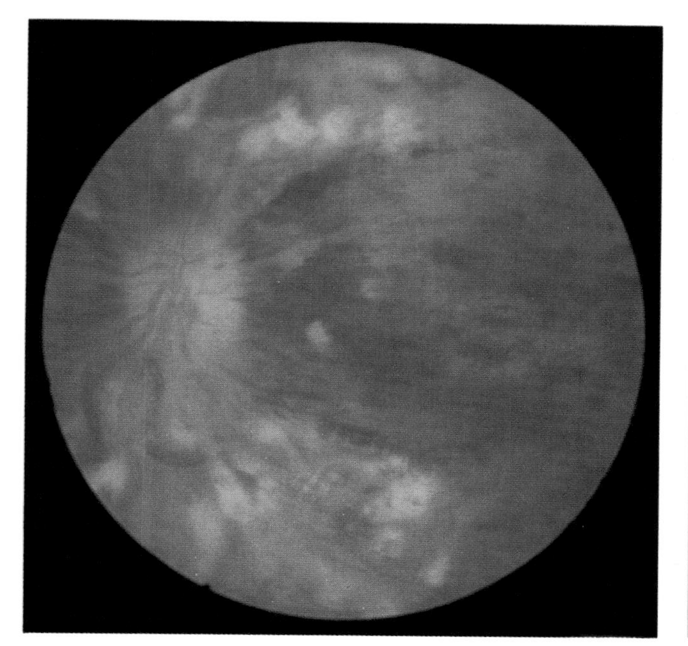

Fig. 8.3 Cotton wool spots and central retinal vein occlusion.

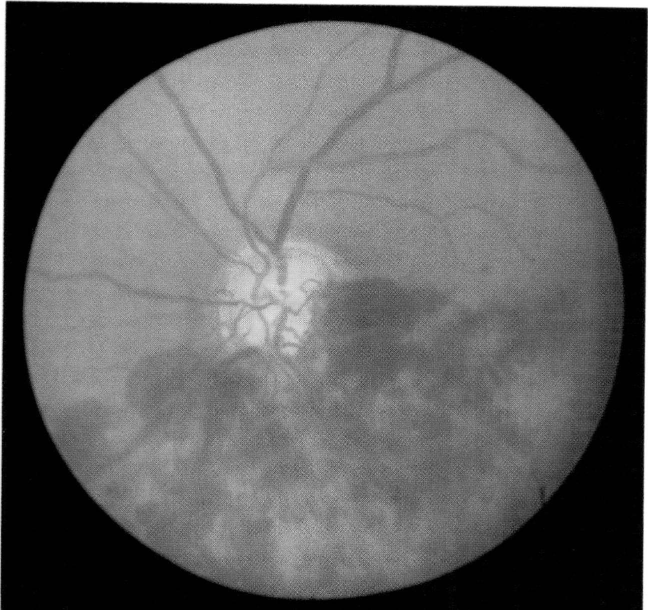

Fig. 8.4 Hemisphere retinal vein occlusion.

disc but may be a predominant feature in the severely ischaemic form (Fig. 8.3).

In the branch form, the same changes occur but are localized in the affected retinal segment. The occlusion usually develops at the first or second arteriovenous crossing outside the disc, and is more common in the superior temporal arcade. The artery in the drainage area of the occluded retinal vein may be markedly narrower than the other retinal arteries.

Occlusion of one of the two major branches of the central retinal vein in or on the optic disc may produce the appearance of an inferior or superior hemisphere occlusion (Fig. 8.4).

(A) INCIPIENT RETINAL VEIN OCCLUSION

This is characterized by (a) alteration in the calibres of the retinal vein and arteries (normally 3:2 to 4:1), and (b) an increase in the calibre of the dark and tortuous veins, accompanied by slight papilloedema and scattered retinal haemorrhages. Other terms to describe this include 'preocclusive retinal vein occlusion' or 'venous statis retinopathy'. The clinical picture is similar to that caused by circulatory changes located proximal to the eye, for example Takayasu's disease and carotid occlusion, or in hyperviscosity syndromes.

Diagnosis of this condition is important, as medical investigation for the cause is urgently needed and treatment at this stage may prevent the development of full-blown retinal vein occlusion. Nevertheless, there are a number of patients with incipient retinal vein occlusion in whom the abnormal retinal appearance reverts spontaneously to normal.

8.3.3 Clinical course

The prognosis of central retinal vein occlusion is generally poor, although spontaneous recovery may occur in rare cases, most likely in adolescents and young adults. Published data suggest that the visual outcome at three months after the occlusive event bears a correlation to that at one year.

After the initial period of leakage, resorption of oedema and haemorrhage takes place. The degree and speed of regression is analogous to the degree of destruction of the capillary network and formation of anastomotic channels, for example between the retinal and ciliary circulation (opticociliary anastomoses). Cotton wool spots tend to resolve early, whereas haemorrhage and retinal oedema may persist for months or even years. The optic disc which is oedematous and hyperaemic may become atrophic and pale in the regression phase. The major complications of retinal vein occlusion are:

1. maculopathy
   (a) macular oedema
   (b) cystoid macular structure
   (c) pigmentary macular dystrophy
   (d) serous retinal detachment
2. neovascularization
   (a) optic disc
   (b) peripheral retina
   (c) iris
3. neovascular glaucoma; due to iris neovascularization
4. recurrence in the previously unaffected eye in 10–15% of patients, if there is no medical intervention.

Macular changes have a major influence on prognosis and treatment. In retinal vein occlusion, poor prognostic features include the development of a cystoid macular structure, a pseudo-hole in the macula, development of pigmentary macular dystrophy, or marked ischaemia. The integrity of the peripheral capillary arcade is also important, and a better outlook is expected when this is intact. The presence of capillary closure at the macula carries a poor prognosis.

Neovascularization occurs following central retinal vein occlusion in 20–30% of patients, although it may occur in the branch form. The new vessels occur in the peripheral retina, but more commonly arise from the optic disc. The main complications of neovascularization are vitreous haemorrhage and, later on, formation of traction bands and glial tissue. The most serious complication is neovascular glaucoma caused by the formation of new vessels on the iris. This is termed '100-day glaucoma', as there is an average latent period of 100 days from the venous occlusion event to the development of glaucoma. The initial appearance of the fundus and level of intraocular pressure do not seem to predict this complication. Similarly, no underlying medical disorder predicts this outcome, but rubeosis does occur in a more elderly population of patients with central retinal vein occlusion (mean age of 70 years).

8.4 UNDERLYING MEDICAL DISORDERS

8.4.1 Common conditions

The most common conditions underlying retinal vein occlusion are show in Table 8.1. Their predomi-

Table 8.1 Medical conditions underlying retinal vein occlusion

	Prevalence (%)	*(n)*
Smoking	35	(208)
Hypertension		
New cases	26	(152)
Established	33	(193)
Total	59	(345)
Diabetes mellitus	10	(61)
Hyperlipidaemia	48	(281)
Chronic renal failure	5	(28)
Myeloma	0.005	(3)
Oestrogen containing preparations	0.02	(10)

From a study of 588 patients collected serially, Birmingham and Midland Eye Hospital.

nance varies according to age (Table 8.2), ethnic group (Table 8.3) and type of occlusion (Table 8.4).

Hypertension seems to be most frequently associated with retinal vein occlusion, particularly when it is limited to the branch form. In affected patients the hypertension is usually poorly controlled and is of the isolated systolic type, mainly essential in aetiology but by no means exclusive of secondary causes.

In young patients hyperlipidaemia rather than hypertension seems to be the major underlying medical condition, indicating that it may also play an important aetiological role. This inference is supported by the positive correlations between concentrations of cholesterol-carrying lipoproteins (LDL in particular) and the extent of retinal damage following venous occlusion.

It is difficult to distinguish between hyperlipidaemia as a primary aetiological factor and any causal relationship between conditions associated with or secondary to it. For example, it has been suggested that the increased prevalence of hyperlipidaemia in patients with retinal vein occlusion might simply reflect widespread atheroma. This premise is refuted by the finding of a significantly higher

Table 8.2 Prevalence of common medical conditions underlying retinal vein occlusion according to age and number of venous events

Patient	*Hypertension*	*Hyperlipidaemia*	*Diabetes mellitus*	*No obvious cause*
Young <50 years	25%	35%	3%	40%
Older >50 years	64%	34%	4–15%	21%
Recurrent (two or bilateral RVO)	88%	47%	3–3%	6%

RVO = retinal vein occlusion.

Table 8.3 Prevalence of medical conditions according to race

	White Europeans	*Asians*	*West Indians*
Number of patients	536	28	24
Prevalence of:			
Hypertension	57.2%	64.1%*	83%~
Hyperlipidaemia	48.3%	50%	33%
Diabetes mellitus	8.2%	29%~	38%~
Chronic renal failure	4.6%	4%	8%
No obvious cause	21.1%	10.7%	8.3%

Study performed at Birmingham and Midland Eye Hospital. *$p < 0.01$, ~$p < 0.001$.

Table 8.4 Prevalence of medical conditions underlying retinal vein occlusion according to type (branch or central form)

Prevalence of:	*Central RVO (n = 235)*	*Branch RVO (n = 305)*
Hypertension	49%	58.3%
Hyperlipidaemia	43%	50%
Diabetes mellitus	12%	8%
Smokers	37%	37%

RVO = retinal vein occlusion. Data from Physicians Clinic, Birmingham and Midland Eye Hospital.

prevalence of hyperlipidaemia in patients with retinal vein occlusion, compared with a closely matched control group with a similar prevalence of clinically detectable macrovascular disease. Data from prospective clinical studies appear to support the hypothesis that retinal venous damage is just one aspect of atherosclerosis affecting both arterial and venous systems.

Retinal vein occlusion is also associated with diabetes mellitus and has even been described as being part of diabetic retinopathy. However, the likely explanation is that diabetic patients are more prone to events of occlusion, owing to the significantly higher prevalence of hypertension and hyperlipidaemia found in diabetes mellitus.

Ethnic factors may play a role. An important but puzzling observation is that retinal vein occlusion is relatively rare in the Asian and West Indian ethnic minority groups in Britain. The different patterns of underlying medical conditions are shown in Table 8.3. Central retinal vein occlusion is rare in West Indians, although in this ethnic group hypertension is common, and tends to be severe and resistant to therapy (factors which are associated with retinal vein occlusion in Caucasians). Several reports have shown a lower prevalence of hyperlipidaemia in Blacks compared with Caucasians; once again, this observation hints at an aetiological role for hyperlipidaemia.

Smoking and alcohol consumption appear related to retinal vein occlusion. Regular alcohol consumption has been implicated, perhaps through the pressor effects of alcohol, which may have a link with hypertension. Alternatively, this relationship may be related to adverse effects on lipid metabolism with elevation of diglyceride-rich particles. The role of smoking is unclear.

In early descriptions, neoplastic disease was thought to be associated with retinal vein occlusion. This worrying finding has not been substantiated in large series, and indeed the mortality rates on follow-up of patients with this condition do not show an excess of mortality from neoplastic disease.

8.4.2 Less common conditions

Retinal vein occlusion is associated with a number of less common disorders, including chronic renal failure, hypothyroidism and the myelomas (see Table 8.1). Inflammatory conditions may also be seen, particularly in young patients, and local causes of external inflammatory activity to the orbit (frontal and maxillary sinusitis) have been reported.

The myelomas are rarely identified; in a recent large series these were seen in less than 1% of patients presenting with retinal vein occlusion. All forms of myeloma have been identified but Waldenstrom's disease and benign gammopathy seem the most frequent.

Retinal vein occlusion may occur in young patients taking contraceptive combined preparations containing oestrogen, and in postmenopausal women on hormone replacement therapy. Multiple single case reports and prevalence in one recent series have emphasized this association (Table 8.1). Whether this is due to an adverse effect of oestrogen on coagulation is only speculative, but it is clear that oestrogen-containing preparations are contraindicated in patients with retinal vein occlusion.

(A) GLAUCOMA

Glaucoma has been traditionally thought of as a major aetiological factor, but this has been questioned by recent data. For example, the underlying medical conditions occur at the same prevalence in patients with retinal vein occlusion, irrespective of the presence of glaucoma. However, it is thought that a hemisphere retinal vein occlusion may be related to raised intraocular pressure.

8.5 MANAGEMENT

Ophthalmic management, particularly of the resulting complications, is carried out concurrently with medical treatment. Management is divided into two categories:

1. Ophthalmic:
   (a) initial examination and diagnosis;
   (b) complications of retinal vein occlusion.

2. Medical:
   (a) identification and treatment of underlying conditions;
   (b) prevention of recurrence;
   (c) initial treatment to improve retinal venous flow.

8.5.1 Ophthalmic management

Patients presenting with retinal vein occlusion require a full ophthalmological examination to eliminate local causes, such as chronic glaucoma or a compressive orbital lesion. Particular emphasis is placed on intraocular pressure, form of occlusion (whether branch or central), visual acuity and appearance of the retina. The degree of macular oedema, retinal haemorrhage and ischaemia should be recorded, preferably by retinal photography. Subsequent management will depend on whether occlusion is in the central retinal vein or in a branch vein, as well as on the severity of the associated retinal ischaemia and other complications.

The principles underlying treatment with laser therapy are now outlined.

(A) BRANCH RETINAL VEIN OCCLUSION (BRVO)

Laser photocoagulation can be extremely helpful in patients with BRVO. The aim of laser treatment is to prevent further visual deterioration from persistent macular oedema or from haemorrhage from new vessels.

The Branch Vein Occlusion Study was a prospective, randomized, multicentre trial that was designed to answer the following questions:

1. Is argon laser photocoagulation useful for improving vision in eyes with 20/40 (6/12) or worse vision secondary to macular oedema caused by branch retinal vein occlusion?
2. Can photocoagulation prevent the development of neovascularization?
3. Can photocoagulation prevent vitreous haemorrhage from retinal neovascularization?

The results of the study showed that for macular oedema those patients treated with a grid of laser burns to the oedematous area, did better at three years follow-up than those that were merely observed. The visual prognosis was also better if the peripheral capillary network was intact.

For neovascularization, laser treatment decreased the risk of vitreous haemorrhage. However, the study results suggested that laser treatment should only be recommended after new vessels have developed (this would prevent the unnecessary treatment of a large number of patients with BRVO who might never develop neovascularization).

The Branch Vein Occlusion Study has proved to have a major influence on management of this condition. A sensible plan of managing patients with BRVO would therefore seem to be:

1. If macular oedema is present on clinical examination with vision 20/40 or worse, wait until haemorrhages have cleared before performing a fundus fluorescein angiogram (FFA) (this may take several weeks/months).
2. If the FFA shows macular oedema, argon green (or krypton red or diode laser) should be applied over the oedematous area, in a grid, avoiding the foveal avascular zone. No laser treatment should be given if there is obvious ischaemia within the macula, which would account for the visual loss.
3. Patients should be examined regularly (approximately every 3 months) for retinal new vessels. If new vessels develop, scatter laser photocoagulation can be applied to the quadrant involved or the non-perfused areas on FFA. Krypton red or diode laser may be useful if there are many haemorrhages as these laser beams are less absorbed than argon. Treatment may need to be repeated.

(B) CENTRAL RETINAL VEIN OCCLUSION (CRVO)

For patients with CRVO there is unfortunately no proven early management that is at present likely to alter the visual prognosis. The main aim of treatment therefore is to identify those patients who have ischaemic damage and are at risk of developing neovascular glaucoma – a particularly devastating and unpleasant complication. On examination the 'ischaemic type' of CRVO is associated with the following characteristics:

1. poor vision (counting fingers or worse)
2. marked afferent pupillary defect;
3. presence of multiple dark, deep intraretinal haemorrhages;
4. presence of multiple cotton wool spots;
5. extensive non-perfusion of retinal capillaries in FFA;
6. moderate or severe macular oedema.

Unfortunately there is, as yet, no exact way of differentiating between the ischaemic and non-ischaemic groups, but the use of electrodiagnostic tests can be helpful. Therefore, it is important to follow up patients with CRVO closely to detect if they are developing new vessels in the anterior chamber angle (detected by gonioscopy) or on the iris (rubeosis iridis). Aggressive periretinal scatter laser photocoagulation has been shown to be successful in preventing these new vessels from developing further. Treatment should be carried out by an experienced person as effective treatment is difficult to perform.

Early periretinal laser photocoagulation or peripheral retinal cryopexy is effective in preventing neovascular glaucoma from developing. For macular oedema associated with CRVO the situation is not so successful and laser photocoagulation in the form of a grid does not seem to influence the visual outcome.

The patient's medical history should be taken and a full examination carried out at an early stage, to allow identification of underlying medical conditions and institute the appropriate therapy.

Key points in the history of patients with retinal vein occlusion are:

1. Symptoms:
   (a) visual loss
   (b) angina
   peripheral vascular disease
   stroke
   (c) nocturia (symptom of hypertension, diabetes, renal disease).
   (d) recent anaesthesia – general; epidural;
2. Past history:
   (a) diabetes mellitus
   (b) hypertension;
3. Familial: premature cardiovascular disease
4. Drugs:
   (a) antihypertensive agents
   (b) oestrogen-containing preparations
   (c) warfarin;
5. Social:
   (a) smoking
   (b) alcohol consumption.

Key signs to look for on physical examination for retinal vein occlusion are:

1. anaemia;
2. blood pressure (hypertension);
3. pulses – peripheral, carotid, rhythm (e.g. atrial fibrillation);
4. hyperlipidaemia – arcus senilis, xanthoma, xanthelasma;
5. heart – rhythm, cardiomegaly, murmurs;
6. alimentary system – hepatomegaly, splenomegaly;
7. respiratory system – coexisting lung disease, cyanosis, polycythaemia;
8. urogenital – palpable kidneys, rectal examination for prostatic state (are there symptoms of prostatic hypertrophy or an elevated serum creatinine)
9. central nervous system – signs of localized orbital lesion: anterior cranial lesion, maxillary and frontal sinuses; peripheral neuropathy.

It is currently under investigation whether medical treatment of retinal vein occlusion is indicated at the time of presentation to medical services, within hours of the occlusive event.

8.5.2 Medical management

Much research has been carried out on this aspect, but the results have been generally disappointing. This may be partly due to the time lapse between the occluding event and presentation of the patient: many venous occlusive lesions spare the macula and therefore do not give rise to immediately apparent visual symptoms.

The avenues explored in initial treatment to improve retinal venous flow are:

1. anticoagulants: heparin;
2. fibrinolytic agents: streptokinase, tissue plasminogen activator;
3. clofibrate;
4. antiplatelet drugs: aspirin, prostacyclin;
5. steroids: prednisolone;
6. haemodilution.

Anticoagulants would seem to be a logical initial treatment, but the results of this approach have been particularly disappointing, owing to their adverse effect on retinal haemorrhage. However, trials of streptokinase therapy have demonstrated a significantly reduced incidence of thrombotic glaucoma complicating central retinal vein occlusion compared with an untreated control group, although the final visual prognosis did not show improvement. A recent trial of tissue plasminogen activator (TPA) in the treatment of experimental retinal vein occlusion in rabbits seems encouraging. Four hours following treatment, previously occluded veins were patent in all eyes treated with TPA, in contrast to 8.3% in those treated with normal saline. Confirmatory evidence in humans is awaited.

Uncontrolled data have suggested that antiplatelet drugs (for example, aspirin, dipyridamole) may be beneficial, but controlled trials are required. The same applies to a more recent report on benefits from immediate prostacyclin infusion, although this effect was compared with that of intravenous heparin administration, which is known to exacerbate retinal haemorrhage and worsen the visual prognosis. Thus, although there is no definitive medical treatment for improving the visual outcome following retinal vein occlusion, prostacyclin, TPA, newer antiplatelet drugs and haemodilution warrant further careful controlled study.

8.5.3 Long term medical management

The following aspects should be considered:

1. Implications of retinal vein occlusion for individual patients, with regard to morbidity and mortality.
2. Prevention as regards an initial vein occlusion, as well as prevention of a further occlusive event which may occur in the unaffected eye.

Retinal vein occlusion appears to be linked with an increase in vascular causes of death (both cardiac and cerebral). In view of the evidence from prospective studies that drug treatment of hypertension reduces the severity of some of its complications, it seems likely that efficient blood pressure control should also influence the mortality of patients with retinal vein occlusion. However, this condition remains a common occurrence in patients receiving single or multiple drug therapy in an attempt to control their hypertension. Whether these disappointing results reflect poor control of hypertension or failure to identify and treat concomitant hyperlipidaemia is an open question.

In view of the high prevalence of hyperlipidaemia, antihypertensive agents known to increase serum lipid levels should be avoided. These include thiazide diuretics and, to a lesser extent, beta-blockers.

Management of hyperlipidaemia is based on conventional lines (section 6.7). Secondary causes such as diabetes mellitus, hypothyroidism and use of thiazide diuretics must be excluded and, where present, appropriately managed. Severe hyperlipidaemia or hyperlipidaemia which is resistant to diet and requires drug therapy, is uncommon. Furthermore, many patients with retinal vein occlusion will be over 65 years of age, and data from the lipid lowering trials in the elderly is scanty. However, current limited evidence supports active treatment in these patients, to prevent recurrence of retinal vein occlusion.

8.5.4 Recurrence

Recurrence develops in 10–15% of patients with a single retinal vein occlusion. Recent data have suggested a means of identifying patients in whom the occlusion is likely to recur. The prevalence rate for associated hypertension and hyperlipidaemia was approximately double that in a well matched group of patients with a single occlusion (Table 8.2). It is therefore inferred that patients with hypertension, hyperlipidaemia and low HDL-cholesterol are at higher risk of recurrence and should receive aggressive medical treatment to prevent it. Preliminary results of this approach are encouraging: 598 patients presenting over a period of six years with a single episode and treated in this manner showed less than 1% recurrence, compared to the 10–15% previously reported.

In a proportion of patients (40% young, 20% middle-aged) presenting with retinal vein occlusion, examination and investigation will be normal and unhelpful. Where the visual outcome is poor, it is our policy to initiate antiplatelet drug therapy (aspirin or dipyridamole) on a long-term basis to prevent recurrence or at least other cardiovascular episodes (such as stroke). Only limited evidence is available regarding the benefits of this approach compared to a control group as has been shown by the report of the Antiplatelet Trialist Collaboration project.

FURTHER READING

Antiplatelet Trialist Collaboration (1994) Collaborative overview of randomised anti-platelet therapy. *Br. Med. J.*, **308**, 81–106.

Branch Vein Occlusion Study Group (1984) Argon laser photocoagulation for macular oedema in branch vein occlusion. *Am. J. Ophthalmol.*, **98**, 271–82.

Branch Vein Occlusion Study Group (1986) Argon laser scatter photocoagulation for prevention of neovascularisation and vitreous haemorrhage in branch vein occlusion. *Arch. Ophthalmol.*, **104**, 34–41.

Dodson, P.M. and Kritzinger, E.E. (1985) Underlying medical conditions in young patients and ethnic differences in retinal vein occlusion. *Trans. Ophthalmol. Soc. UK*, **104**, 114–9.

Dodson, P.M. and Kritzinger, E.E. (1987) Management of retinal vein occlusion. *Br. Med. J.*, **295**, 1434–5.

Dodson, P.M., Kubicki, A.J., Taylor, K.G. and Kritzinger, E.E. (1985) Medical conditions underlying recurrence of retinal vein occlusion. *Br. J. Ophthalmol.*, **69**, 493–6.

Dodson, P.M., Kritzinger, E.E. and Clough, C.G. (1992) Diabetes mellitus and retinal vein occlusion in patients of Asian, West Indian and White European Origin. *Eye*, **6**, 66–8.

Dodson, P.M., Clough, C.G., Downes, S.M. and Kritzinger, E.E. (1993) Does type II diabetes predispose to retinal vein occlusion? *Eur. J. Ophthalmol.*, **3**(3), 109–13.

Keenan, J.M., Dodson, P.M. and Kritzinger, E.E. (1993) Management of retinal vein occlusion. *Br. Hosp. J. Med.*, **49**, 268–73.

Keenan, J.M., Dodson, P.M. and Kritzinger, E.E. (1993) Are there medical conditions specifically underlying the development of rubeosis in Central Retinal Vein Occlusion. *Eye*, **7**, 407–10.

Morrell, A.J., Thompson, D.A., Gibson, J.M. *et al.* (1991) Electro-retinopathy as a prognostic indicator for neovascularisation in CRVO. *Eye*, **5**, 362–8.

9 *Inflammatory retinal disease*

Clinical Retinopathies. Paul M. Dodson, Jonathan M. Gibson and Erna E. Kritzinger.
Published in 1995 by Chapman & Hall, London. ISBN 0 412 35930 8

9.1 INTRODUCTION

Inflammation of the retina and retinal blood vessels is an important cause of visual morbidity, especially in the younger age group. The findings of inflammatory changes in the eye together with involvement of the retinal blood vessels provides a large spectrum of clinical manifestations. Retinal vasculitis itself may occur as an isolated phenomenon or as a feature of systemic inflammatory disease. The latter may enable the physician or ophthalmologist to make a diagnosis of significant systemic disease by recognizing different patterns.

Ocular inflammation is most commonly associated in the eye with the uveal tract. Uveitis may affect the anterior components of the tract (the iris and ciliary body) giving rise to iritis, cyclitis or if both structures are involved, iridocyclitis. Inflammation of the posterior part of the uveal tract, the choroid, causes choroiditis and this may be associated with inflammatory changes of the retina and retinal blood vessels, termed retinitis and retinal vasculitis. Particular systemic conditions may have a predilection to be associated with either anterior or posterior uveitis, or, the inflammation may be generalized giving rise to a panuveitis. Retinal vasculitis may give rise to inflammation of the veins or retinal periphlebitis (Fig. 9.1).

Although inflammatory retinal disease constitutes important ophthalmological signs, as such it may not indicate a specific disease entity, reflecting many infective, toxic and immunological states. This chapter will deal with inflammatory conditions affecting the retina and choroid. Other chapters deal with the infective and toxic causes. A separate detailed description of cranial arteritis is also included.

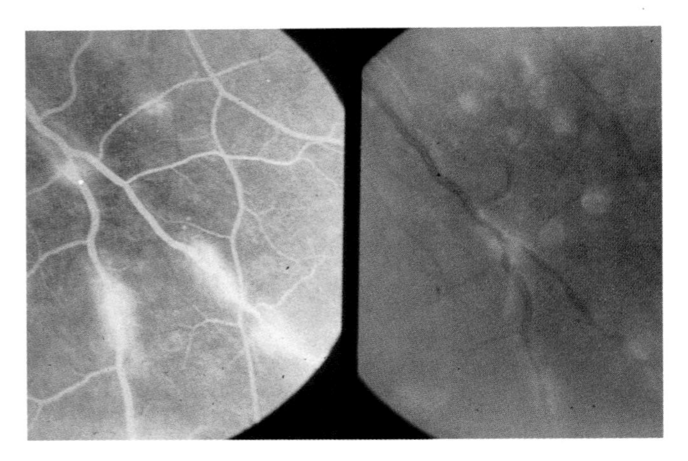

Fig. 9.1 A fundus photograph and fluorescein angiogram showing venous sheathing and periphlebitis (focal staining of the veins on fluorescein) seen in idiopathic retinal vasculitis. The discrete white patches on the fundus photographs are artefactual.

9.2 PATHOLOGY

The major structural changes in inflammatory eye disease are:

1. Retinal vasculitis:
   perivascular cuffing with lymphocytes;
   hyalinization of the vein (sheathing);
   thickening of internal limiting membrane and media;
   endothelial cell hypertrophy;
   vessel lumen obstruction;
   secondary capillary closure;
   neovascularization;
   granulomata (rare, sarcoid).
2. Arteritis:
   isolated arteriolitis;
   multiple retinal arterial occlusion;
   scarring and pigmentation.
3. Choroiditis:
   inflammatory lesions, atrophy and pigmentation
4. Vitreous involvement:
   inflammatory cell infiltrate (vitritis);
   aggregation of cells to form a membrane-like structure.
5. Papillitis:
   optic nerve head swelling;
   optic atrophy.

These include inflammatory changes affecting the vessels (vasculitis), the choroid (choroiditis), optic nerve head (papillitis), and the vitreous gel (vitritis). Changes of isolated arteritis are rare but may appear as an isolated arteriolitis, or multiple retinal arterial occlusions.

The typical signs of inflammation of the retina are commonly those of vasculitis. Clinical features include sheathing or cuffing of the blood vessels, which is visible on ophthalmoscopy (Fig. 9.1). Changes in the vessel walls allow the passage of serous exudate into the retina which may eventually lead to cystoid macular oedema. As retinal vasculitis progresses, vascular obstruction may occur and give rise to retinal ischaemia. This may present as cotton wool spots (infarcts of the nerve fibre layer) or capillary closure.

New vessel formation may occur on the retina secondary to this and may also occur on the iris (iris neovascularization). Severe vascular deficiency can progress to retinal atrophy and scarring associated in the long term with deposition of pigment. Choroiditis may be a specific feature of inflammatory eye disease. In the active phase there are ill-defined white lesions arising in the choroid. These may later give rise to choroidal atrophy, surrounded by patches of pigmentation (Figure 9.2). Some cases may lead to choroidal detachments, or large bulbous shaped space occupying lesions which bulge forwards into the vitreous.

The vitreous may be involved as an inflammatory cell infiltrate which with aggregation of cells may form a membrane-like structure. Inflammatory disease of the optic nerve head may be an isolated finding or may be present with other features of inflammatory eye disease. The changes are due to inflammation of the optic nerve head and may progress to optic atrophy. Initially the optic disc is hyperaemic and swollen, and may be difficult to distinguish from papilloedema associated with other causes (see optic nerve disorders, Chapter 12).

9.3 CLINICAL FEATURES AND RETINAL APPEARANCES

9.3.1 Retinal vasculitis

Retinal vasculitis occurs when there is coincident inflammation of the eye and involvement of the retinal blood vessels. The inflammatory changes may partly involve the arteries, veins or capillaries, producing a wide spectrum of clinical presentation. Retinal vasculitis may occur as an isolated phenomenon (idiopathic retinal vasculitis) or as part of a systemic inflammatory disease.

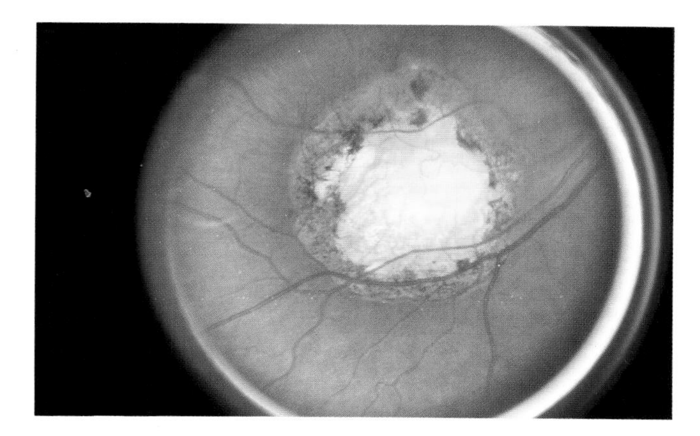

Fig. 9.2 Choroidal atrophy and increase in pigmentation type of longstanding inactive choroiditis.

The aetiology of retinal vasculitis is:

Common:
- autoimmune (idiopathic)
- systemic lupus erythematosus
- sarcoidosis
- Behçet's disease

Rare:
- polyarteritis nodosa
- Loeffler's syndrome
- multiple sclerosis
- Whipple's disease
- Goodpasture's syndrome
- malignant disease
- ischaemic disease
- infective causes
  - tuberculosis
  - viral
  - syphilis
  - fungus infections

This aetiology of retinal arteritis is:
- idiopathic
- systemic lupus erythematosus
- polyarteritis nodosa
- Wegener's granulomatosis
- Goodpasture's syndrome
- Loeffler's eosinophilic syndrome
- giant cell arteritis
- Takayasu's arteritis

Typically retinal vasculitis occurs in young adults who are often otherwise apparently healthy. The vision tends to be good to begin with because the major lesions are in the peripheral retina. Patients commonly complain of black spots, floaters and blurred vision. Field defects rarely occur. Examination of the retina may show changes ranging from mild perivascular sheathing of small peripheral veins to frank vascular occlusion and secondary neovascularization. A retinal haemorrhage may occur, which may extend into the vitreous. Retinal vasculitis tends to have relapses and remissions, but massive vitreous haemorrhage may occur which may leave marked visual impairment. Neovascularization (retinitis proliferans) may lead to fibrous traction bands forming between retina and vitreous which may lead to retinal detachment.

In idiopathic retinal vasculitis, sheathing of peripheral veins and leakage from small capillaries is the commonest vascular abnormality. This may occur particularly in the macular area producing macular oedema, which is an important cause of visual loss (Fig. 9.3). Secondary glaucoma and cataract may accompany this condition. Fifty per cent of patients with retinal vasculitis have the idiopathic

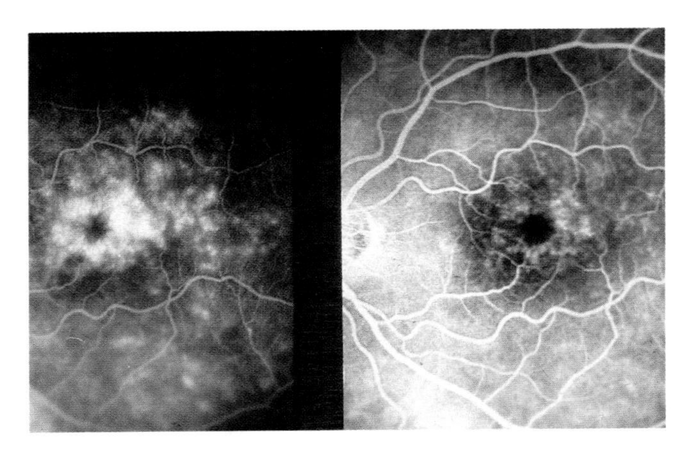

Fig. 9.3 Fluorescein angiogram demonstrating macula oedema of inflammatory origin.

variety, the remainder presenting with symptoms referable to an underlying systemic inflammatory disorder.

9.3.2 Choroiditis

This condition typically presents with visual disturbances including floating specks, distortion of objects, defective visual acuity and scotoma. The inflammation is primarily of the choroid, but may also involve the adjacent retina (choroidoretinitis). If the lesion involves the macular region, there may be distortion of the shape of objects, which may appear smaller or larger, and there may also be photophobia. If the lesion is remote from the macula there may be no symptoms although slight blurring of vision can occur. Choroiditis may be due to infective causes which are described in a later chapter, but another cause is sarcoidosis.

The fundus shows a localized patch of inflammatory exudate derived from the choroid which forms yellow patches with fluffy margins. It is often barely visible through the inflammatory haze in the overlying vitreous.

In the long term, atrophy of the choroido-retinal lesion will occur. This may lead to the exposure of white sclera, together with retinal pigment epithelium proliferation (Fig. 9.2). the areas involved are usually irregular, and if bilateral, rarely symmetrical. Severe impairment of vision may occur in the acute attack of choroiditis due to vitreous exudation, particularly if the macular area is involved. Once a chronic lesion is formed, impairment of vision is usually stationary, but areas of choroiditis may be asymptomatic and identified as an incidental lesion on ophthalmoscopy.

9.3.3 Optic nerve swelling (papillitis)

Inflammation or degenerative foci of the choroid and optic nerve head may arise from a variety of causes:

Choroiditis:
- syphilis
- toxoplasmosis
- *Toxocara*
- histoplasmosis
- sarcoidosis

Papillitis:
- multiple sclerosis
- Behçet's syndrome
- giant cell arteritis
- Devic's disease
- Leber's disease
- viral (measles, whooping cough, other exanthema)

These foci may be placed near the anterior end of the nerve with engorgement visible ophthalmoscopically on the optic disc. This gives rise to the appearance of papillitis which may closely resemble papilloedema resulting from raised intracranial pressure. In both conditions the optic disc is hyperaemic and swollen, but in papillitis visual acuity is always severely reduced whereas in papilloedema visual acuity is usually normal, although the blind spot is enlarged. If the inflammation is posterior in the optic nerve head, the optic disc may be normal. Optic neuritis behind the globe is termed retrobulbar neuritis.

Fundoscopy will either reveal a normal optic disc (retrobulbar neuritis), or there may be papillitis. It may progress to optic atrophy. The direct pupillary responses to light are sluggish and consensual reflexes are generally unchanged. However, there may later be evidence of a Marcus Gunn pupil, detected by the swinging flash light test (Chapter 3). The pupil on the affected side may even be moderately dilated. In cases of retrobulbar neuritis, movement of the eye on the affected side evokes pain because of pressure of the contracting muscle on the inflamed nerve. Enlargement of the blind spot or sectorial scotoma may be demonstrated.

9.4 AETIOLOGY

9.4.1 Retinal vasculitis

The aetiology of retinal vasculitis is still obscure. Ophthalmological evidence suggest that it has an immunological background. Fifty per cent of patients with retinal vasculitis have the idiopathic form which predominantly affects patients in the third and fourth decades with equal sex incidence. Fifty per cent are related to systemic diseases, the causes of which are listed in section 9.3.1. The idiopathic variety appears to be a T-cell dependent immune reaction, which can be induced by several substances either injected into the eye, intravenously or intraperitoneally. These include endotoxins or lipopolysaccharides of Gram-negative bacteria and superoxide generating mixtures of xanthine oxidase.

Retinal-S antigen, which has been described more recently, stimulates an intense inflammatory response when injected with adjuvant at a site far from the eye. This material has been characterized as a glycoprotein with a molecular weight of 55 000 Daltons, and is specifically located in the outer rod segments of the photoreceptor cells and pineal gland. Retinal-S antigen has been implicated in the aetiology of only certain types of vasculitis. It is still unclear whether the presence of Retinal-S antigen in human serum relates to prognosis or whether it is involved in the pathogenesis.

In this context, it is worthy of note that lymphocytes are not usually in a great abundance in the eye but are attracted by antigen. It may be that once exposure to retinal antigens has occurred resulting in antibody formation, subsequent exposure to the same antigen will result in renewed antibody production and inflammation. Hence the chronic relapsing state is often encountered. Lymphocytic reactivation within the eye has been attributed to the presence of memory cells. Thus recurrent uveitis and vasculitis probably represents an immune response to antigens that might not even originate within the eye.

Another avenue that has been extensively explored is the association between the HLA system and retinal vasculitis. The established associations are shown in Table 9.1. For example, HLA B8 is associated with sarcoidosis and systemic lupus erythematosus. These B lymphocyte antigens are located on chromosome 6. This genetic region might not only control immune responses, but may also play an important role in cell interaction with antigens, which could be causally related.

Table 9.1 HLA associations and conditions causing retinal vasculitis

Condition	*HLA association*
Sarcoidosis	B8
Behçet's disease	B27 (arthritic), B5, B12 (muco-cutaneous)
Systemic lupus erythematosus	B8, DR2
Rheumatoid arthritis	DR4, D4, B27 Juvenile

Table 9.2 Eye diagnosis in relation to systemic inflammatory disease

Type of vessel affected	*Disease*	*Retinal vasculitis*	*Optic nerve disease*
Arterial	Giant cell arteritis	–	++
	SLE	Ischaemic cotton-wool spots	+
	Wegener's granulomatosis	+	+ (Rare)
	PAN	Ischaemic choroidal vasculitis	+
Capillary	Sclerodema	Ischaemic choroidal vasculitis	+
	Ankylosing spondylitis	+ (rare)	–
Venous	Sarcoidosis	++	+
	Behçet's disease	++	+
	Multiple sclerosis	+	++

SLE = Systemic lupus erythematosus.
PAN = Polyarteritis nodosa.

9.4.2 Inflammatory disorders and retinal vasculitis

Retinal vasculitis may reflect a wide variety of systemic inflammatory disease. Table 9.2 shows the degree to which retinal vasculitis may occur, as well as associated ischaemic changes and optic nerve abnormalities in these disorders. A description of each individual condition will now be undertaken.

9.5 BEHÇET'S DISEASE

Professor Halusi Behçet first described the clinical triad of hypopyon iritis, thrombophlebitis and orogenital ulceration in 1937.

It is a multisystem disease affecting young adults, more common in males and presenting in the second and third decades of life. Important clinical manifestations are arthritis, headache and diplopia secondary to involvement of the central nervous system. Diarrhoea may occur with gastro-intestinal involvement.

To summarize, the features of Behçet's syndrome are:

Major features:
- oral ulceration
- genital ulceration
- skin lesions:
  - erythema nodosum
  - pustules
  - ulceration
  - hypersensitivity
- eye:
  - uveitis
  - retinal vasculitis

Minor features:
- arthritis
- vasculitis
- gastrointestinal ulceration
- CNS:
  - brain stem syndrome
  - meningoencephalitis
  - headache, coma
  - epilepsy
  - psychoses
- cardiovascular involvement
- pulmonary

The underlying histopathological lesion in all organ systems is vasculitis. This includes perivascular infiltrates of mononuclear cells, swelling and proliferation of endothelial cells leading to partial obliteration of small vessels and fibrinoid degradation.

The eye is involved in 70% of patients. The ocular manifestations are clinically important, as up to 25% of patients may go blind. Mortality from Behçet's syndrome is rare at 3–4% of patients. The disease usually burns itself out, leaving a blind or partially sighted patient. Early diagnosis is essential as active management can prevent the spread of the condition to other unaffected systems. Ocular involvement includes:

1. Inflammation. Uveitis with hypopyon is frequently described in association with Behçet's disease but is rarely seen nowadays (Fig. 9.4).
2. Posterior involvement. There may be extensive formation of posterior synechiae with serious complications, of occlusion of the pupil and secondary glaucoma. Cataract formation is common. Inflammation of the vitreous is usually present and frequently obscures the retinal details.

Inflammation of the retina and posterior segment of the eye has the following features:

1. A generalized vasodilation of the retinal vessels is a common finding with increased vascular permeability giving rise to retinal oedema and cystoid macular oedema. On ophthalmoscopy, these changes may be masked by recurrent vitreous haemorrhage and other gross pathological changes (Fig. 9.5).
2. Obliterative vasculitis may occur, first involving the veins and then the arteries, the former giving rise to retinal branch vein occlusion.
3. The most severe retinal changes occur as a consequence of retinal arterial occlusion. This gives rise to large areas of retinal infarction and atrophy with intense secondary vitritis.

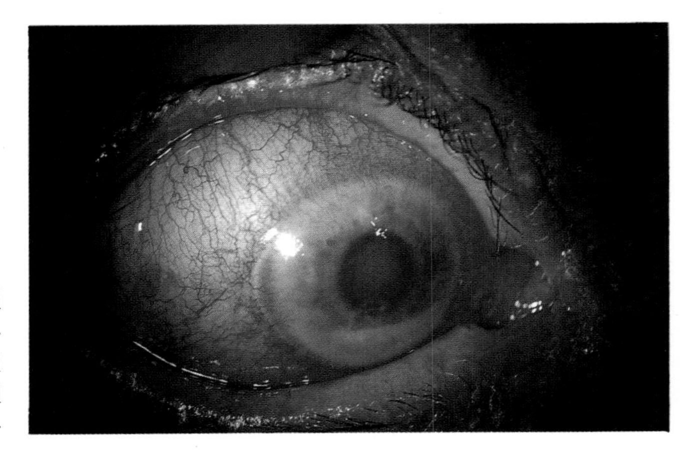

Fig. 9.4 A hypopyon as a result of Behçet's disease.

4. Hyperaemia of the optic disc signifies involvement of the optic nerve head (papillitis) which may develop subsequent optic atrophy (Fig. 9.6).

Branch vein occlusion is a frequent finding in Behçet's disease and usually occurs in the mid-periphery of the retina. These occlusions commonly involve the infero-temporal vessels and macular oedema ensues. In contrast to other causes of branch vein occlusion, retinal neovascularization is comparatively rare. The picture of a branch vein occlusion in the presence of severe uveitis is virtually diagnostic of Behçet's disease. Retinal infiltration usually occurs, presenting as deep pale areas in the retina surrounded by haemorrhages. A combination of retinal infiltration and branch vein occlusion are also specific pathognomonic features of the retinopathy of Behçet's disease.

It must be stressed that if ocular Behçet's disease is left untreated, retinopathy develops with devastating visual loss. Previous treatment regimens in the last decade have shown that 75% of patients go blind in both eyes within four years of ocular diagnosis. Fortunately the advent of new treatment regimens have altered this prognosis.

9.5.1 Diagnosis

The diagnosis of Behçet's disease is essentially clinical although there are a wide variety of immunological abnormalities shown in this condition.

International criteria for diagnosis of Behçet's disease are:

- recurrent oral ulceration
- and two other features of:
  - recurrent genital ulceration
  - eye lesions
  - skin lesions
  - positive pathargy test

There is a high prevalence of HLAB5 in ocular Behçet's disease, with HLAB27 being found in the arthritic type and HLAB12 in the mucocutaneous type. Immune complexes are found in patients with exacerbations of Behçet's disease along with increased IgG and IgM, and a decrease of IgG complexes.

9.5.2 Treatment

Behçet's disease does appear to respond to steroids (initial dose of prednisolone 30–60 mg daily) in combination with azathioprine (150 mg daily). Other drugs which are helpful include chlorambucil as an additional immunosuppressive. Recent trials have clearly shown the benefit of combination therapy in this disease. Bone marrow depression is the most common side-effect requiring regular monitoring of the blood count. Non-steroidal inflammatory drugs should not be used as they may exacerbate the orogenital ulceration.

9.6 SARCOIDOSIS

Sarcoidosis is a multisystem disorder of unknown aetiology. It most commonly affects young adults.

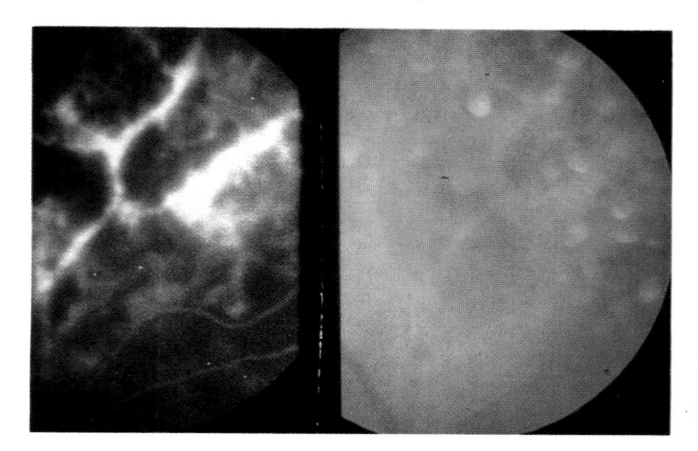

Fig. 9.5 A colour fundus and fluorescein angiographic example of Behçet's disease demonstrating widespread haemorrhage, severe phlebitis and retinal leakage.

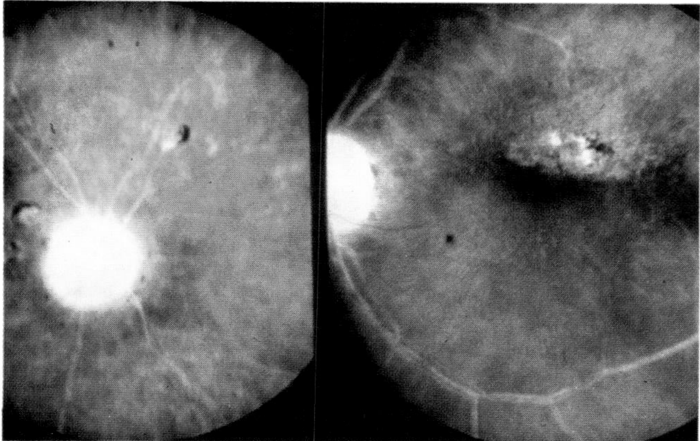

Fig. 9.6 A fundus photograph of end stage Behçet's disease demonstrating occluded vessels and optic atrophy.

Speculation exists that sarcoidosis begins in the respiratory system as pulmonary involvement is found in 75–95% of cases.

9.6.1 Pathology

The disease is characterized by non-caseating granuloma formation consisting of epitheloid and giant cells and macrophages. These changes may be found in the eyes, lungs, skin, joints and liver but there may also be central nervous system and cardiac involvement.

Sarcoid may involve the posterior segment of the eye, with the cardinal change of retinal periphlebitis. In this the retinal veins are sheathed especially at arteriovenous crossings which may be segmental. The pathology of these areas shows that the veins are cuffed with lymphocytes and other inflammatory cells associated with areas of focal leakage, suggesting damage to endothelial cells. Severe periphlebitis may result in vein occlusion or peripheral capillary closure. Disc oedema occurs in sarcoid due to direct infiltration of the optic nerve head by granulomata or in association with severe posterior uveitis (Fig. 9.7). Lesions may occur in the pigment epithelium which may evolve from yellow fluffy lesions to areas of pigment epithelial atrophy. Sub-pigment epithelial granulomata may also occur. Neovascularization is unusual in sarcoid though new disc vessels may develop either spontaneously or secondary to a major vein occlusion.

9.6.2 Clinical features

Sarcoidosis usually presents in the 20–40 year age group. The major clinical features associated with ocular involvement which occurs in about 25% of patients with sarcoidosis are:

Intrathoracic involvement	75%
Reticulo-endothelial:	
lymphadenopathy	27%
splenomegaly	12%
Skin plaques	36%
Erythema nodosum	26%
Hypercalcaemia	26%
CNS (central nervous system) involvement	15%
Facial palsy	12%
Parotid	10%
Bone	8%
Lacrimal	7%

The disease has two main patterns, the acute or chronic forms. The chronic pattern occurs commonly in West Indian subjects and is characterized by chronic uveitis, lupus pernio and pulmonary fibrosis. White Caucasians commonly have the acute form which presents with hilar lymphadenopathy, arthritis, erythema nodosum and acute uveitis. Posterior segment involvement occurs in 25% of patients with ocular sarcoid. The condition therefore, may present to a multitude of specialists according to appropriate symptoms and signs.

9.6.3 Investigation of suspected ocular sarcoid

A diagnosis of sarcoidosis can be suspected from general medical examination and ophthalmic features. The major tests that will aid and confirm the diagnosis are:

1. chest x-ray
2. Kveim test
3. tuberculin skin test
4. serum calcium
5. serum ACE level
6. biopsy of affected tissues, e.g.
   lymph node
   bronchus (alveolar lavage)
   liver
   salivary gland
   conjunctiva
   gingiva

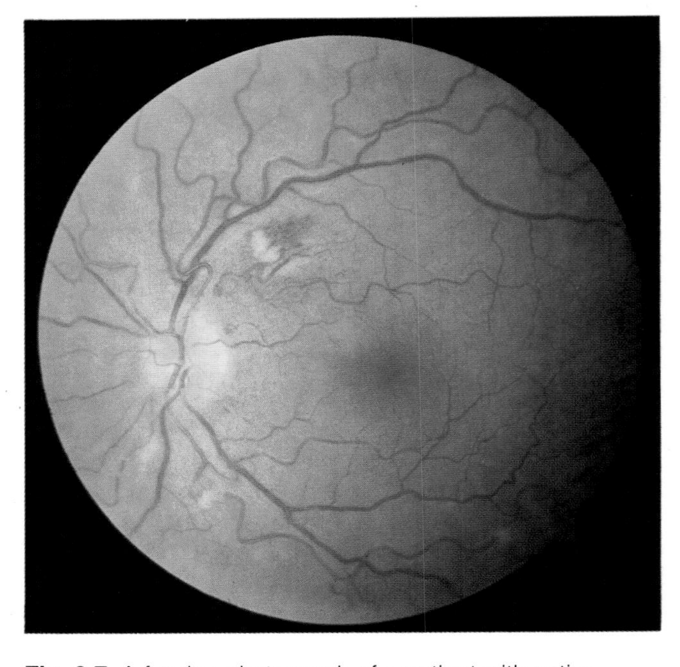

Fig. 9.7 A fundus photograph of a patient with active sarcoidosis showing cotton wool spots, haemorrhage and phlebitis.

Chest x-ray in white Caucasians is likely to be abnormal in at least 75% of patients with ocular presentation. The Kveim test is positive in 75% of patients with active sarcoid but there are problems with a false negative rate of 3% as well as recent debate about HIV contamination of the Kveim material. The Mantoux test is often negative suggesting depression of the hypersensitivity reaction. Hypercalcaemia and hypercalciuria are well recognized features of sarcoid. Fifty per cent of patients with sarcoidosis are likely to have one of these features, although hypercalciuria is more frequent than hypercalcaemia.

Serum angiotensin converting enzyme (SACE) levels are elevated in 60% of patients with active sarcoidosis and may be used as a marker of disease activity but this investigation gives a false positive result in 10% of patients without sarcoidosis.

A major diagnostic tool is biopsy. Biopsy of lymph nodes may be rewarding as may transbronchial biopsy and alveolar lavage. There is a 50% positive yield from transbronchial biopsy and if multiple biopsies are taken the yield may be much higher. Biopsy of other tissues, for example liver, salivary glands, conjunctiva and gingiva may be helpful. Abnormalities may also be noticed in measurement of prolineuria and hyperuricaemia.

9.6.4 Immunology

In sarcoidosis there is a depression in cell mediated immunity suggested by reduction in the number of circulating T-cells. There are impaired responses of these cells to polyclonal mitogens and antigens. There is also heightened B-cell activity with elevation of serum immunoglobulins and the presence of autoantibodies and circulating immune complexes.

Abnormal immunoglobulin levels are shown in approximately 80% of patients with sarcoidosis. IgG may be increased in 50% of patients, whereas an increase in IgA or IgM is less common. The increase in IgG levels is particularly associated with West Indian subjects. In acute sarcoidosis there is activation of the complement system due to circulating immune complexes. When they are detectable the sedimentation rate is generally high.

9.6.5 Clinical features of neurological and ocular sarcoid

(A) NEUROSARCOIDOSIS

Neurological involvement occurs in approximately 7% of patients presenting with sarcoidosis. It is strongly associated with ocular disease in 60% of patients. These patients present between 20 and 50 years of age and the manifestations include peripheral neuropathy, meningitis, space-occupying brain lesions, myopathy, epilepsy, cerebellar ataxia, hypopituitarism and diabetes insipidus. Neurosarcoidosis carries a mortality of 10%, and is more likely to occur in younger patients with a very acute onset.

(B) OCULAR INVOLVEMENT

The most common ocular lesions are anterior uveitis, posterior uveitis, conjunctival lesions and scleral plaques.

Posterior involvement comprises choroidal nodules, papilloedema, haemorrhages and retinal perivasculitis. Choroidal nodules are usually scattered, discrete, off-white, waxy exudates which may be associated with retinal venous constriction and periphlebitis. The retinal veins may appear sheathed (Fig. 9.7).

The acute retinopathy of sarcoid is unusual but consists of swelling of the optic disc, haemorrhage, vascular occlusion, and extensive perivascular cuffing. This may be associated with acute neurological changes, bilateral hilar lymph adenopathy and erythema nodosum.

Papilloedema occurs, particularly in females, in association with facial palsy. Diagnosis of neurological sarcoid should be sought particularly if there is evidence of cranial nerve palsies or unusual sensory symptoms.

The pattern of disease with sarcoidosis has been dramatically changed with the advent of corticosteroid therapy. The disease tends to be self-limiting although there are unusual patients who relapse several years after diagnosis and require further treatment.

9.6.6 Management

The mainstay of treatment for sarcoidosis is corticosteroids. Topical corticosteroids should be administered for iridocyclitis but oral corticosteroids are indicated if local treatment does not lead to a rapid response. The presence of posterior uveitis indicates treatment with oral steroids. Other agents which may be useful include oxyphenbutazone, chloroquine or methotrexate.

9.7 IDIOPATHIC RETINAL VASCULITIS

The aetiology of this form of retinal vasculitis is still obscure. Pathological evidence suggests that it has an immunological background and may be a response to an antigen although its precise nature is unknown.

As previously discussed, retinal-S antigen may be important. The absence of a systemic inflammatory disease is found in 50% of patients with retinal vasculitis; hence the term idiopathic retinal vasculitis. It typically affects patients in the third and fourth decade. The pathology and the aetiology of this condition have been discussed earlier.

9.7.1 Clinical features

The retinovascular changes occurring in idiopathic retinal vasculitis range from mild perivascular sheathing of small peripheral veins to frank vascular occlusion and secondary neovascularization. In 83% of patients there is evidence of diffuse capillary leakage and in 25% there is evidence of capillary closure and neovascularization. In contrast to Behçet's disease, there is no evidence of damage to the branch veins and in contrast to sarcoidosis, no evidence of peripheral periphlebitis.

9.7.2 Diagnosis

Evidence of systemic inflammatory disease should be sought by performing investigations such as a chest X-ray, ESR, C-reative protein, autoimmune profile and immunoglobulins. The absence of a systemic inflammatory disease on full examination and investigation, in the presence of retinal vasculitis, will allow the diagnosis of the idiopathic form. However, non-specific changes may be seen in immunological parameters. In particular IgA levels may be elevated in conjunction with the finding of elevation of circulating immune complexes and retinal antibodies.

9.7.3 Treatment of idiopathic retinal vasculitis

The majority of cases are asymptomatic and have good visual acuity despite the presence of active vitritis and peripheral vascular sheathing. The major cause of visual loss in this condition is macular oedema or vitreous haemorrhage. The inflammation is treated with systemic steroids which may be needed in large doses. In refractory cases, azathioprine may be helpful particularly as it has an excellent steroid-sparing effect. Photocoagulation may be necessary in patients with disc new vessels which do not resolve.

9.8 SYSTEMIC LUPUS ERYTHEMATOSUS

Systemic lupus erythematosus is a well established autoimmune disease in which ocular involvement is uncommon. In particular, uveitis is a rare association. By contrast, retinal vasculitis (arteritis) is an established finding and may occur in 5–10% of the cases.

The retinal features are due primarily to arterial occlusion and the characteristic finding is cotton wool spots (cytoid bodies) (Fig. 9.8).

Pathological studies suggest that arterioles are completely occluded by thrombi and in some cases the vessel lumen is reduced through expansion of the vessel wall due to inflammatory tissue. Choroidal changes may occur due to active vasculitis in the choroidal vessels. In addition to cotton wool spots, large retinal infarcts, optic disc infarction and embolic occlusion from cardiac vegetations may occur. A particular feature of the retinopathy of systemic lupus erythematosus is that the veins are not involved, in contrast to sarcoidosis and Behçet's disease. Rarer features may include papillitis sometimes proceeding to optic atrophy and occasional Sjögren's syndrome giving rise to dry eyes.

9.8.1 Other clinical features of SLE

SLE is principally a disease of women of child-bearing years, with a female to male ratio of 9:1. The

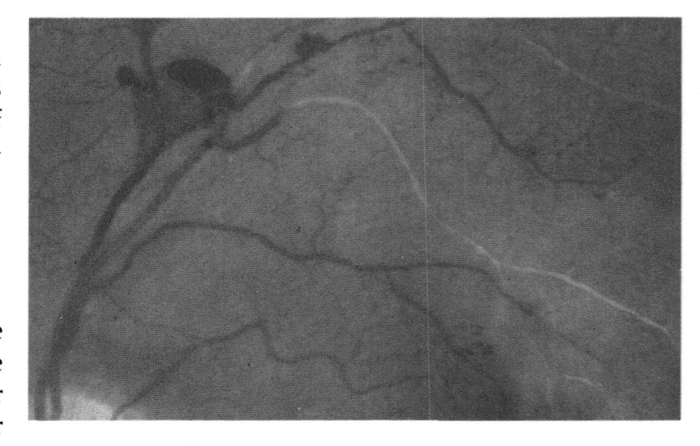

Fig. 9.8 A typical fundus photograph of systemic lupus erythematosus, demonstrating arteriolar occlusion with multiple cytoid bodies.

disease is more common in Negro populations. The presenting features of systemic lupus erythematosus in clinical practice are:

Common features:

- constitutional – fever, fatigue, weight loss;
- musculo-skeletal symptoms;
- rashes – butterfly, discoid, photosensitivity, cutaneous vasculitis;
- peripheral synovitis.

Less common features:

- pyrexia of unknown origin;
- pericarditis;
- pleurisy;
- renal disease;
- neuropsychiatric manifestations;
- thrombocytopenic purpura.

Musculo-articular manifestations are present in 95% of patients whereas renal involvement is present in 53% and cardiac disease with endocarditis present in 38%. Examination may reveal neurological syndromes including epilepsy, motor neurone lesions or abnormal movements as well as a peripheral neuropathy. The spleen may be palpable.

The diagnosis of systemic lupus depends on recognizing the characteristic pattern of clinical laboratory abnormalities, which has been defined by the American Rheumatism Association. They have suggested that four or more criteria are required for the diagnosis of systemic lupus:

- malar rash
- discoid rash
- photosensitivity
- oral ulceration
- non-erosive arthritis
- pleurisy or pericarditis
- persistent proteinuria (>0.5 g/day)
- seizures or psychosis
- haemolytic anaemia/leukopenia/lymphopenia/thrombocytopenia
- Positive LE cells/anti-DNA/anti-Sm/false +ve VDRL
- ANA +ve

The immunoflourescent test for anti-nuclear antibody is a valuable screening test and has therefore replaced the LE cell test in most laboratories. ANA is frequently found in other connective tissue disease, and in approximately 5% of the normal population. Antibodies to Anti-Sm are present in 10%, anti-Ro in 40%, and anti-La in 10% of patients with systemic lupus.

Laboratory diagnosis of systemic lupus erythematosus involves:

- erythrocyte sedimentation rate (C-reactive protein often normal)
- normochromic normocytic anaemia
- leukopenia, lymphopenia, thrombocytopenia
- LE cells
- hypergammaglobulinaemia
- anti-nuclear antibodies 95%
  to: DNA 70%
  nucleoprotein 70%
  soluble ribonucleoproteins 70%
  (nRNP, Sm, Ro, La)
- rheumatoid factor positive (40%)
- positive Coombs' test
- false positive VDRL
- serum complement levels (low C3 and C4)
- (renal biopsy)

9.8.2 Treatment

Management is based around general measures during active disease with avoidance of sun exposure and symptomatic measures. Many patients do not require systemic steroids. Non-steroidal anti-inflammatory agents may be used although systemic steroids are usually used in the presence of retinal vasculitis. Other agents which may be useful include the anti-malarial group, and immunosuppressive agents such as azathioprine. Drugs known to precipitate a lupus syndrome should be avoided. A small proportion of patients may develop renal failure at any stage, requiring chronic dialysis. Renal transplantation is not contraindicated in systemic lupus.

The prognosis in systemic lupus has improved dramatically with a current 10-year survival rate of 90%.

9.9 RARER CAUSES OF RETINAL VASCULITIS: WEGENER'S GRANULOMATOSIS AND POLYARTERITIS NODOSA

It is likely that these two conditions represent different clinical spectrums of the same disease.

Polyarteritis nodosa (PAN) is an inflammatory condition of small and medium sized arteries leading primarily to aneurysm formation, thrombosis and infarction. Fortunately it is a rare condition. It is more common in males with a 4:1 male:female ratio. The aetiology is largely unknown but up to 30% of patients possess the hepatitis B antigen. Immunoglobulin deposits are found in blood vessels in patients with polyarteritis and recently IgM, IgG and complement have been demonstrated within the smaller and medium sized arterioles in conjunctiva and skin lesions. It is suggested that the immune complexes damage the vessel walls causing destruction and corrosion. Rupture, haemorrhage, thrombosis, or healing follows.

Wegener's granulomatosis is characterized by a necrotizing granulomatous vasculitis which involves multiple organ systems. Again its cause is unknown but it may be a consequence of hypersensitivity to an unidentified antigen.

Circulating immune complexes are present in a proportion of patients with this disorder and immune related compounds have been found on biopsy. However, it is not clear whether these immune complexes have a primary role in tissue damage. Histologically Wegener's disease involves primarily collagen and blood vessels. Vascular lesions include phlebitis, granulomatous vasculitis, and necrotizing vasculitis similar to polyarteritis nodosa.

The major clinical features are shown in Table 9.3. Renal involvement is a significant feature in both diseases as is joint involvement. However, lung involvement is present in 90% of patients with Wegener's granulomatosis but in only 30% of those with polyarteritis nodosa. Typically Wegener's also affects the sinuses and nose with rhinitis and nasal ulceration, which are not features of polyarteritis nodosa.

9.9.1 Ocular manifestations

Retinopathy is one of the more commonly associated complications of polyarteritis. The major features are of retinal ischaemia and oedema, cotton wool spots and irregular calibre of retinal vessels. Retinal vascular occlusion and retinal haemorrhages are frequently found. The former changes may relate to severe hypertension or changes secondary to a renal disease.

Wegener's granulomatosis may involve the posterior segment with retinitis and venous congestion, uveitis and optic neuropathy. Adenexal involvement may be manifested by orbital lesions, and nasal and lacrimal ducts may obstruct.

9.9.2 Diagnosis

Diagnosis of PAN is based on a combination of clinical features and the finding of a necrotizing arteritis on biopsy or arterial aneurysms on angiography. Biopsy of a clinically involved site, such as kidney, skin or nerve, can be helpful but blind biopsy may be performed in kidney, rectum, muscle, liver or testes. The diagnosis of Wegener's granulomatosis is based on the combination of characteristic clinical features and the typical findings on biopsy of necrotizing granulomata and vasculitis. In this situation nasal biopsy may be useful in the diagnosis but open lung biopsy may occasionally be necessary.

Table 9.3 Clinical features of polyarteritis nodosa (PAN) and Wegener's granulomatosis

	PAN	*Wegener's*
Renal involvement (haematuria, renal failure, nephrotic syndrome)	85%	80%
Joint involvement	65%	65%
Neuropathy (mononeuritis multiplex)	40%	32%
Skin involvement (nodules, digital gangrene)	50%	45%
Lung involvement (asthma/pneumonitis, haemoptysis)	30%	90%
Cardiovascular (hypertension, heart failure, ischaemic heart disease)	20%	20%
Intestinal infarction	45%	20%
Ophthalmic (vasculitis, proptosis)	15%	50%
Sinuses (sinusitis, rhinitis, nasal ulceration)		95%

9.9.3 Treatment

(A) PAN

Vigorous treatment to suppress the disease is required, as without treatment the eventual prognosis is poor. Steroids in the form of prednisolone are required and, in patients who respond to this treatment, aneurysm resolution may be seen.

Other recent reports have suggested that cytotoxic agents (e.g. cyclophosphamide) can be used in combination with corticosteroids. Plasma exchange has been reported as a useful adjunctive therapy. Corticosteroids have demonstrated an improvement of the five-year survival from 15 to 50%. Poor prognostic features include severe renal disease, older age group at onset or intestinal infarction.

(B) WEGENER'S GRANULOMATOSIS

Steroids have been used but have not been shown to improve overall mortality in this condition. Oral cyclophosphamide has now proved to be effective and is the treatment of choice in this disease. Steroids may, however, be required for skin vasculitis, retinal vasculitis or pericarditis.

(C) CHURG-STRAUSS SYNDROME

This is a syndrome in which patients have systemic vasculitis which differs from those with classical PAN in some features. These include a previous allergy history, particularly of asthma, blood eosinophilia and the presence of extravascular granulomata. It is rare and mainly affects middle-aged males.

The condition predominantly affects the respiratory tract. The respiratory symptoms are usually the earliest feature with a history of asthma associated with eosinophilia. Systemic and retinal vasculitis may occur. The pattern of organ involvement is predominantly in the chest with chest x-ray abnormalities of patchy infiltrates. Renal involvement is less prominent than in PAN. Treatment consists of corticosteroids. The prognosis is better than for PAN, with a five-year survival exceeding 70%.

9.10 OTHER RARE CONDITIONS

A few patients with disseminated sclerosis may have involvement of the posterior chamber of the eye, with a posterior uveitis and perivenous sheathing. Retinal vasculitis may be associated rarely with tuberculosis giving rise to a posterior uveitis with florid retinal periphlebitis with venous occlusion and haemorrhages. Syphilis is also a known but rare cause of arteritis.

Herpes zoster, herpes simplex and cytomegalovirus have all been implicated (Chapter 10). *Toxocara* and *Toxoplasma* may lead to a retinal vasculitis with secondary macular oedema. Goodpasture's syndrome, characterized by haemoptysis, anaemia and proteinuria, is associated with venous and arteriolar retinal occlusion, haemorrhages, exudates and serous retinal detachments. Whipple's disease consisting of arthralgia, polyseritis, diarrhoea and weight loss is associated with a posterior uveitis. This includes a retinal vasculitis and a tetracycline is the treatment of choice.

9.11 POLYMYALGIA RHEUMATICA AND GIANT CELL ARTERITIS

The two conditions of giant cell arteritis (GCA) and polymyalgia rheumatica (PMR) are considered as a spectrum of the same disease affecting a similar population and frequently occur together in the same individual.

Polymyalgia rheumatica is a clinical syndrome of the middle-aged and elderly patient causing pain and stiffness in the neck, shoulder and pelvic girdles. This may be accompanied by general systemic symptoms such as a fever, fatigue and weight loss. The eryhrocyte sedimenation rate is usually elevated and a dramatic response is observed with steroid therapy.

Giant cell arteritis is a term used to describe temporal arteritis, cranial arteritis or even granulomatous arteritis.

The mean age of onset of these conditions is approximately 70 years, with women affected twice as commonly as men. The onset of the disease can be dramatic as well as insidious. Systemic symptoms including fatigue, anorexia, weight loss or depression, are present in a large number of patients. In polymyalgia rheumatica symptoms are commonest in the shoulder region and neck which is symmetrically involved.

Stiffness is a predominant feature, particularly severe after rest and may prevent the patient getting out of bed in the morning. Movement accentuates the pain. Muscle strength is usually unimpaired. There is tenderness of involved structures with restriction of shoulder movement. An improvement of the range of movement of the shoulder is rapid with oral steroid therapy.

9.11.1 Pathology

Giant cell arteritis and polymyalgia rheumatica are due to a granulomatous arteritis focused on the media of the artery and associated with smooth muscle and internal elastic membrane destruction. The presence of giant cells is inconsistent and not necessary to make the diagnosis, particularly on temporal artery biopsy. Non-specific inflammatory changes may occur adjacent to areas of granulomatous inflammation. In severe disease, a panarteritis may occur, leading to inflammatory, thrombotic or fibrotic occlusion of the vessel lumen.

9.11.2 Giant cell arteritis and ophthalmic manifestations

There is a wide variety of symptoms but headache is the most common and is present in two-thirds of patients. It is an early feature and is the most common presenting symptom. The pain is usually severe, localized to the temporal region, but may be occipital or less well defined. It may be precipitated by brushing the hair or touching the scalp. Scalp tenderness is common particularly in the temporal and occipital arterial territory and may disturb sleep.

Visual disturbances may be present in 25–50% of cases although the incidence of visual loss is now less than 10%. This may be due to early recognition and active treatment. Blindness may be the initial presentation of giant cell arteritis but tends to follow other typical symptoms which have not been recognized and treated.

Other symptoms include pain on mastication due to claudication of the muscles for mastication, and this occurs in up to two-thirds of patients. Paraesthesia in the tongue, loss of taste and pain in the mouth and throat may also occur. A few patients may describe transient visual symptoms prior to the onset of visual loss. These range from typical amaurosis fugax to nonspecific visual symptoms. Amaurosis fugax in association with retro-orbital pain signifies a precarious vascular supply to the eye and requires urgent treatment. Diplopia is a relatively frequent symptom from patients with giant cell arteritis. Visual hallucinations have also been described.

9.11.3 Ophthalmological signs

Visual loss may occur in up to 50% of patients with giant cell arteritis. This is predominantly due to an ischaemic optic neuropathy due to occlusion of the posterior ciliary arteries which supply the optic nerve and choroid. Occlusion of the central retinal artery itself may account for 5% of patients with visual loss. Typically a dense inferior altitudinal field defect associated with a afferent papillary defect is present. On ophthalmoscopy the optic disc is pale and swollen with attenuated arterioles (Fig. 9.9). Infrequently haemorrhages may occur around the disc and subsequent to this cotton wool spots may appear.

Central retinal artery occlusion produces total blindness and complete loss of the visual field, with a classical fundus picture of attenuated arterioles, pale oedematous retina and a cherry red spot at the macula (Chapter 7).

9.11.4 Non-ophthalmological physical signs

Examination of the temporal arteries should be performed, feeling for enlargement, overlying erythema and tenderness. Tenderness on combing hair or scalp tenderness may be a prominent feature. The temporal pulses may still be present or be completely absent. The facial arteries should also be palpated to check for absence. This sign may be related to jaw claudication. Polymyalgia rheumatica on the other hand has few physical signs with the predominant features being symptoms.

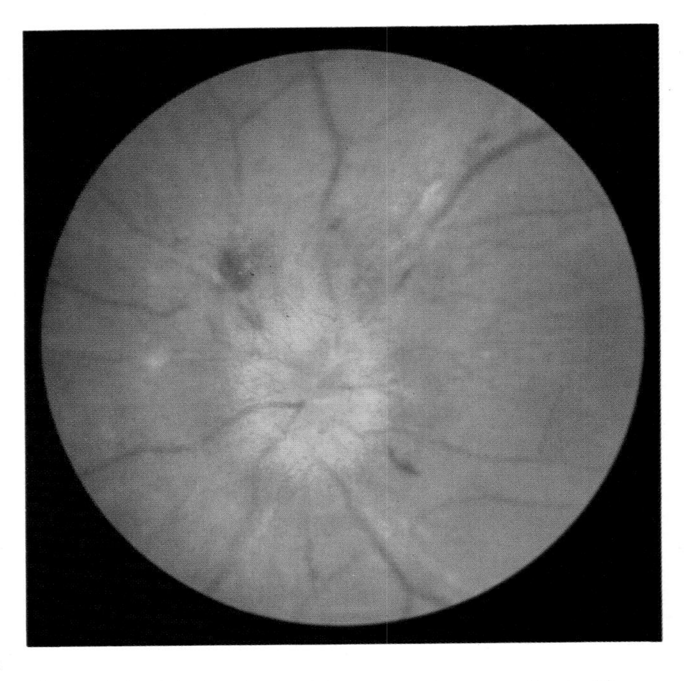

Fig. 9.9 Ophthalmological features of giant cell arteritis including a swollen optic disc and attenuated arterioles.

9.11.5 Diagnosis

The differential diagnosis of polymyalgia rheumatica and giant cell arteritis is wide:

1. neoplastic disease
2. joint disease
   - cervical spondylosis
   - rheumatoid arthritis
   - systemic collagen disease
3. multiple myeloma
   leukaemia
   lymphoma
4. muscle disease
   - polymyositis
   - myopathy
5. hypothyroidism

However, the diagnosis of giant cell arteritis should be considered in any patient over the age of 50 with recent onset of headache, particularly if associated with transient or sudden loss of vision. The arteries of the head, neck and limbs should be examined for tenderness, enlargement, thrombosis and bruits.

The erythrocyte sedimentation rate (ESR) is the primary laboratory measure which often exceeds a fall of 70 mm in the first hour. However, plasma viscosity is used in many centres and from published data appears to be of similar sensitivity. Cases may occur with a normal ESR and plasma viscosity. C-reactive protein is also a sensitive measure. There is frequently a normochromic normocytic anaemia and a non-specific increase in gammaglobulins.

TEMPORAL ARTERY BIOPSY

The role of temporal artery biopsy in the diagnosis of giant cell arteritis is debatable. It is clear that temporal artery biopsy is not necessary in patients with polymyalgia rheumatica as blindness is very rarely associated with this condition in isolation. However, with cranial arteritis it is recommended that temporal artery biopsies are performed. In our experience it is helpful particularly for follow-up as well as aiding in diagnosis. However, the biopsy may be falsely negative owing to the presence of arteritic skip lesions and also the inadequacy of the length of biopsy obtained. Another factor is the large number of slices required in a temporal artery biopsy to maximize the detection of diagnostic changes.

To perform a biopsy, the branch of the temporal artery anterior to the main trunk should be selected. A segment of 3–5 cm should be chosen particularly if it is inflamed or tender. Cross sections of the artery at 0.25 to 0.5 mm intervals should be stained. The biopsy may be taken within 24 hours of commencing prednisolone without change in its diagnostic potential.

9.11.6 Prognosis

With prompt steroid treatment, the prognosis for giant cell arteritis is excellent. Many reports have suggested more emphasis on symptoms other than ESR in monitoring patients during follow-up, as the presence or absence of symptoms give a better relationship to outcome.

In 50% of patients the disease becomes inactive with 18 months of steroid therapy but 50% of patients may become chronically steroid dependent in the long term.

The major cause of mortality in giant cell arteritis is vertebral ischaemia, which usually signifies the severe form of the disease. A worse prognosis is also evident in those patients who require a dose of prednisolone >10 mg per day to control symptoms in the longer term.

9.11.7 Management

Initial management of giant cell arteritis or polymyalgia rheumatica is with high dose steroids. Most physicians use between 40 and 60 mg a day whereas ophthalmologists may tend to use a dose as high as 120 mg. Intravenous hydrocortisone may be used if there is either threatening or profound visual loss. The dose of prednisolone is then slowly tailed over several months according to ESR and symptoms. Importance should be attached to symptomatic relief. However, some patients may remain asymptomatic but the ESR may rise. Interpretation of this may produce clinical difficulties.

There is no reliable method of predicting those patients most at risk of arteritic relapses after 18 months therapy. Relapse however is unusual after 18 months therapy in patients with polymyalgia rheumatica alone. Temporal artery biopsy does not help in prediction. The risks of continuing treatment with steroids are those of steroid related complications. Approximately 20% may experience serious side-effects unless a maintenance dose of prednisolone of 7.5 mg or less is achieved. Azathioprine can be used to exert a steroid sparing effect.

Once eighteen months to two years of therapy is completed, reduction of prednisolone dosage may be undertaken by 1 mg a month. An alternative is to reduce the dose on alternate days. The addition of a non-steroidal inflammatory agent may be helpful in reducing minor muscular symptoms that patients develop on steroid withdrawal. Monitoring for relapse should continue for at least six months after stopping steroids.

FURTHER READING

Allison, M.C. (1988) Temporal artery biopsy. *Br. Med. J.*, **297**, 933–4.

Barnes, C.G. (1991) Behçet's syndrome. *Topical Reviews* (Reports on Rheumatic Diseases Series 2), **18**, 1–6.

Brittain, G.P.H, McIlwaine, G.G., Bell, J.A. and Gibson, J.M. (1991) Plasma viscosity or erythrocyte sedimentation rate in the diagnosis of giant cell arteritis? *Br. J. Ophthalmol.*, **75**, 656–9.

Clearkin, L.G. and Watts, M.T. (1990) Ocular involvement in giant cell arteritis. *Br. J. Hosp. Med.*, **43**, 373–6.

Forrester, J.V. (1992) Sarcoidosis and inflammatory eye disease. *Br. J. Ophthalmol.*, **76**, 193–4.

Graham, E., Holland, A., Avery, A. and Ross-Russel, R.W. (1981) Prognosis in giant cell arteritis. *Br. Med. J.*, **282**, 269–71.

Graham, E.M., Sanders, M.D., James, D.G. *et al.* (1985) Cyclosporin A in the treatment of posterior uveitis. *Trans. Ophthalmol. Soc. UK*, **104**, 146–51.

Graham, E.M., Stanford, M.R., Sanders, M.D. *et al.* (1989) A point prevalence study of 150 patients with idiopathic retinal vasculitis 1. Diagnostic value of ophthalmological features. *Br. J. Ophthalmol.*, **73**, 714–21.

Isenberg, D.A. (1992) Mechanisms of auto-immunity. *Topical Reviews* (Reports on Rheumatic Disease Series), **22**, 1–7.

James, G. Treatment of sarcoidosis. *Prescribers J.*, **32**(1), 9–14.

Lanham, J.G. (1992) Churg-Strauss syndrome. *Br. J. Hosp. Med.*, **47**(9), 667–73.

Murray, P.I. and Rahi, A.H.S. (1985) New concepts in the control of ocular inflammation. *Trans. Ophthalmol. Soc. UK*, **104**, 152–7.

Saboor, S.A. and Johnson, N.M. (1992) Sarcoidosis. *Br. J. Hosp. Med.*, **48**(6), 293–302.

Sanders, M.D. (1987) Retinal arteritis, retinal vasculitis and auto-immune retinal vasculitis. *Eye*, **1**, 441–65.

Spalton, D.J., Graham, E.M., Page, N.G.R. and Sanders, M.D. (1981) Ocular changes in limited forms of Wegener's granulomatosis. *Br. J. Ophthalmol.*, **65**, 553–63.

Stanford, M. (1990) Systemic inflammatory disease and the eye. *Br. J. Hosp. Med.*, **44**, 100–5.

Yaziki, H., Pazarli, H., Barnes, C. *et al.* (1990) A controlled trial of azathioprine in Behçet's syndrome. *New Eng. J. Med.*, **322**, 281–5.

10 Infections and the retina

Clinical Retinopathies. Paul M. Dodson, Jonathan M. Gibson and Erna E. Kritzinger.
Published in 1995 by Chapman & Hall, London. ISBN 0 412 35930 8

10.1 INTRODUCTION

Although the retina can be the primary focus of inflammation, most infections involving the retina start within the posterior uveal tract or the vitreous. Most forms of inflammation therefore are not pure retinitis but are more correctly termed chorioretinitis, retinochoroiditis or endophthalmitis. This may be asymptomatic or be associated with decreased visual acuity as the only symptom. The inflammation of the choroid and retina may be purulent or granulomatous. The acute, purulent forms are usually forms of bacterial or fungal endophthalmitis.

The most common causes of acute purulent endophthalmitis are as follows:
Following surgery:

- *Staphylococcus epidermidis*
- *Staphylococcus aureus*
- *Pseudomonas aeruginosa*
- *Propionibacterium acnes*
- various fungi.

Associated with penetrating trauma:

- *Bacillus cereus* and other *Bacillus* species

Haematogenous spread:

- *Streptococcus pneumoniae*
- *Staphylococcus aureus*
- *Neisseria meningitidis*
- *Candida* species
- *Aspergillus* species.

More commonly, however, chorioretinitis of infectious origin is granulomatous and characterized by focal collections of macrophages, lymphocytes and plasma cells forming nodules in the choroid. There is a number of infectious causes of this syndrome the frequency of which depends upon age, geography and the patient's immunological defence mechanisms.

Certain forms of infectious uveitis are now being seen with increasing frequency as a result of the extensive use of immunosuppressive drugs and the appearance and spread of the worldwide epidemic of acquired immunodeficiency syndrome (AIDS).

The diagnosis of infectious uveitis may be difficult as it is rare for the infection to be disseminated and hence the aetiological organism itself is rarely detected except after enucleation of the eye or at autopsy. Even culture of aspirated vitreous or aqueous humour is rarely helpful except in cases of fungal or bacterial endophthalmitis. Diagnosis is usually made on the basis of skin and blood tests although these tests generally only indicate previous systemic exposure to a particular pathogen. Evidence of local production of specific antibody by the plasma cells within the uveal tract is much more helpful and may be obtained by demonstrating such antibodies in the aqueous humour. If such antibodies are present in a concentration that cannot be explained by increased permeability of the blood aqueous barrier then their presence can be of considerable diagnostic value.

10.2 *TOXOCARA*

10.2.1 Aetiology and pathology

The common roundworms of dogs and cats, *Toxocara canis* and *T. cati* respectively, have a worldwide distribution and are a frequent parasitic cause of endophthalmitis in humans. The adult *Toxocara* live in the gut of dogs and cats and eggs are excreted into the soil. After a few weeks the eggs become infective and may be eaten by another dog (or cat). The larvae hatch and usually migrate via the lungs, trachea, and posterior pharynx to the bowel where they mature into adults. Other larvae migrate to the muscles and remain dormant but alive. If the eggs are eaten by other animals (including humans), the second stage larvae cannot complete their life cycle in the gut but do migrate into various tissues. The process of migration in humans is called visceral larva migrans (VLM). The life cycle of *T. canis* is, however, unique. In the pregnant bitch, hormonal changes stimulate the development of the dormant larvae in the muscles which then migrate transplacentally to the fetal puppies, where they then mature to adults within the bowel. Prenatal infection of cats with *T. catis* does not occur; cats become infected by ingesting larvae in the tissues of mice and other 'accidental' hosts.

In humans infective eggs of *Toxocara canis* are usually ingested in soil by young children with a history of pica. The prevalence of infection is variable and depends upon socioeconomic factors and contact with contaminated soil in gardens, parks and rural areas. In one study in the United States more than half of a rural community had serological evidence of asymptomatic toxocaral infection (Jones *et al.*, 1980). The larvae penetrate the bowel wall and migrate through the liver and the systemic circulation to the tissues, where they reach a capillary too small to pass. They penetrate the vessel, enter the tissue and either die or become dormant; they are surrounded by an eosinophilic granulomatous response which may later calcify.

10.2.2 Clinical features

Most cases of VLM occur in preschool children and are asymptomatic. In some, probably depending upon the number of larvae ingested, there may be any number of a variety of symptoms (cough, wheeze, fever, abdominal pain, nausea, anorexia, headache, behaviour disturbances, etc). Other more specific features depend upon the organs involved in the granulomatous process. Hepatomegaly and pulmonary infiltrates are frequent and a peripheral blood eosinophilia is characteristic and often marked.

(a) OCULAR LESIONS

Ocular manifestions of *Toxocara* infection are:

Common:

- posterior pole granuloma
- peripheral granuloma in quiet eye

Rare:

- diffuse chronic endophthalmitis
- vitreous abscess
- papillitis
- vitreous haemorrhage
- iridocyclitis

Studies undertaken in the 1960s showed toxocariasis to be responsible for about 10% of cases of uveitis in children and that about 2% of 1000 eyes enucleated from children under 15 years of age had evidence of toxocaral endophthalmitis. It tends to occur in slightly older children (their average age is about 8 years) than those who suffer from VLM and may be due to relatively light infections with less immunological response. Hence, eye involvement in toxocariasis often unfortunately occurs in the absence of any other visceral features and without an eosinophilia (Schantz *et al.*, 1979).

The child rarely notices any visual problem, but loss of vision and disuse may produce a noticeable squint. At other times it is only detected after routine acuity testing has prompted ophthalmological examination.

The usual presentation is with a 'cold' single, large, white granulomatous lesion at the posterior pole of the eye (Fig. 10.1) perhaps with a cloudy vitreous and/or posterior synechiae. The differential diagnosis is often retinoblastoma. Sometimes a crescentic darker area can be seen in the centre of the mass; this is the parasite.

In other cases of toxocariasis the inflammatory process is much more active at presentation and the lesions are in the peripheral pars plana region. They appear as smaller, peripheral dense yellowish-white lesions, sometimes with membranes or cells in the vitreous. Traction bands can be a serious problem. In long-standing infections there is a white area of retinal scarring.

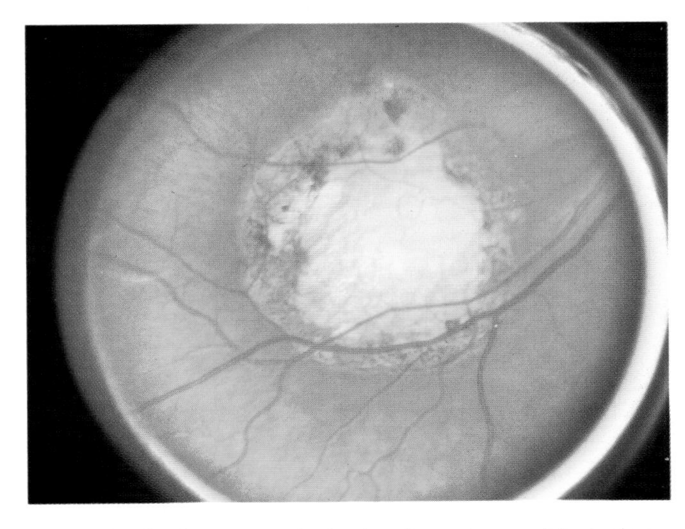

Fig. 10.1 Ocular toxocariasis showing a large white lesion (choroidoretinitis) at the posterior pole of the eye. Courtesy of Dr P.M. Dodson.

10.2.3 Management

(a) DIAGNOSIS

The definitive diagnosis of VLM can be attempted by direct visualization of larvae in tissue (usually most conveniently, liver) biopsy specimens but this is only rarely successful; some other cases may show granulomatous reactions containing large numbers of eosinophils which supports but does not prove the diagnosis of VLM. A blood eosinophilia is a useful pointer if present but in many ocular cases this feature is absent. The diagnosis of toxocariasis is, therefore, usually dependent upon serology using an enzyme-linked immunosorbent assay (ELISA). This test has a sensitivity and specificity greater than 90% in non-ocular VLM but patients with ocular larva migrans sometimes have negative or low titres. In order to confirm the diagnosis of ocular *Toxocara* infection it may be necessary to examine the aqueous humour and reveal eosinophils and elevated toxocaral ELISA titres. This test is widely used in Europe but is rarely undertaken in the UK.

(b) THERAPY

There is no evidence of any benefit of therapy for ocular toxocariasis. The drugs that are used for the treatment of VLM are diethylcarbamazine (DEC) and thiabendazole and although these may improve symptoms, there are no controlled studies. Furthermore, therapy is often accompanied by an increase in the inflammatory reaction (as judged by eosinophilia). There is, therefore, a risk that DEC or thiabendazole therapy for ocular toxocariasis may be hazardous by provoking more inflammation. For inactive disease, therefore, therapy is usually not advised and the child should be regularly reviewed in case a retinal detachment should occur. For more active disease there are often misgivings about the use of antihelminthic drugs but if oral DEC (3 mg/kg 8 hourly for 21 days) or thiabendazole (50 mg/kg daily for 5 days) is used for ocular infection then it probably should be given together with an anti-inflammatory drug (usually a corticosteroid) to reduce the intraocular inflammation that accompanies death of the *Toxocara* larva.

(c) PREVENTION

The risks of infection could be minimized by regular worming of infected pets, avoiding the handling by children of puppies that have not been dewormed, and reducing the pollution by dog and cat excreta of environments frequented by young children.

10.3 TOXOPLASMOSIS

10.3.1 Epidemiology and aetiology

Toxoplasmosis is probably the most common infectious disease involving the retina. *Toxoplasma gondii* is a sporozoan parasite with a two-host life cycle. In members of the cat family there is a sexual cycle in the epithelium of the intestine. Gametocytes are produced followed by the production of oocysts which are excreted in the cat's faeces. The oocysts then sporulate in the soil over a period of several days and are eaten by any one of a large number of species of birds or mammals (including humans). In the intermediate host there is an acute infection associated with the replication of tachyzoite forms of the organism, but after a few days and the development of immunity, these organisms encyst within the tissues (particularly muscles and brain) and chronic infection ensues. By preying upon the intermediate hosts, cats ingest the tissue cysts and the life cycle is completed.

Human infection can result from oocyst contamination of soil or water or from the ingestion of undercooked meat containing tissue cysts. Transplacental transmission can also occur in 30–40% of women when primary infection is contracted during pregnancy. Transplacental infection is prevented by the development of immunity although rare instances of transmission to the foetus have been recorded in immunosuppressed women.

The prevalence of toxoplasmosis can be assessed by serological surveys and varies widely in different geographic localities depending upon the density of cats and the eating of undercooked or raw meat products. The incidence of infection is also age dependent: it is acquired in childhood in many parts of the Tropics and in late teens and early adult life in other parts of the world. In Europe the French have a very high incidence among young adults, probably due to their custom of eating undercooked lamb.

10.3.2 Pathology

In humans the ingested parasites leave the gut and disseminate haematogenously, probably within macrophages, to various organs. The tachyzoites multiply within any nucleated cell, and within a few days cause cellular necrosis; in acute infections almost any tissue can show patchy inflammation. With developing immunity tissue cysts are formed, particularly in the muscles, brain and retina. The tissue cysts remain viable during chronic infection.

Occasionally such tissue cysts can rupture – what ensues depends upon the immunity of the individual. In the normal individual there is a local hypersensitivity reaction leading to tissue necrosis and chronic inflammation and death of the released trophozoites. This reaction is self-limiting but is important in the retina where even a small area of inflammation can cause serious visual disturbance. In the immunosuppressed individual the trophozoites released from ruptured tissue cysts multiply and produce progressive focal lesions, usually in the brain, retina or lung.

10.3.3 Clinical features

(a) CLINICAL SYMPTOMS

On average about 10% of congenitally infected infants have neonatal signs of a generalized infection with hepatosplenomegaly, fever, central nervous system involvement, lymphadenopathy, chorioretinitis, etc. Most of these children are mentally retarded. Infected neonates who appear normal at birth, however, develop reactivation of disease: 75–90% develop chorioretinitis in later childhood or early adult life and many of these children will have severe impairment of vision.

Acquired acute toxoplasmosis, whether contracted from oocysts or tissue cysts, usually produces symptoms, with 90% of persons having fever, 85% headache and firm, non-tender lymphadenopathy, 60% myalgia, and some rash or arthralgia. Chorioretinitis is an uncommon finding during acute infection.

In the immunocompromised patient, particularly those with AIDS or other defects in cellular immunity, toxoplasmosis can be more severe. Primary infections can result from naturally acquired infection or following transmission of organisms in transplanted organs or transfused blood. These infections are generalized and are similar to, but more severe than, those described above. Most cases in the immunocompromised host, however, are relapses of chronic infection. Approximately 25% of toxoplasma antibody-positive persons with AIDS will develop reactivation of *T. gondii*. This is usually intracerebral producing single or multifocal space-occupying lesions. Chorioretinitis can occur as a manifestation of either form of toxoplasmosis in the immunocompromised patient. Ocular toxoplasmosis is associated with cerebral involvement in about one-third of infected AIDS patients.

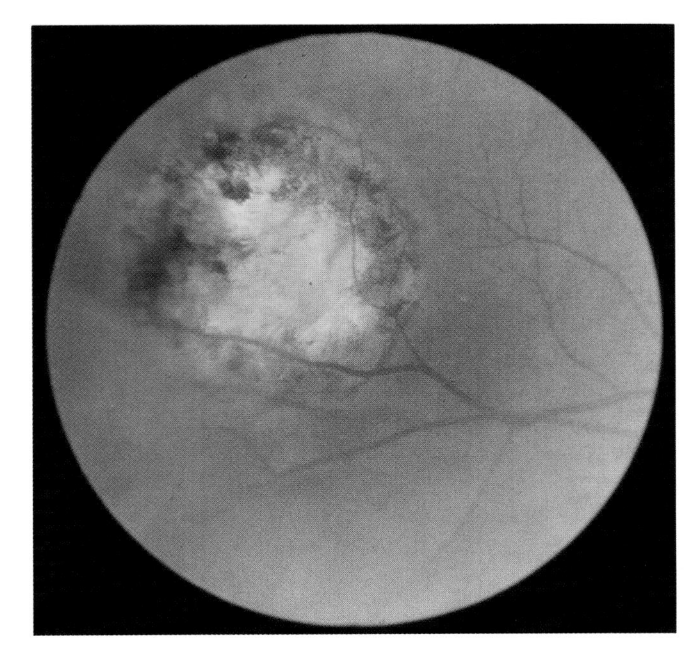

Fig. 10.2 Well defined scar surrounded by pigment in ocular toxoplasmosis, presumed to be due to reactivation of congenital infection. Courtesy of Professor G.J. Johnson, Institute of Ophthalmology, London.

Most symptomatic cases of ocular toxoplasmosis in Europe (Perkins, 1973) occur in the second or third decade of life and are thought to result from reactivation of congenital disease. The evidence for this is largely epidemiological: less than 2% of persons with *Toxoplasma* lymphadenopathy have ocular disease and, furthermore, although the prevalence of acquired toxoplasmosis rises with age, ocular disease is rare after the age of 40. In other geographical areas, notably southern Brazil, ocular toxoplasmosis seems to be a sequela of postnatal rather than congenital infection (Glasner *et al.*, 1992). The ocular symptoms of toxoplasmosis are marked blurring of vision due to the vitreous inflammatory exudate, scotoma and central visual loss when the lesion involves the macula. There is rarely any pain.

The usual appearances of ocular toxoplasmosis are those of a focal destructive chorioretinitis which leaves well-defined heavily pigmented scars surrounded by normal appearing retina (Fig. 10.2). In active disease, as is usually found in the congenitally infected neonate or the early stages of acquired toxoplasmosis, the lesions are yellow-white, about the size of the disc with indistinct borders and there is an intense overlying vitreous haze. In neonates the foci tend to be bilateral and in the macular region, although any part of the fundus may be involved. In children or adults the disease is typically unilateral. As the activity of the disease diminishes, the lesions become atrophic and develop black pigment, and the vitreous haze disappears. Lesions may appear to be quiescent but have a tendency to become reactivated, producing a new fluffy white retinal lesion at the edge of an area of previous scarring. The possible complications of ocular toxoplasmosis are:

- retinal vasculitis
- vitreous haemorrhage
- retinal oedema
- optic neuritis
- retinal detachment
- glaucoma
- cataract

In ocular toxoplasmosis occurring as part of acquired acute toxoplasmal infection, the inflammation does not usually involve the choroid or pigment-producing cells so there is no pigmentation and little vitreous haze. In patients with AIDS, too, the lesions of ocular toxoplasmosis are invariably not associated with a pre-existing retinochoroidal scar (Fig. 10.3), suggesting the lesions are a manifestation of acquired rather than congenital disease.

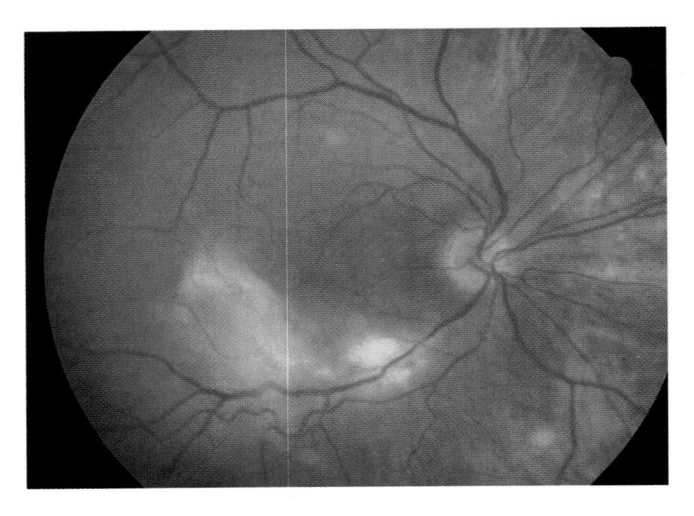

Fig. 10.3 Retinal toxoplasmosis in a patient with AIDS. Note the lack of a pre-existing retinochoroidal scar and pigment. By courtesy of Dr J.J. Gonzalez-Guijarro, Hospital de la Princesa, Madrid, Spain.

10.3.4 Management

(a) DIAGNOSIS

Although *T. gondii* can be demonstrated histologically in biopsy or autopsy specimens this is not a feasible way of diagnosing ocular disease. For most cases reliance has to be upon serological techniques.

IgG and IgM antibodies to *T. gondii* can be detected and distinguished by immunofluorescent antibody tests, ELISA tests or by immunosorbent assays. The Sabin and Feldman dye test is the accepted reference assay: it requires live organisms and is predominantly a test for specific IgG antibodies. In acute toxoplasmosis the initial antibody reaction is IgM. IgG antibodies appear within 1–2 weeks of acute infection, rise to a peak after 2–3 months and then remain in declining titres for many years.

For acute systemic toxoplasmosis a fourfold or greater rise in IgG titre (usually to levels above 1:1000), or the presence of specific IgM, is diagnostic. This is useful in those rare instances where chorioretinitis accompanies acute infection. In the neonate a very high IgG titre or positive dye test may support the diagnosis of congenital infection but in order to rule out the possibility of transplacental transfer of antibodies from the mother IgM antibody needs to be detected.

Most patients with toxoplasmal chorioretinitis, however, do not show rising or high antibody levels since the disease is reactivation of chronic infection. In such patients a completely negative IgG antibody test makes toxoplasmosis very unlikely but if the dye test is positive at any titre then the diagnosis is possible and, in the presence of typical ophthalmological appearances, likely. High antibody levels in the aqueous humour can be taken to indicate local production and active disease but, in the UK at least, this investigation is rarely performed.

In recrudescent infection in the immunocompromised patient, particularly those with AIDS, the antibody titres are extremely variable and it is often not possible to detect a fourfold rise in IgG levels or the appearance of any specific IgM. In those patients with encephalopathy a positive diagnosis can often be made by biopsy although evidence for local production of toxoplasmal antibodies within the CSF may also be sought.

(b) TREATMENT

Few ophthalmologists treat all cases of active ocular toxoplasmosis, the decision depending upon the presence of decreased visual acuity, vitreous inflammation, whether the disease is acquired or reactivation of congenital infection and whether the patient is immunocompromised (Dutton, 1989; Engstrom *et al.*, 1991). The best therapy for ocular toxoplasmosis is controversial. The drug combination usually recommended is oral sulphadiazine (500 mg 6-hourly) and pyrimethamine (50 mg 12-hourly for 3 days and then 25–50 mg/day). The respective doses for children are 25–35 mg/kg 6 hourly and 1 mg/kg/day, reducing to 0.5 mg/kg/day after 3 days. (Much higher doses of sulphadiazine may be needed to treat *Toxoplasma* encephalitis in AIDS patients.) The controlled clinical trials have, however, given conflicting results regarding the efficacy of this regimen and a number of other regimens are used (Rothova *et al.*, 1989). Clindamycin, 300 mg 6-hourly, is also effective against *Toxoplasma*. It can also be used, alone or together with pyrimethamine, in patients who are allergic to sulphonamides. Therapy should be given for a total of 4–6 weeks. With such therapy an improvement can be seen within 10 days in 70% of cases and healing takes a mean of 9–10 weeks (Fig. 10.4). Pyrimethamine has effects upon human folic acid metabolism and hence may cause bone marrow depression. To overcome this, folinic acid (NOT folic acid) needs to be given in a dose of 3–10 mg daily (1 mg/day for children); this decreases the toxicity of pyrimethamine without impairing the anti-toxoplasmal activity. Checks upon platelet and white blood cell counts need to be performed at least weekly. If the platelet count falls below 100 000/mm^3, or the white

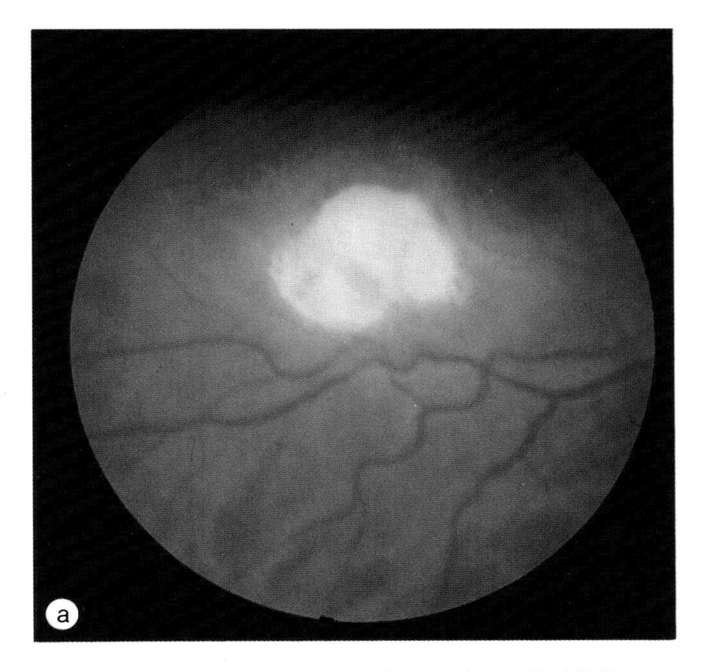

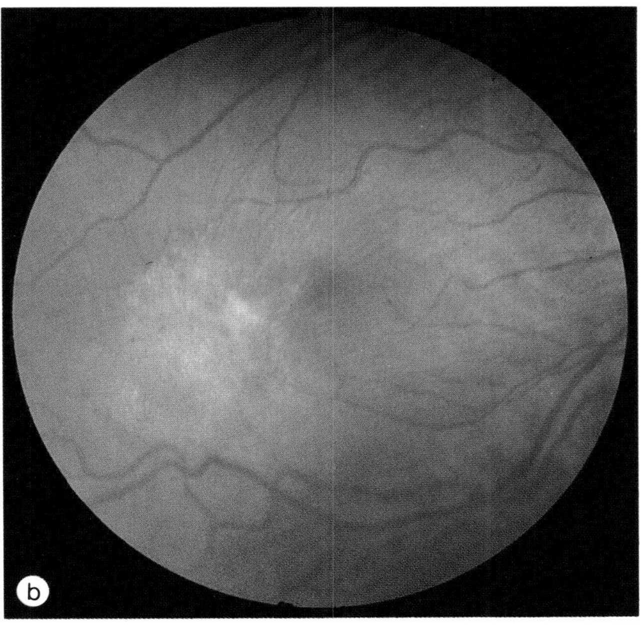

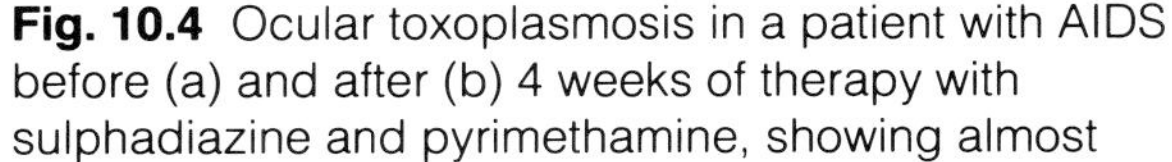

Fig. 10.4 Ocular toxoplasmosis in a patient with AIDS before (a) and after (b) 4 weeks of therapy with sulphadiazine and pyrimethamine, showing almost complete healing of the lesion. By courtesy of Professor P. Pivetti-Pezzi, University of Rome, 'La Sapienza', Italy.

blood cell count falls below 4000/mm^3, then pyrimethamine therapy should be discontinued (and clindamycin substituted). Pyrimethamine may also cause vomiting, headache and a nasty taste in the mouth.

Corticosteroids are also recommended when ocular toxoplasmosis threatening the macula or optic nerve head is treated with chemotherapy. This reduces the inflammatory hypersensitivity reaction that occurs when the *Toxoplasma* are killed. Prednisolone 60 mg/day is given for 5 days (or until signs of vitreous inflammation have disappeared) and then tailed off over a period of 2 weeks. Steroids are probably best avoided in the treatment of toxoplasmosis in AIDS patients since their use has been associated with the development of cytomegalovirus (CMV) retinitis.

The treatment of ocular toxoplasmosis in the pregnant woman is potentially hazardous because of the teratogenicity of conventional chemotherapy. Treatment is primarily given to protect the vision of the mother and most would use sulphonamides, clindamycin or spiramycin, without pyrimethamine. Spiramycin is a macrolide with minimal toxicity but is only available for compassionate use in the UK.

The efficiency of cotrimoxazole (sulphamethoxazole and trimethoprim) in toxoplasmosis is uncertain but it has been used when sulphadiazine is not available and it may have fewer side-effects. Sulphamethoxazole is, however, less active than other sulphonamides against *T. gondii in vitro*. Other drugs that show promise in animal models of toxoplasmosis and which are being studied in immunocompromised individuals with toxoplasmal encephalitis are the new macrolide antibiotics azithromycin and clarithromycin.

Patients with AIDS are likely to remain profoundly immunosuppressed for the rest of their lives and since the present chemotherapeutic regimens do not kill tissue cysts, there is a strong likelihood (about 80% in the case of toxoplasmal encephalitis) of recrudescence of toxoplasmosis even after apparently successful therapy of the disease. Such patients therefore require permanent prophylaxis against toxoplasmosis after the acute therapy is finished. Such prophylaxis is probably best given with 2 g of sulphonamide and 25–50 mg pyrimethamine daily for three days each week or with Fansidar (sulphadoxine and pyrimethamine) two tablets once weekly. During maintenance treatment the 24-month relapse rate of ocular toxoplasmosis in AIDS patients is about 20%, possibly with higher failure rates in patients given clindamycin.

10.4 ONCHOCERCIASIS

10.4.1 Aetiology and pathology

Onchocerciasis or 'river blindness' is a filarial infection caused by the nematode *Onchocerca volvulus*. It is widespread in much of tropical West and Central Africa, where 30 million or so people are infected, and is also found in parts of Arabia and Central and South America. The life cycle is simple, involving only man. The microfilarial larvae are transmitted by the bite of an infected blackfly of the *Simulium* genus (in Africa, *S. damnosum*). The larvae enter the wound when the fly bites and develop over a year or two in the subcutaneous tissues into mature worms. The males are about 3 cm and the females 40 cm long and they often lie coiled up in fibrous nodules that may be felt over bony prominences. Female worms live for 15 to 20 years, producing several thousand larvae (microfilariae) each day. These microfilariae, which are about 300 μm long, migrate into the skin, eyes and lymphatic tissues and may be taken up by biting blackflies (and hence complete the life cycle by being transmitted to infect new hosts). The flies breed in streams and rivers and when onchocerciasis is prevalent 90% or more of the population may be infected and much of the prime farming land in the neighbourhood is rendered uninhabitable.

The adult worms cause no problems other than the unsightly, non-tender, 3–5 cm diameter, nodules which can usually be felt in the subcutaneous tissues. Live microfilariae also do not cause any significant problems but if they are not taken up by vector blackflies then, after about one year, the microfilariae die and induce a serious inflammatory reaction. The dead microfilaria is surrounded by eosinophils and a granulomatous reaction and ultimately phagocytosed. In the skin there is inflammation in the upper dermis and, after chronic infection, the dermis becomes thickened and leathery with loss of pigmentation; this is probably due to the destruction of elastic tissue by toxins and is often most pronounced on the shins – the main target for blackfly bites. A chronic regional lymphadenitis ensues.

The involvement of the immune system in killing the microfilariae varies from individual to individual but in general those with active skin disease are killing more microfilariae.

It is the inflammatory response to the death of the microfilariae in the eye that produces the most serious effects. The role of the immune system in the ocular lesions is still unclear but corneal and fundal damage both occur. The pathogenesis of the chorioretinal changes is probably directly related to the number of microfilariae in the retina: it may be caused either by occlusion of the small blood vessels or by soluble toxins released by dying microfilariae.

10.4.2 Clinical features

The clinical features of onchocerciasis vary depending upon the intensity and duration of infection and the immune response (Gibson *et al.*, 1988). Heavy infections are limited to those brought up in hyperendemic areas and are rarely seen in Europe or North America. Infected expatriates tend to have limited cutaneous disease and minimal ocular signs. The patient has an itchy papular rash with slight thickening over the affected parts, typically one leg. In heavy infections the skin becomes intensely itchy, particularly over the lower body, associated with a papular rash and altered skin pigmentation. In chronic infections the skin becomes thin, wrinkled and aged in appearance. Nodules can be found in almost any area of the body and many patients have lymphadenitis and a characteristic 'hanging groin' appearance.

In the eye, the earliest sign is the appearance of live microfilariae seen by slit-lamp examination. In the cornea dead microfilariae may be surrounded by an opaque inflammatory infiltrate to produce a punctate keratitis with 'snowflake' opacities. Progressive sclerosing keratitis may develop until the cornea is opaque. Anterior uveitis is variable in severity but can produce secondary glaucoma, cataracts and blindness. The most frequent choroidal change is atrophy of the retinal pigment epithelium associated with intraretinal pigment clumping and hypertrophy. Subretinal fibrosis appears as well-defined white patches with overlying pigment (Fig. 10.5). Fundal changes are usually bilateral and symmetrical. Optic atrophy and optic neuritis are also common complications of onchocerciasis.

Blindness is the most serious complication of onchocerciasis. The blindness may result from either anterior segment disease (sclerosing keratitis or complications of anterior uveitis) or retinal pigment epithelium atrophy and optic neuropathy (Fig. 10.6).

10.4.3 Management

(a) DIAGNOSIS

Blood eosinophilia is found in onchocerciasis but, as yet, there are no useful serological tests to establish the diagnosis. Diagnosis is, therefore, established by microscopic examination of excised nodules in which tangles of adult filariae are seen or, more simply, by examination of 'skin snips'. These are obtained by slicing off a tiny bloodless portion of skin which has been elevated by piercing the skin with a fine needle to no greater depth than is necessary for the skin just to be tented by raising the needle tip. The ophthalmic scleral-corneal punch is an ideal alternative instrument for obtaining skin snips. Snips are placed on a microscopic slide in a drop of saline and examined under low power after an hour or two. If the skin is infected microfilariae will be seen wriggling in the saline.

The ophthalmologist can diagnose onchocerciasis by visualizing microfilariae in the anterior chamber with a slit-lamp and using an intense oblique beam. (A useful trick to increase the number of microfilariae in the anterior chamber is to ask the patient to sit with his head between his knees for two minutes prior to the examination.)

(b) TREATMENT

Treatment of onchocerciasis is indicated for those with sight-threatening disease. It is beneficial in punctate keratitis but is less useful for sclerosing keratitis or chorioretinal disease. Until recently, onchocerciasis was treated with a course of diethylcarbamazine (DEC) and suramin. This therapy was associated with severe, occasionally fatal, host reactions that included worsening of the eye disease. Ivermectin is now the drug of choice for the treatment of onchocerciasis (Gibson *et al.*, 1988). This is a newer microfilaricidal drug which has the advantage of not provoking the severe reactions seen with DEC. Side effects requiring aspirin do occur in those who are heavily infected but these reactions are not life threatening. After therapy the microfilariae disappear from the eye within 6–10 weeks and the progression of ocular and skin disease is halted. The microfilarial counts remain low for up to one year as ivermectin also suppresses microfilarial production by the adult females. Neither ivermectin nor DEC kills the adult worms and the surgical removal of those adults that can be discovered may limit the source of fresh microfilariae. The dose of ivermectin is 150 μg/kg which may be repeated every 6–12 months.

The other drug which may be used is suramin which needs to be given intravenously and which has marked toxicity. It does, however, have the advantage of killing both microfilariae and adult worms and a radical cure of onchocerciasis may be achieved.

The World Health Organization (WHO) has

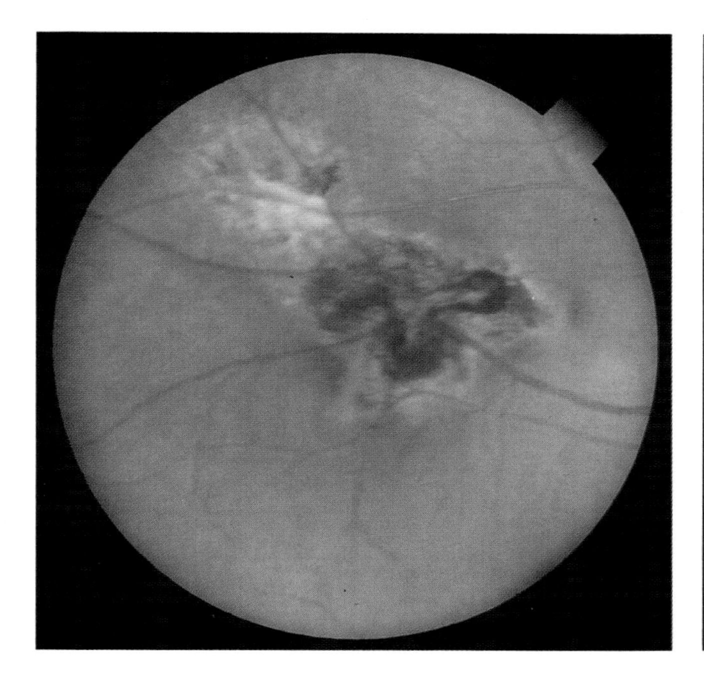

Fig. 10.5 An area of subretinal fibrosis with overlying pigment in a patient with onchocerciasis. Courtesy of Dr Henry Newland, Flinders Medical Centre, Australia.

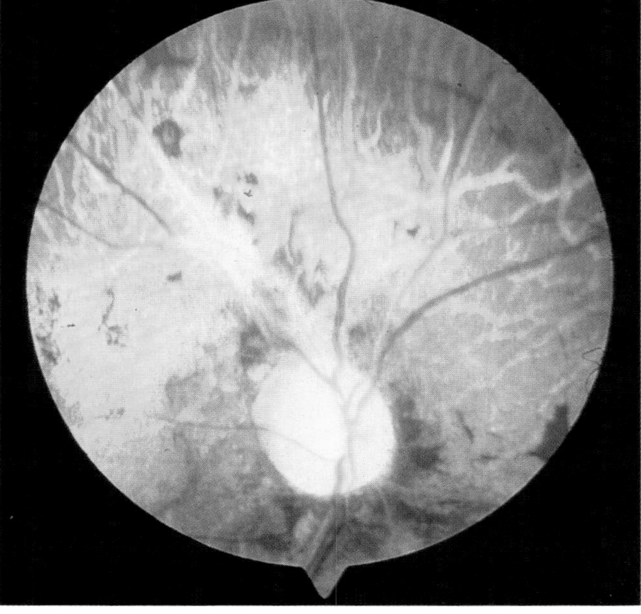

Fig. 10.6 Onchocerciasis, showing areas of pigment hypertrophy and pigment epithelium atrophy and optic atrophy. Courtesy of Professor Dr J.S. Stilma, Academisch Ziekenhuis, Utrecht, Holland.

attempted vector control with insecticides in the rivers in which blackflies breed but this has not been as successful as was once hoped (Gibson *et al.*, 1988).

10.5 CYTOMEGALOVIRUS

10.5.1 Epidemiology

Cytomegalovirus (CMV) is a typical herpes virus in that primary infection is followed by persistence of the virus in the body, in a latent form, for the remainder of life. Naturally occurring reactivation of the virus takes place particularly in young women during the later stages of pregnancy and virus is then excreted into urine, saliva, cervical secretions and breast milk. Congenital or perinatal infection of the baby can occur and there is rapid acquisition of CMV infection during the first 2 years of life. In countries where populations live in crowded and unhygienic conditions, 90–100% of infants have had primary infection by 5 years of age but in North America and Western Europe up to 50% of the population, dependent upon socio-economic factors, escape CMV infection during childhood and adolescence.

Virus is also spread by sexual contact in both heterosexual and homosexual populations. The prevalence of latent CMV infection in homosexual men is very high, particularly in those who engage in anal-receptive intercourse, and excretion of CMV in the semen occurs much more frequently among homosexuals than in heterosexual men. Studies in North America, for instance, have shown CMV in the semen in up to a third of homosexual men compared to 1% of heterosexual men of similar age. The reason for this difference in excretion between homosexual and heterosexual men is unclear. Almost 100% of homosexual men with HIV infection have serological evidence of active CMV replication and more than 50% are shedding CMV in their semen.

Acute infection with cytomegalovirus (CMV) beyond the neonatal period is asymptomatic in about 90% of cases and in the rest causes an infectious mononucleosis-like syndrome. Although the primary infection is asymptomatic, the virus remains latently present, however, and if cell-mediated immunity is impaired then CMV may reactivate to produce a variety of clinical syndromes, including retinitis. This may be seen in patients being treated for haematological malignancies but retinitis is particularly likely to occur in renal transplant recipients and patients with AIDS. CMV retinitis occurs in up to 10% of patients with AIDS (and is the index diagnosis in about 1–2%). Retinal CMV infections in otherwise healthy adults are very rare.

Spread of CMV to the retina is probably haematogenous via the retinal vasculature. It may be particularly common in patients with AIDS because the retinal vessels have been damaged by the HIV

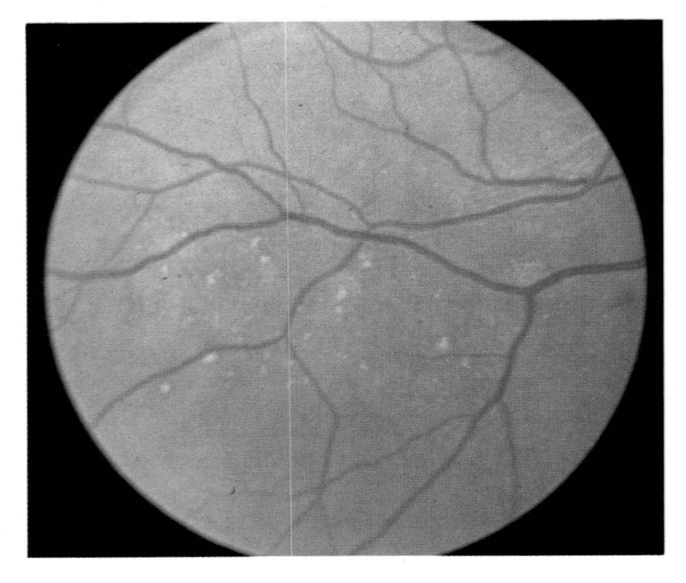

Fig. 10.7 Early granular lesions of cytomegalovirus retinitis in a patient with AIDS. Reproduced from Farrar *et al.* (1992) by courtesy of Gower Medical Publishing.

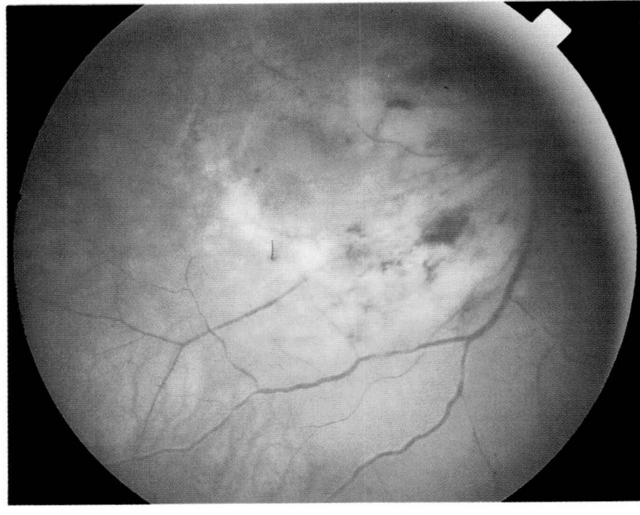

Fig. 10.8 CMV retinitis in a patient with AIDS, showing areas of retinal exudates, haemorrhage and sheathing of vessels.

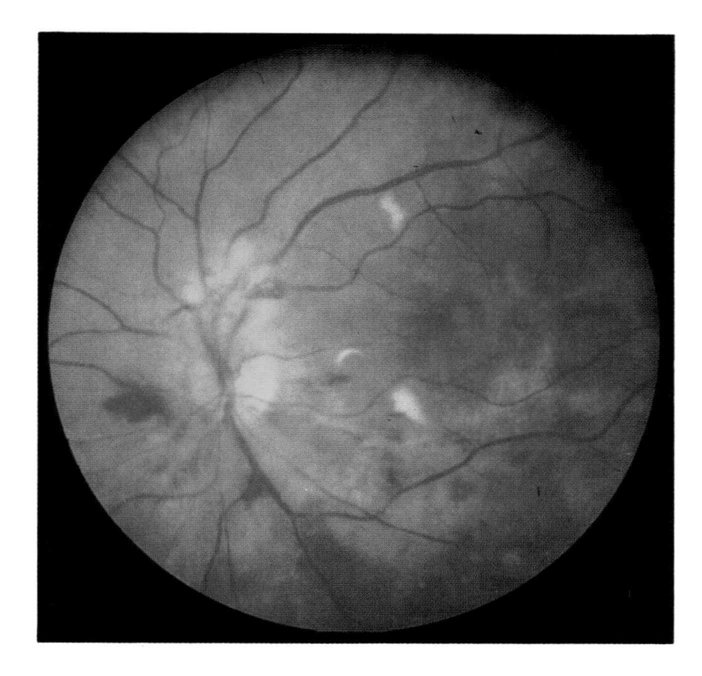

Fig. 10.9 Severe CMV retinitis with widespread retinal necrosis and haemorrhages. Note also the presence of several small white 'cotton wool spots' of HIV retinopathy. Courtesy of Dr J.J. Gonzalez-Guijarro, Hospital de la Princesa, Madrid, Spain.

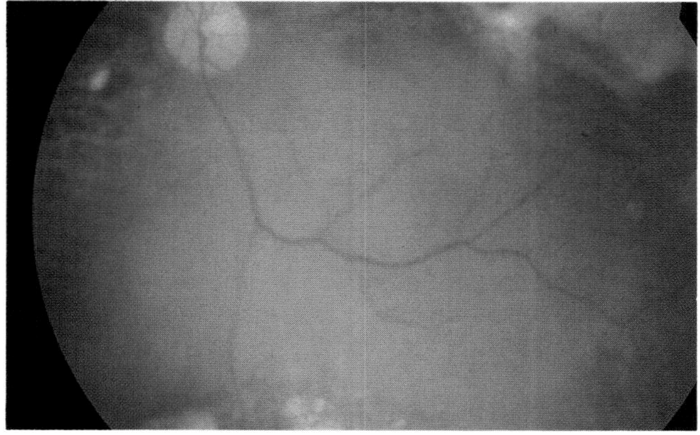

Fig. 10.10 Retinal detachment complicating cytomegalovirus retinitis in a patient with AIDS. Courtesy of Dr J.J. Gonzalez-Guijarro, Hospital de la Princesa, Madrid, Spain.

retinopathy that is commonly seen in AIDS patients (see below). The retinal cells are swollen with intracellular inclusions and *in situ* hybridization confirms that they are infected with CMV. The end result of infection is full thickness retinal necrosis.

10.5.2 Clinical features

CMV retinitis presents either insidiously or acutely with visual field loss, blurred vision or decreased visual acuity, often initially unilateral but later becoming bilateral, severe and progressive (Palestine, 1988). There is no pain.

The fundal changes initially comprise small white granular lesions on the retina of one or both eyes (Fig. 10.7). As the infection progresses the lesions enlarge and coalesce to form fluffy white exudates with associated retinal oedema, scattered haemorrhages and attenuation and sheathing of vessels (Fig. 10.8). Often lesions are initially peripheral, later involving the fovea. In severe forms the haemorrhages and retinal necrosis produce in the fundus the so-called 'pizza pie' or 'tomato sauce and salad dressing' appearance (Fig. 10.9). Histopathology reveals full thickness coagulation necrosis with mononuclear cell infiltration. Pathological studies, however, have failed to provide any evidence of CMV infecting the retinal endothelial cells.

The natural history of untreated CMV retinitis in non-AIDS patients is for the lesions to expand while the immunosuppression persists and the entire retina becomes involved within about 6 months. In patients with CMV retinitis complicating organ transplants a reduction in immunosuppressive drugs leads to healing of the infection, leaving an atrophic scar. Most patients with CMV retinitis and AIDS have received medical therapy but in a small group given no specific therapy, none survived more than 6 weeks after the retinitis was diagnosed. The atrophy and scarring that occurs with CMV retinitis may lead to rhegmatogenous retinal detachment (Fig. 10.10) and this leads to sudden total loss of sight in the affected eye. This may occur even after the active retinitis appears to be healing.

10.5.3 Management

(a) DIAGNOSIS

The diagnosis of CMV retinitis is essentially a clinical one as it is often impracticable to obtain tissue or fluid from the eye for CMV culture or DNA probing.

CMV can be cultured from the blood or urine in almost all the patients with CMV retinitis but CMV viraemia may be detected in 50% of patients with AIDS with or without clinical CMV infection.

(b) OPHTHALMOLOGICAL MANAGEMENT

Differentiating early CMV retinitis from the cotton-wool spots of HIV retinopathy (see below) may be difficult and in questionable cases it is important to re-examine the fundus every other day in order to detect progression of lesions or other features that would suggest the need for therapy for presumed CMV disease.

Once therapy for CMV retinitis has been commenced serial ophthalmological photographs are a means by which disease progression can be accurately assessed.

(c) MEDICAL MANAGEMENT

Untreated CMV retinitis is usually progressive and sight threatening. It must, therefore, be treated urgently. Two drugs have been used with some success; ganciclovir, an acyclic thymidine analogue that inhibits CMV replication, and foscarnet (phosphonoformate), a DNA and RNA polymerase inhibitor.

Ganciclovir is given intravenously in a dose of 7.5–15 mg/kg/day in divided doses. Retinal lesions stabilize and CMV can no longer be cultured from blood or urine in about 80% of those treated with a 21-day course of ganciclovir. Visual acuity stabilizes but rarely improves dramatically from pretreatment levels. Initial therapy must be followed by maintenance therapy to delay relapses during the remainder of the period of immunosuppression (lifelong in the case of AIDS patients). In the study of Holland *et al.* (1987) continuation of ganciclovir for longer than 3 weeks did not prevent, but merely delayed, relapses: if therapy was stopped after an initial response reactivation of disease occurred within 8 weeks (median 3 weeks) while in those continued on ganciclovir the time to relapse ranged from 3 to 17 weeks. This relapse is not associated with the development of resistance to ganciclovir. The dose of ganciclovir for maintenance therapy is usually 5–6 mg/kg/day given as a single iv infusion 5–7 days per week. The median survival of patients with ganciclovir-treated retinitis in the era of zidovudine therapy and prophylaxis for *Pneumocystis* infection has recently been estimated as 9 months with about 40% still alive at year one.

The major toxicity of ganciclovir is bone marrow suppression causing neutropenia and thrombocytopenia. Neutropenia eventually develops in more than 50% of individuals receiving ganciclovir and this seriously limits its use in patients receiving zidovudine (which is also myelosuppressive). Indeed it is often necessary to stop zidovudine altogether during the induction phase of treatment of CMV disease in AIDS patients.

Intravitreal ganciclovir has been tried but its efficacy and safety are compromised by retinal detachment.

When foscarnet was initially introduced, therapy was given as a continuous infusion over 24 hours of 200 mg/kg/day. It has now been shown to be equally as effective, however, given either as a 1-hour infusion in a dose of 60 mg/kg every 8 hours or as 2-hour infusions of 100 mg/kg twice daily. With these regimens a clinical response can be expected in more than 90% of patients, although there appears to be a dissociation between the clinical and virological efficacy of foscarnet since 20–40% of patients continue to shed CMV in the blood or urine. Two comparative studies of ganciclovir and foscarnet as initial therapy for AIDS-associated CMV retinitis have both shown that the two drugs were equally effective therapies for CMV retinitis. One study (Studies of Ocular Complications of AIDS Research Group, 1992) suggested, however, that patients given foscarnet survived for significantly longer than did those given ganciclovir and this has led to authorities in the USA recommending that foscarnet may be the better drug for the initial treatment of CMV retinitis in AIDS patients. One explanation for this perceived advantage is that foscarnet has some effects against HIV itself. Another may be related to the lack of myelotoxicity of foscarnet and hence the ability to continue other (haematotoxic) drugs commonly used in AIDS such as zidovudine or cotrimoxazole in most foscarnet-treated patients. The major side-effect of foscarnet is nephrotoxicity, including acute tubular necrosis, but the risk of this can be minimized by keeping the patient well hydrated with infusions of 2 l of isotonic saline daily. Even so up to 50% of persons develop a rising serum creatinine concentration. Foscarnet inhibits renal tubular phosphate reabsorption and there are often changes in the serum calcium concentration, which may fall (to produce tetany) or rise. Penile ulcers have also been seen relatively frequently, particularly in the uncircumcised.

Maintenance therapy with foscarnet is probably best given as infusions (preferably via a central venous catheter and with concomitant hydration with isotonic saline) of 120 mg/kg daily throughout the entire week.

10.6 PRESUMED OCULAR HISTOPLASMOSIS SYNDROME

Infection with the yeast form of *Histoplasma capsulatum* is the most common fungal infection of humans in the USA. The organism lives in the soil that is polluted by the excrement of birds or bats. It is endemic in the Mississippi river valley of the central USA and is also found in scattered foci of many other parts of the tropical and temperate zones of the world.

Inhalation of the spores of the fungus causes an illness termed acute pulmonary histoplasmosis during which the organisms multiply within macrophages prior to the development of hypersensitivity. Most organisms are then killed, tissue necrosis and caseation occur, and there is fibrosis and calcification of foci in the lungs and lymph nodes. Ocular disease does not occur.

In some instances, particularly in those with defects in cellular immunity, persisting *Histoplasma* in macrophages multiply and cause a disseminated infection. The infected macrophages can be found in almost any tissue of the body. The symptoms and signs depend upon the degree to which the macrophages of the reticuloendothelial system are infected and the extent of the immunosuppression. During this form of infection ocular granulomata containing *H. capsulatum* have occasionally been recorded but the eye problems are usually a minor part of the spectrum of clinical manifestations and the diagnosis is usually made from culture of blood or biopsies from liver or other obviously involved tissues.

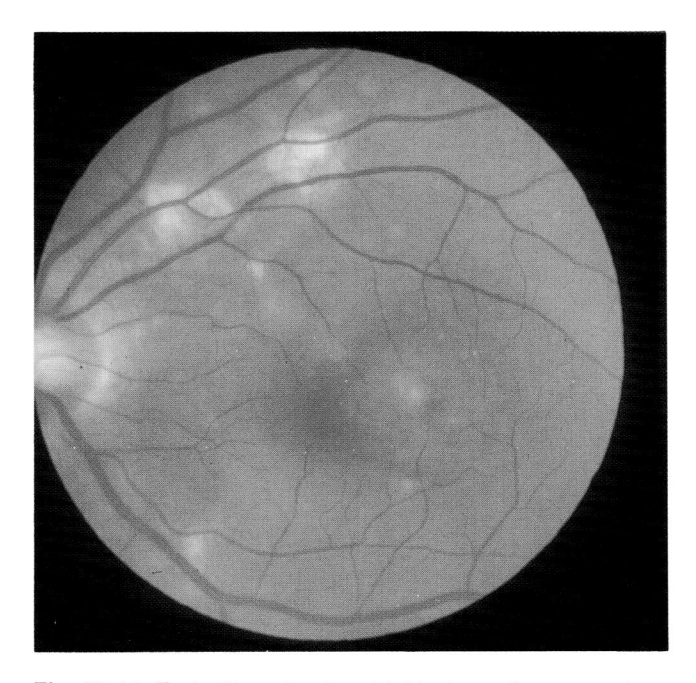

Fig. 10.11 Early discrete choroidal lesions of presumed ocular histoplasmosis syndrome. Reproduced from Farrar *et al.* (1992) by courtesy of Gower Medical Publishing.

The 'presumed ocular histoplasmosis syndrome' (POHS) has never been proved to be caused by *Histoplasma*. It is characterized by the presence of small multiple yellow punched-out spots visible in the fundus (Fig. 10.11) and histologically situated in the choroid, peripapillary atrophy and a haemorrhagic maculopathy. The vitreous is free of inflammation. If the maculopathy is present then visual acuity is affected, but in a significant minority of persons there is later some spontaneous improvement.

Only rarely has *H. capsulatum* been identified in the ocular lesions of a patient with no signs of active histoplasmosis elsewhere. The name of the syndrome is based upon an association between the clinical features and a positive skin test to histoplasmal antigens. The correlation is, however, not absolute and the typical ocular appearances can occur in those with negative skin tests and no history of travel to an area where histoplasmosis is endemic – the 'pseudo-presumed ocular histoplasmosis syndrome'!

The debate about the aetiology of POHS continues. If it is caused (even only occasionally) by *Histoplasma*, however, then it is likely to be a late manifestation of previous acute histoplasmosis and there is no evidence that there is any active fungal infection still present. Hence, there is no place for anti-histoplasmal drugs. Corticosteroids and laser photocoagulation have both been advocated for the prevention of visual loss but it is far from clear whether any therapy is effective (or needed).

10.7 UVEAL TUBERCULOSIS

Although *Mycobacterium tuberculosis* can cause disease in almost any organ in the body, it is extremely rare for tuberculosis to affect the retina. When it does affect the posterior segment of the eye it is usually as part of uveal tract disease consequent upon haematogenous dissemination to the eye. The pathological features of tuberculosis depend upon the degree of hypersensitivity and the amount of bacterial antigen present. If the antigen load is low then, once tissue hypersensitivity develops, granulomatous lesions are formed with containment of the infection. If there is a large antigen load, then the response is exudative with marked tissue necrosis due to enzymes produced from macrophages. Haematogenous dissemination of mycobacteria to the eye can occur very early in the course of tuberculous infection. This preallergic dissemination is usually occult, but, particularly in the young, once hypersensitivity develops, acute miliary tuberculosis can supervene. Haematogenous spread can also occur later in life, usually when ageing or other factors (particularly, in recent years, human immunodeficiency virus (HIV) infection) compromise cellular immunity and hypersensitivity.

10.7.1 Clinical features

In young children miliary tuberculosis is an acute illness with fevers, night sweats and weakness. The chest x-ray usually shows a typical miliary pattern of shadowing, the tuberculin skin test is positive and, in two-thirds of cases, there are symptoms or signs of meningitis. A similar condition may occur in adults, particularly those with underlying illnesses, but in many elderly patients the tuberculin test is negative and the patient may present with a fever of unknown origin. The ocular signs of miliary tuberculosis are the presence of choroidal tubercles (Fig. 10.12). These are small yellow-white nodules with indistinct borders and between one-sixth and one-half of the diameter of the optic disc. Other forms of tuberculous uveitis that occur are: an exudative tuberculous retinitis, which usually presents as a solitary posterior pole tuberculoma – a yellowish raised lesion larger than the choroidal tubercles and often with serous elevation of the surrounding retina (Fig. 10.13); massive acute destructive endophthalmitis; and tuberculous chorioretinitis with perivasculitis (Fig. 10.14).

10.7.2 Treatment

Studies have clearly shown that successful treatment of tuberculosis can be undertaken with six-month regimens based upon an initial two-month four-drug phase and four more months with rifampicin and isoniazid. The standard regimen is a combination of isoniazid (300 mg) plus rifampicin (600 mg) given once daily and combined with pyrazinamide (25–35 mg/kg/day) and ethambutol (15 mg/kg/day) for the first two months. Treatment should be supervised by a physician with experience of tuberculosis therapy.

10.8 SYPHILIS

Treponema pallidum, the causative agent of syphilis, is a slim spirochaete, 5–15 μm long. It is an exclusively human pathogen and infection is acquired either from direct sexual contact or via transplacental

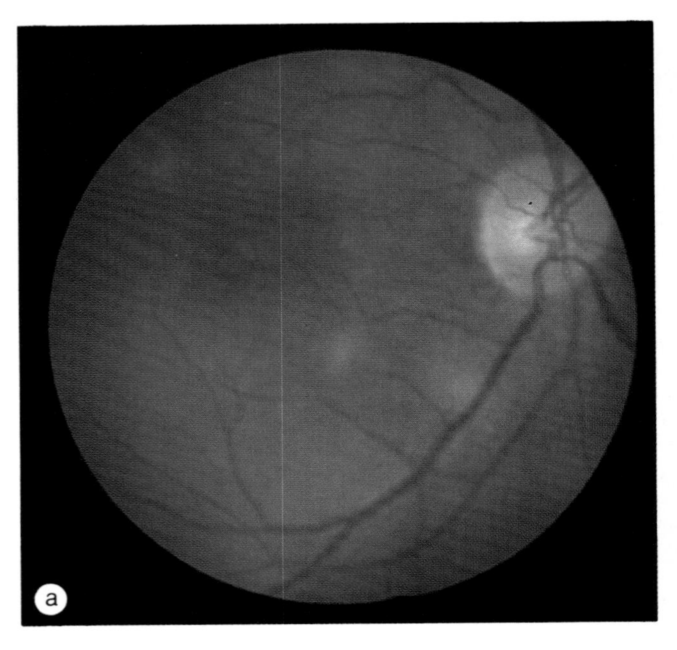

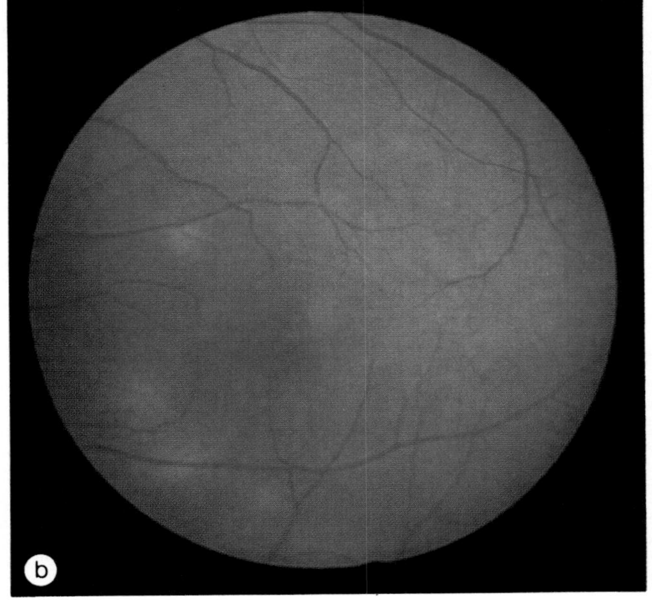

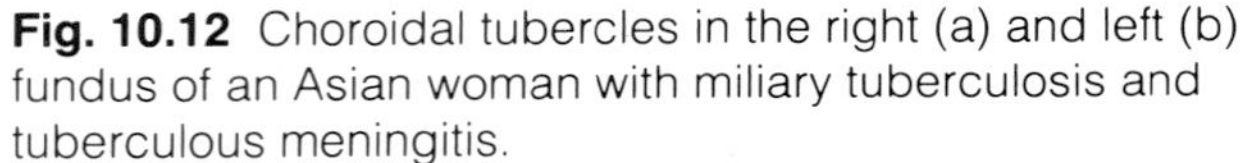
Fig. 10.12 Choroidal tubercles in the right (a) and left (b) fundus of an Asian woman with miliary tuberculosis and tuberculous meningitis.

spread to the foetus. The disease, having been a major public health problem in the first half of the 20th century, declined markedly in the Western world between 1955 and 1985 but the incidence has increased rapidly again, probably related to increased sexual activity linked to illegal drug use. The spirochaete multiplies locally in the subepithelial tissues and spreads rapidly to local lymph nodes and thence via the bloodstream.

10.8.1 Clinical features

The primary lesion is an indurated painless chancre at the site of initial inoculation; it usually heals within a few weeks. There is then an asymptomatic period of several weeks before the secondary stage develops. This is a disseminated illness with fever, lymphadenopathy, patchy alopecia, a skin rash and erosions of the mucous membranes, and warty condylomata lata in moist areas of skin. Virtually any organ in the body, including the eye (see below), can be involved during this phase. After the secondary stage the disease may become latent, with positive treponemal antibody tests but no further clinical manifestations. In a proportion of patients, however, the tertiary manifestations of syphilis develop 2–20 years later. These are granulomatous lesions associated with endarteritis and affect the skin, bones and joints, cardiovascular system, liver or central nervous system (including the eye). Congenital syphilis may present with any of the major manifestations of secondary or tertiary disease.

Neurological disease can occur at any time after primary syphilis and may be symptomatic or asymptomatic (with abnormalities of the cerebrospinal fluid (CSF) only). The chorioretinal manifestations of syphilis may occur as part of syphilitic meningitis during the late secondary phase or as an isolated finding during the tertiary phase of acquired disease, or as part of congenital infection. The characteristic retinal sign in congenital disease is a bilateral 'salt and pepper' appearance. This is a reflection of healed chorioretinal inflammation with gliosis, and necrosis and atrophy of some (with hypertrophy of the remaining) choroidal pigment-producing cells. Sometimes the chorioretinitis is more circumscribed with large plaques of atrophy and clumps of pigment that might be confused with the appearances of retinitis pigmentosa.

In acquired syphilis the classical retinal appearances are those of a diffuse chorioretinitis (Forster's chorioretinitis). There are diffuse yellowish-grey exudates in the midzone of the fundus (which may produce a partial or complete ring scotoma), with a fine punctate vitreous haze and perivascular sheathing, which may be accompanied by flame-shaped retinal haemorrhages and retinal oedema. After

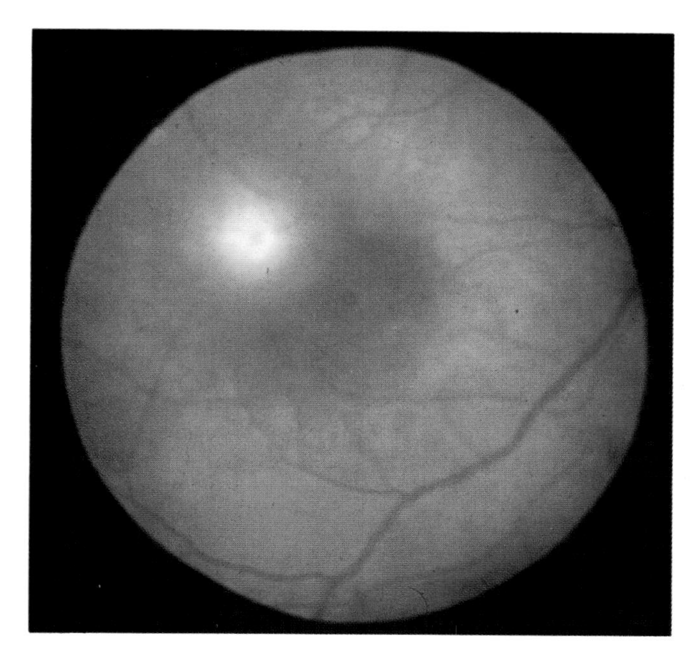

Fig. 10.13 A solitary posterior pole tuberculoma in a patient with miliary tuberculosis. By courtesy of Dr J.A. Innes.

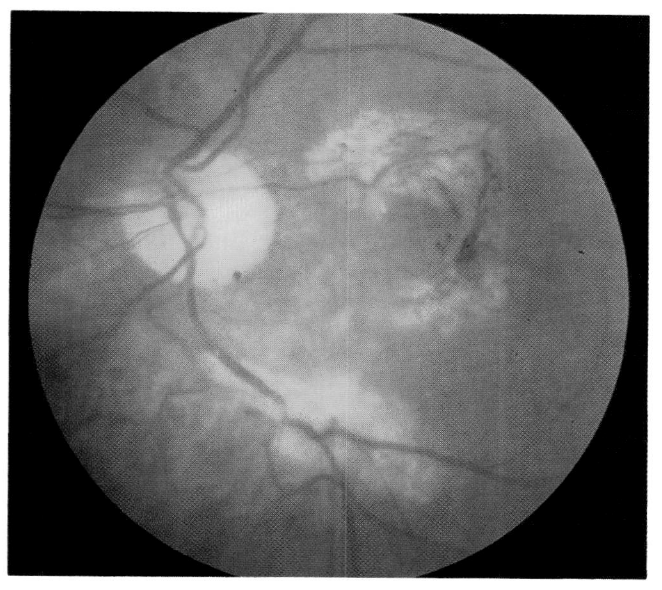

Fig. 10.14 Tuberculous retinochoroiditis and perivasculitis together with optic atrophy in a patient with disseminated *M. tuberculosis* infection and AIDS. Courtesy of Dr J.J. Gonzalez-Guijarro, Hospital de la Princesa, Madrid, Spain.

healing, there is choroidal atrophy and pigment changes. The chorioretinitis may be accompanied by optic atrophy, particularly in patients with parenchymous tertiary neurosyphilis (tabes dorsalis).

10.8.2 Diagnosis

Serological tests are used for the diagnosis of other than primary syphilis. For screening, quantitative, nontreponemal reaginic tests such as the Venereal Disease Research Laboratory (VDRL) test are used. Antibodies measured by these tests reach very high levels during secondary disease but may decline naturally during the latent stages. The specific treponemal tests such as the fluorescent treponemal-antibody absorption (FTA-ABS) test or the microagglutination assay for *T. pallidum* (MHA-TP) are used to confirm reaginic tests but remain positive for life and cannot be used to confirm active disease. In tertiary neurosyphilis the serum reaginic tests may be negative but neurological involvement can be confirmed by a reactive CSF VDRL test.

10.8.3 Management

Penicillin remains the treatment of choice for syphilis but the preparation used and the duration of therapy differ depending upon the stage of disease being treated. The details of the various regimens are outside the scope of this account but for ocular disease, or any form of neurological syphilis, it is now recognized that the previously used course of benzathine penicillin may be inadequate. The recommended therapy now is 10–14 days of either high-dose intravenous penicillin G or a combination of intramuscular procaine penicillin and oral probenecid. No alternative regimens have been sufficiently studied for the treatment of neurosyphilis in a patient with penicillin allergy.

10.9 *PNEUMOCYSTIS CARINII* CHOROIDITIS

Pneumocystis carinii is an opportunistic pathogen (once thought to be a protozoan but now classified as a fungus) that causes pneumonitis in more than 80% of patients with AIDS. The pneumonia is generally treated with systemic cotrimoxazole or pentamidine but, because relapse is very common, lifelong secondary prophylaxis must follow.

Scattered yellow-white choroidal lesions due to disseminated *Pneumocystis carinii* infection have been described in patients with AIDS (Rao *et al.*, 1989). The patients have usually suffered from previous *P. carinii* pneumonia (PCP) and have been maintained on prophylaxis with nebulized pentamidine rather than with oral cotrimoxazole or dapsone. It is presumed that such nebulized therapy, which produces low blood drug concentrations, may suppress PCP but fails to prevent dissemination of the organism and hence the development of retinal lesions.

Histological examination of eyes containing such lesions shows normal retinal tissues but frothy eosinophilic choroidal infiltrates containing *P. carinii* organisms.

10.9.1 Clinical features

There is often little visual impairment and the lesions are detected at routine ophthalmological examination. There are numerous, bilateral, flat or slightly elevated, yellow-white lesions ranging in size from 0.5 to 2 disc diameters (Fig. 10.15). There is no evidence of intraocular inflammation. With time the lesions tend to become more discrete and deeper orange in colour.

In an immunocompromised host these ophthalmoscopic features are usually diagnostic of disseminated *P. carinii* infection although a number of other conditions can cause similar fundal appearances. These are:

- reticulum cell sarcoma
- metastatic carcinoma
- *Mycobacterium avium-intracellulare* infection
- Vogt-Koyanagi-Harada syndrome
- sarcoidosis

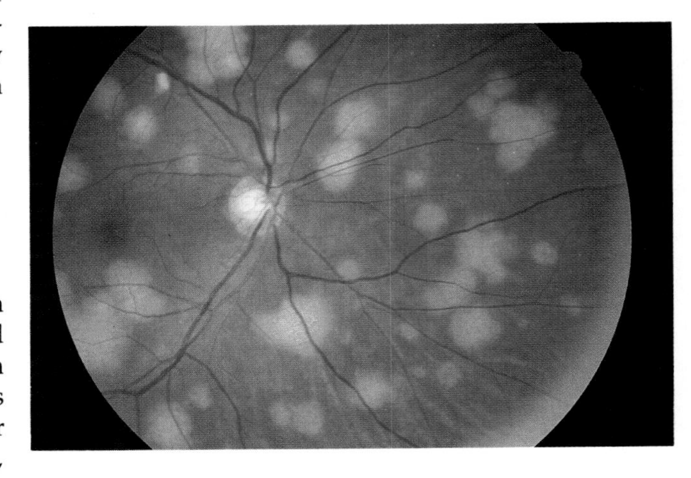

Fig. 10.15 Pneumocystis choroiditis. Courtesy of Thomas A. Deutsch, MD, Rush-Presbyterian-St Luke's Medical Center, Chicago, USA.

Confirmatory evidence of disseminated *P. carinii* infection may be obtained from microscopy of bone marrow, liver or splenic biopsies.

Initial reports suggested that such evidence of disseminated pneumocystis infection carried a poor prognosis with death within a few weeks. With new therapies and perhaps greater awareness of the condition the choroidal lesions can resolve and the patients remain alive for many months.

10.9.2 Management

The treatment of *P. carinii* infections in AIDS patients is with cotrimoxazole or pentamidine and these two drugs are equally effective in PCP. Cotrimoxazole is usually given as 15–20 mg/kg/day of the trimethoprim component (in 3–4 divided doses), either intravenously or orally and pentamidine as the isethionate, 4 mg/kg/day intravenously. Therapy is continued for 3 weeks. One of the major problems with therapy in AIDs is the high frequency of adverse reactions to cotrimoxazole that are often severe enough to require discontinuation of the drug. Even so, cotrimoxazole is usually preferred as the initial therapy because of its oral bioavailability and ease of administration. If toxicity develops then a favourable response can usually be expected with pentamidine. Either therapy should be given for presumed disseminated *Pneumocystis* infection with retinitis, although it is not known whether therapy of patients with chorioretinitis will improve their long-term survival. Some improvement in ocular signs and vision can be obtained after several months (Sneed *et al.*, 1990). If the acute disseminated infection is successfully treated, then it is important to continue permanent prophylaxis with systemic drugs rather than with inhaled pentamidine: dapsone or thrice-weekly cotrimoxazole are suitable choices.

10.10 ACUTE RETINAL NECROSIS SYNDROME

The acute retinal necrosis syndrome (ARN) was first described in Japan in 1971 and is characterized by an initial anterior uveitis followed by panuveitis, vitritis, retinal vaso-occlusive arteritis and full-thickness necrosis of the retina (Fisher *et al.*, 1982).

10.10.1 Aetiology and pathology

The role of the herpes viruses in ARN was demonstrated in the early 1980s. Histological examination of enucleated eyes shows eosinophilic intranuclear inclusion bodies and electron microscopy has demonstrated virus particles morphologically characteristic of the herpes viruses. Varicella zoster virus (VZV) antigens and viral DNA have been demonstrated within the retinal cells and VZV has occasionally been cultured from the vitreous. Epidemiological studies have confirmed that ARN may follow either primary varicella (chickenpox) or reactivation of VZV causing shingles, not necessarily herpes zoster ophthalmicus. Herpes simplex virus has also been implicated as a cause of ARN by both immunofluorescent techniques and by viral isolation. Such cases have occurred in conjunction with herpes simplex skin lesions and also simultaneously with HSV encephalitis. Cytomegalovirus and Epstein-Barr virus have also been implicated in the pathogenesis of ARN.

The route by which the virus reaches the retina is uncertain. It is unlikely to be along the ophthalmic nerve from the trigeminal ganglion and it seems most likely that spread is either haematogenous or down a bilateral neural pathway from the central nervous system.

Initially there is a mild anterior uveitis but a panuveitis follows. There is a vaso-occlusive retinal arteritis and large areas of the retina become necrotic. There is a sharp border between the necrotic and normal retina suggesting that the viruses cause ARN by direct cell-to-cell spread and subsequent cytolysis throughout the retina. The choroid is thickened with a lymphocytic infiltrate. The vitreous becomes turbid and traction on the retina commences; as fibrous organization of the vitreous develops retinal traction may lead to detachment.

10.10.2 Clinical features

(a) SYMPTOMS AND SIGNS

Patients are often previously healthy with no past ocular disease but ARN can also be seen in immunocompromised individuals (including those with AIDS). Overall, the sexes are equally affected. In about one third of cases the disease is bilateral, with the second eye becoming involved within a few weeks of the onset of disease in the first eye. The onset of disease is often insidious with mild blurring of vision and floaters. Once panuveitis ensues the progression of visual loss is often dramatic with reduction to counting fingers within a few days or weeks.

Examination of the visual fields shows reduced

sensitivity with patchy areas of visual loss. There may be a few cells in the anterior chamber.

In the early stages there may be evidence of arteritis with occlusion of peripheral or central retinal vessels. As the disease progresses the peripheral retina consists of large areas of cloudy white retinal necrosis which coalesce and may extend throughout 360° (Fig. 10.16). With evolution to the late phase the necrotic retinal areas regress to form sharply demarcated zones with patchy pigmentation extending towards the equator. There is considerable vitreous debris and a dense posterior vitreous infiltrate. There may be signs of retinal detachment with or without evidence of retinal breaks at the junction between normal and necrotic retina.

In between 50% and 75% of cases there is rhegmatogenous and traction retinal detachment (Fig. 10.17) and there may also be macular oedema and optic nerve damage secondary to vascular insufficiency. The disease consequently has devastating effects upon vision. Three-quarters of individuals have residual visual acuity less than 6/60.

(b) MILD ACUTE RETINAL NECROSIS SYNDROME

Japanese authors have now described a milder form of ARN following herpes infections including chickenpox (Matsuo *et al.*, 1988). In these patients there are peripheral retinal exudates with perivasculitis but the lesions are slowly progressive and are self limiting. Retinal detachment does not occur.

10.10.3 Management

The diagnosis of ARN is essentially clinical. The place of serological investigations in determining the aetiology of ARN is limited since antibodies against VZV and against herpes simplex virus are ubiquitous in the normal adult population. High anti-VZV or anti-HSV concentrations within the vitreous (evidence supporting local antibody production intraocularly) can sometimes be found but such titres are difficult to interpret since they could reflect leakage and concentration of antibody secondary to the retinal vasculitis.

In most cases there has been little proof of benefit from either medical or surgical intervention. Since recent reports have implicated herpes simplex (HSV), varicella zoster virus (VZV) and Epstein-Barr virus (EBV) in the aetiology, acyclovir therapy has been used with limited success. Intravenous acyclovir (5–10 mg/kg 8-hourly for 7–10 days), if given during the early stages, will probably limit the retinal necrosis but has no effect upon the vitritis and progression to retinal detachment. Steroids may well reduce the intraocular inflammation and anti-platelet drugs have been used in an attempt to reduce the arterial occlusion. Unfortunately, early initiation of therapy has not been shown to influence the final visual outcome, which seems to be largely governed by the age of the patient and the severity of the disease at presentation.

Attempts have been made to identify patients in whom a poor outcome is likely and to adopt a more

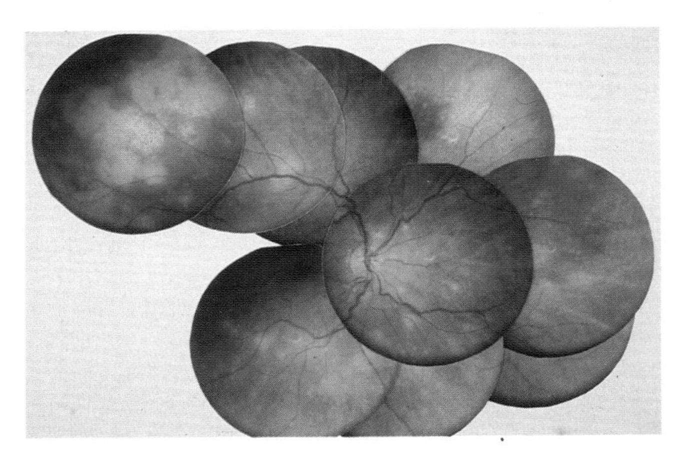

Fig. 10.16 Montage of fundal photographs showing acute retinal necrosis. Courtesy of Dr J.J. Gonzalez-Guijarro, Hospital de la Princesa, Madrid, Spain.

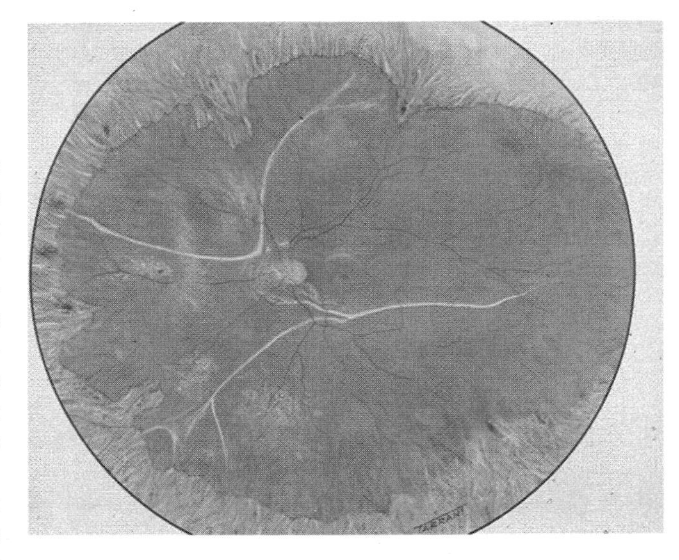

Fig. 10.17 Retinal drawing of typical late phase acute retinal necrosis, showing peripheral pigmentary mottling and subtotal retinal detachment due to retinal breaks at the junction of healthy and necrotic retina. Reproduced with permission of Mr D.S. Gartry and Editors of British Journal of Ophthalmology from Gartry *et al.* (1991).

constructive, interventional approach. Prophylactic laser photocoagulation at areas between necrosis and normal retina has been reported as useful to prevent detachment but these patients were also given acyclovir, steroids and antiplatelet drugs and which measure(s) may have been helpful is unclear. It has also been suggested that prophylactic scleral buckling together with intravitreal acyclovir might improve the outcome.

Conventional surgical retinal detachment procedures may need to be performed, but surgery is often technically very difficult.

10.11 RETINAL CHANGES IN AIDS

The retinal manifestations of advanced HIV infection include a non-infectious microangiopathy (HIV-related retinopathy), opportunistic infections, other non-opportunistic infections and optic neuropathy and atrophy.

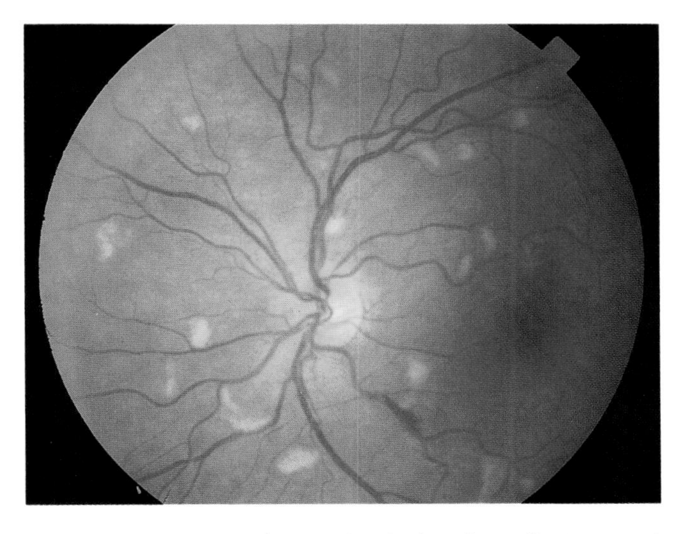

Fig. 10.18 Numerous areas of retinal oedema ('cotton wool spots') and a retinal haemorrhage in a patient with human immunodeficiency virus retinopathy.

10.11.1 HIV-related retinopathy

Clinical manifestations of HIV-related retinopathy are seen in about 40% of patients with AIDS-related complex and in two-thirds or more of those with AIDS. It is equally frequent in homosexuals and heterosexuals with HIV infection. It is not often (*c.* 1–2%) seen in individuals with asymptomatic HIV infection and seems to correlate with the clinical stage of HIV infection.

Cotton wool spots (Fig. 10.18) are the characteristic feature seen on ophthalmoscopy. They are usually located at the posterior pole and are areas of focal microinfarcts in the retinal nerve fibre layer. They are not specific for HIV infection and are seen in a variety of other conditions (Section 2.7). If fluorescein angiography is performed then there is evidence of thickened and occluded capillaries with micro-aneurysms, telangiectasia, and focal areas of non-perfusion. Intraretinal haemorrhages and Roth spots are less common and are associated with more advanced HIV infection.

It was thought that HIV-related retinopathy was caused by the deposition of circulating immune complexes with subsequent vasculitis: immunoperoxidase staining has shown deposition of immunoglobulin within the vessels and high levels of circulating immune complexes have been detected in the majority of AIDS and ARC patients (Pepose *et al.*, 1985). Subsequently, however, HIV has been associated with the retina of patients with AIDS and HIV antigens were detected within retinal epithelial cells and neuroretinal cells, probably of glial origin (Pomerantz *et al.*, 1987). It is possible therefore that the retinal lesions seen in HIV-related retinopathy are caused by virus-induced vascular alterations.

The signs of HIV retinopathy are transient with most lesions tending to disappear within a month or two.

10.11.2 Opportunistic and other infections

There are a number of infectious agents that produce retinal manifestations in AIDS. These are:

- cytomegalovirus
- *Pneumocystis carinii*
- *Toxoplasma gondii*
- *Cryptococcus neoformans*
- *Mycobacterium avium-intracellulare*
- *Mycobacterium tuberculosis*
- *Treponema pallidum*
- *Histoplasma capsulatum*
- *Candida*

Some of these are true opportunistic pathogens but others cause retinal disease in normal individuals – in HIV-infected persons the manifestations may be more severe. Details of most of these have been given above.

Cytomegalovirus infection (see above) is by far the most common, being reported in between 25% and 50% of patients with AIDS in the USA and Europe. It is the AIDS defining infection in only 2–3% of individuals. It seems to be less common in African patients with AIDS, occurring in only 5% of AIDS patients in Ruanda but it is not clear whether this reflects lack of intensive therapy for HIV-related infections and hence shorter survival of patients in Africa or a lower incidence of CMV retinitis in heterosexuals than in homosexual men. Besides CMV, other retinal infections each occur in less than 1% of individuals with HIV infection or AIDS.

Despite the frequency of *Candida* oesophagitis and *Toxoplasma* infection of the central nervous system, retinal infections with these organisms are infrequent. Cryptococcal infection usually involves the central nervous system but intraocular involvement may occur as an isolated feature or as part of disseminated disease. Discrete yellow chorioretinal lesions are seen. Similar lesions may also be seen as part of disseminated *Mycobacterium avium-intracellulare* infection in AIDS patients. In either of these conditions the diagnosis is usually obvious from cultures, serological tests or biopsies of other involved organs.

10.11.3 Optic neuropathy

Optic neuropathy, with visual loss and optic atrophy, is seen in 2–3% of AIDS patients and can be secondary to cryptococcal meningitis or to syphilis. Papilloedema also occasionally occurs secondary to cryptococcal infections (Fig. 10.19).

10.12 ENDOPHTHALMITIS

Endophthalmitis is the most serious of all ocular infections and is a suppurative infection of the intraocular tissues. The infection may affect only specific tissues within the eye or may involve the intraocular contents generally. It usually results as a complication of ocular surgery or other trauma but it may also develop as a metastatic manifestation of septicaemia or fungaemia, often in immunocompromised patients. Most cases of endophthalmitis following surgery or non-surgical trauma to the eye present with visual disturbances, severe ocular pain and signs principally affecting the anterior segment of the eye (hypopyon and severe anterior uveitis, conjunctival hyperaemia and corneal oedema). Vitreous infection and focal chorioretinitis occur but are part of a general panophthalmitis.

Haematogenous spread of infection from an endogenous septic focus produces a similar clinical picture to postoperative endophthalmitis except that the posterior segment of the eye is more likely to be affected, fungi are more likely to be pathogens and the patients are often immunocompromised.

10.12.1 Bacterial endophthalmitis

(a) POSTSURGICAL

Endophthalmitis following ocular surgery is uncommon, probably occurring in 0.1–0.5% of cases. The most common bacteria involved (Section 10.1) are staphylococci (particularly *Staphylococcus epidermidis*), streptococci and *Pseudomonas aeruginosa* and about half of the cases occur more than 7 days after the operation (Shrader *et al.*, 1990). In this series 20% of the patients did not develop clinical evidence of infection until more than one month after potential exposure. If the diagnosis of endophthalmitis is suspected urgent ophthalmological referral is mandatory so that intraocular specimens can be taken for microbiological examination. Specimens from the aqueous humour are as reliable as aspiration of the vitreous unless infection is limited to the posterior segment of the eye. Aggressive antibiotic therapy with broad spectrum agents given systemically, topically and by intravitreal injections is needed (Forster *et al.*, 1980) and the majority of patients will require at least one vitrectomy. Even with this aggressive approach 50% or more of patients will suffer major visual loss.

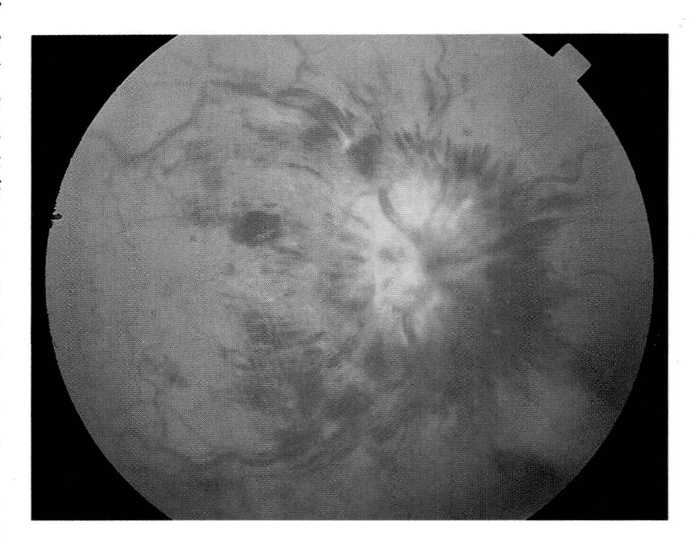

Fig. 10.19 Severe papilloedema in a patient with cryptococcal meningitis complicating AIDS.

(b) HAEMATOGENOUS SPREAD

When endophthalmitis occurs in an eye that has not recently been traumatized, there are usually signs of a septic focus elsewhere in the body (Greenwald *et al.*, 1986). Almost any bacterium may be responsible but the most commonly implicated pathogens are *Streptococcus pneumoniae, Staph. aureus* and the meningococci. In endogenous endophthalmitis the organisms have reached the eye via the retinal or choroidal circulation and the blood retina barrier has, hence, been disrupted. The systemically administered antibiotics achieve therapeutic levels within the eye more easily and intravitreal administration may not be necessary (Greenwald *et al.*, 1986).

(c) SUBACUTE BACTERIAL ENDOCARDITIS

The aetiological agents of bacterial endocarditis are usually of low virulence and the ocular signs associated with haematogenous spread to the eye are minimal. Roth spots, retinal haemorrhages with white centres, are characteristic but not pathognomonic and represent septic emboli.

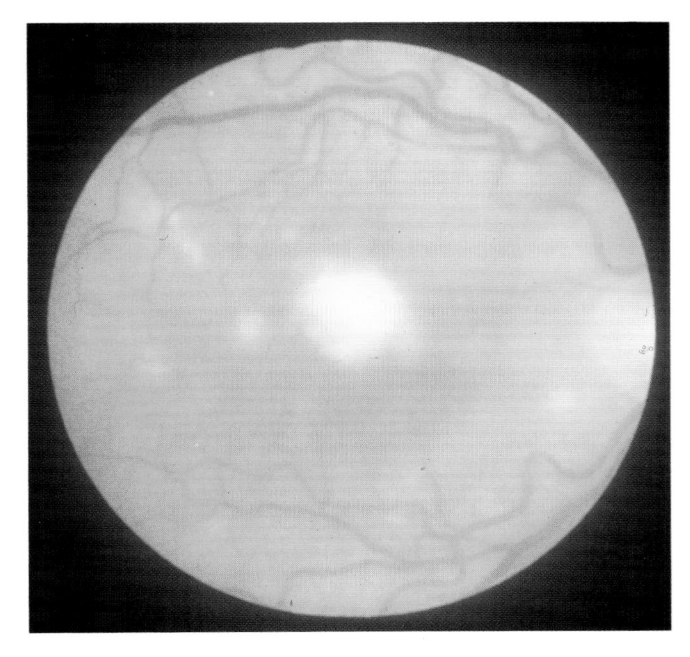

Fig. 10.20 Candida retinitis. Large fluffy white lesion and several smaller lesions with overlying vitreal haze in a patient with disseminated candidiasis. By courtesy of Professor A.M. Geddes.

10.12.2 Fungal endophthalmitis

Fungal endophthalmitis may also result from trauma (either surgical or non-surgical) or from endogenous sources. After trauma the appearance of symptoms and signs is often delayed for much longer than for bacterial infections (often several weeks) and the course is more indolent. *Candida albicans* is the most common cause of haematogenous fungal endophthalmitis, occurring in about 5% of patients with disseminated candidiasis. It is associated with the use of intravascular catheters, immunosuppression, the use of broad spectrum antibiotics and intravenous drug addiction. Disseminated candidiasis is increasing in frequency but is often difficult to diagnose premortem: blood cultures are usually negative in neutropenic patients with disseminated disease. A finding of ocular lesions is thus an important indicator of underlying, potentially lethal infection. Reduction of vision is the earliest symptom but many patients are too ill to report this. In about half of the patients who are found to have candidal endophthalmitis blood cultures will have been positive for *Candida*, often two to three weeks previously. It is important, therefore, in patients with known or suspected candidaemia, to perform periodic fundoscopic examinations. The first sign is a small yellow-white chorioretinal exudate that, especially given the population at chief risk, may be mistaken for a lesion of diabetic retinopathy, acute leukaemia or systemic lupus erythematosus. The lesion then extends to the vitreous and an overlying haze appears that gradually enlarges to form a fluffy white ball extending into the vitreous (Fig. 10.20). Retinal scarring may lead to a severe loss of vision or even loss of the eye. Progression to the anterior chamber may occur.

Topical antifungal therapy is required together with systemic amphotericin B and, in view of the poor vitreal penetration of amphotericin B, oral 5-flucytosine. Intravitreal amphotericin B is often added: even so recovery of vision may not be complete.

Other fungal infections that may be associated with endophthalmitis as part of disseminated disease include aspergillosis, cryptococcosis, and coccidioidomycosis.

REFERENCES

Dutton, G.N. (1989) Recent developments in the prevention and treatment of congenital toxoplasmosis. *Int. Ophthalmol.*, **13**, 407–13.

Engstrom, R.E., Holland, G.N., Nussenblatt, R.B. and Jabs, D.A. (1991) Current practices in the management of ocular toxoplasmosis. *Am. J. Ophthalmol.*, **111**, 601–10.

Farrer, W.E., Wood, M.J., Innes, J.A. and Tubbs, H. (1992) *Infectious Diseases: Text and Color Atlas*, Second edition, Gower Medical, London.

Fisher, J.P., Lewis, M.L., Blumenkranz, M.S. *et al.* (1982) The acute retinal necrosis syndrome. Part 1. Clinical manifestations. *Ophthalmol.*, **89**, 1306–16.

Forster, R.K., Abbott, R.L. and Gelender, H. (1980) Management of infectious endophthalmitis. *Ophthalmol.*, **87**, 313–9.

Gartry, D.S., Spalton, D.J., Tilzey, A. and Hykin, P. G. (1991) Acute retinal necrosis syndrome. *Br. J. Ophthalmol.*, **75**, 292–7.

Gibson, D.W., Duke, B.O.L. and Connor, D.H. (1988) Onchocerciasis: a review of clinical, pathologic and chemotherapeutic aspects, and vector control program. *Prog. Clin. Parasitol.*, **1**, 57.

Glasner, P.D., Silveira, C., Kruszon-Moran, D. *et al.* (1992) An unusually high prevalence of ocular toxoplasmosis in southern Brazil. *Am. J. Ophthalmol.*, **114**, 136–44.

Greenwald, M.J., Wohl, L.G. and Sell, C.H. (1986) Metastatic bacterial endophthalmitis: a contemporary reappraisal. *Surv. Ophthalmol.*, **31**, 81–101.

Holland, G.N., Sidikaro, Y., Kreiger, A.E. *et al.* (1987) Treatment of cytomegalovirus retinopathy with ganciclovir. *Ophthalmol.*, **94**, 815–23.

Jones, W.E., Schantz, P.M., Foreman, K. *et al.* (1980) Human toxocariasis in a rural community. *Am. J. Dis. Child.*, **134**, 967–72.

Matsuo, T., Nakayama, T., Koyama, T. *et al.* (1986) A proposed mild type of acute retinal necrosis syndrome. *Am. J. Ophthalmol.*, **102**, 701–9.

Palestine, A.G. (1988) Clinical aspects of cytomegalovirus retinitis. *Rev. Infect. Dis.*, **10** (suppl. 3), S515–21.

Pepose, J.S., Holland, G.N., Nestor, M.S. *et al.* (1985) Acquired immune deficiency syndrome: pathogenic mechanisms of ocular disease. *Ophthalmol.*, **92**, 472–84.

Perkins, E.S. (1973) Ocular toxoplasmosis. *Br. J. Ophthalmol.*, **57**, 1–17.

Pomerantz, R.J., Kuritzkes, D.R., de la Monte, S.M. *et al.* (1987) Infection of the retina by human immunodeficiency virus type I. *New Engl. J. Med.*, **317**, 1643–7.

Rao, N.A., Zimmerman, P.L., Boyer, D. *et al.* (1989) A clinical, histopathologic, and electron microscopic study of *Pneumocystis carinii* choroiditis. *Am. J. Ophthalmol.*, **107**, 218–28.

Rothova, A., Buitenhuis, H.J., Meenken, C. *et al.* (1989) Therapy in ocular toxoplasmosis. *Int. Ophthalmol.*, **13**, 415–9.

Schantz, P.M., Meyer, D. and Glickman, L.T. (1979) Clinical, serologic and epidemiologic characteristics of ocular toxocariasis. *Am. J. Trop. Med. Hyg.*, **28**, 24–9.

Shrader, S.K., Band, J.D., Lauter, C.B. and Murphy, P. (1990) The clinical spectrum of endophthalmitis: incidence, predisposing factors, and features influencing outcome. *J. Infect. Dis.*, **162**, 115–20.

Sneed, S.R., Blodi, C.F., Berger, B.B. *et al.* (1990) *Pneumocystis carinii* choroiditis in patients receiving inhalted pentamidine. *New Engl. J. Med.*, **322**, 936–7.

Studies of Ocular Complications of AIDS Research Group, in Collaboration with the AIDS Clinical Trials Group. (1992). Mortality in patients with the acquired immunodeficiency syndrome treated with either foscarnet or gangiclovir for cytomegalovirus retinitis. *New Engl. J. Med.*, **326**, 213–20.

11 *Retinopathy and haematological disorders*

Clinical Retinopathies. Paul M. Dodson, Jonathan M. Gibson and Erna E. Kritzinger.
Published in 1995 by Chapman & Hall, London. ISBN 0 412 35930 8

11.1 INTRODUCTION

Fundus examination by ophthalmoscopy is an important part of the assessment of haematological disorders. It may yield information about the diagnosis and course of the disease and is of crucial importance in detecting ophthalmic complications that could be sight threatening. It is easy to forget, however, when we examine the retinal vessels, that the blood itself which is contained within those vessels can have a profound effect on the retinal vascular appearance. In fact as the walls of healthy retinal arterioles and veins are normally transparent, it is the actual blood column that we see.

Several features of the blood can be affected and these need to be considered. Abnormalities can occur in the blood flow, the coagulability, the rheology and in the actual cellular components in the blood which can cause characteristic fundus changes. Blood rheology is the study of the deformation and flow of blood in the circulation. It can be conveniently divided into blood viscosity and its determinants, and cellular and other factors in the blood. It is important to realize that for small vessels, such as retinal capillaries, the flow of blood will to a great extent depend on the deformability and shape of the red and white cells themselves. These abnormalities will now be considered in relation to the important haematological disorders.

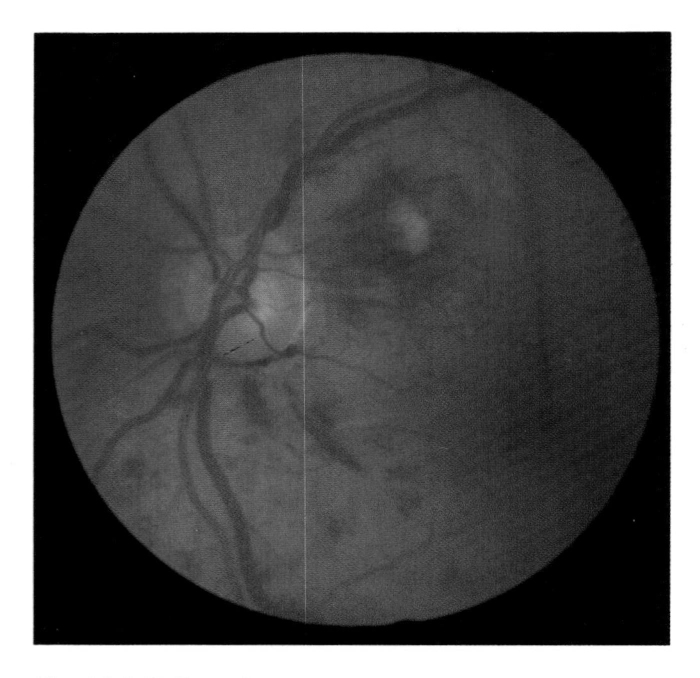

Fig. 11.1 Roth spot.

11.2 ANAEMIA

In most chronic or mild anaemias no abnormality is visible on fundoscopy. If the anaemia is prolonged the earliest common abnormality is a general dilatation of retinal arterioles and veins due to a compensatory increased blood flow through the circulation. In more severe cases the fundus may appear paler than normal but this is notoriously difficult to judge because of the remarkable variation in retinal and choroidal pigmentation that occurs in healthy patients.

In more severe or acute causes of anaemia abnormalities in the fundus are more likely. These include flame-shaped haemorrhages within the nerve fibre layer of the retina, white centred haemorrhages (so called Roth's spots, Fig. 11.1), pre-retinal haemorrhages, cotton wool spots, retinal venous tortuosity and dilatation and exudate formation within the retina. As a rough rule, retinal haemorrhages and cotton wool spots are unlikely to occur unless the red cell number drops below 50% of the normal value. However, the cause of the anaemia with the accompanying haematological abnormalities such as leukaemia, thrombocytopenia and hyperviscosity are probably more important in the production of retinal abnormalities than the absolute level of haemoglobin or red cell number. A list of common causes of anaemia is shown in Table 11.1, and a list of useful investigations in making haematological diagnosis is given in Table 11.2.

Patients with retinopathy due to anaemia are unlikely to have any visual symptoms unless haemorrhage occurs at the macula. There have been reports of complete loss of vision in patients with severe blood loss associated with retinal and optic nerve ischaemia. In anaemic retinopathy many of the superficial flame-shaped haemorrhages are surprisingly large, and situated in the peripapillary area. Roth's spots have been described in patients with septic embolization. Roth, a German physician, first described haemorrhages and white lesions in patients with sepsis in 1872, and a few years later, white centred haemorrhages in septic endocarditis were termed 'Roth's spots', a term which has subsequently remained in use. They are more usually seen in cases of anaemia from any cause, in particular pernicious anaemia, leukaemia, and in AIDS. The white centred area within the area of haemorrhage is thought to be due to either retinal ischaemia, as in cotton wool spots, or fibrin related to the infected embolus.

Causes of white centred haemorrhages (Roth's spots) are:

Table 11.1 Common causes of anaemia

1. Deficiencies:	Iron B_{12} or folate Vitamin C Protein
2. Aplastic anaemia	e.g. Drug induced
3. Marrow infiltration:	Metastatic carcinoma Leukaemia Lymphoma Myeloma Myelofibrosis Tuberculosis
4. Anaemia of chronic disease:	e.g. Collagen disease Renal failure Malignancy Thalassemia (other haemoglobinopathies)
5. Sideroblastic anaemia	(hypochromic anaemia with large number of normoblasts containing many iron granules in the marrow)
Refractory normoblastic anaemia	(Pyridoxine deficiency, Lead poisoning)
6. Endocrine:	Hypothyroidism Hypopituitarism
7. Haemorrhage:	Trauma Gastro-intestinal Uterine Renal
8. Haemolysis:	Haemoglobinopathies Auto-immune a) Idiopathic b) Viral or mycloplasma infection Myeloproliferative disorders Systemic Lupus Erythematosus Malaria
9. Drugs and chemicals:	e.g. Non-steroidal anti-inflammatories, Lead, Methyl Dopa

- infective endocarditis
- pernicious anaemia
- other anaemias
- leukaemia
- AIDS

11.3 POLYCYTHAEMIA

Polycythaemia (Fig. 11.2) causes retinal ischaemia by increased viscosity and interference with blood flow. In milder forms venous dilatation is the only recognizable change. In polycythaemia secondary to congenital heart disease, the vessels can become hugely dilated with associated optic disc swelling, but normal visual acuity.

In polycythaemia rubra vera, vascular dilatation and tortuosity together with deep and superficial haemorrhages can cause a fundus picture which is identical to central retinal vein occlusion (CRVO) the latter is due to venous stasis retinopathy. This is one reason why all patients with a CRVO should have a full blood count, haemoglobin and plasma viscosity performed, to exclude such an underlying haematological abnormality.

Table 11.2 Useful investigations in the diagnosis of haematological conditions

1. Full blood count	Haemoglobin Red cell morphology and number Packed cell volume White cell differential and count Platelet count
Blood film	Size, shape and abnormal cells Microcytosis (e.g. Iron deficiency) Macrocytosis (e.g. B_{12} or folate deficiency) Target cells Blast cells (myeloproliferative disease)
2. Haemolytic anaemias	Haemoglobin electrophoresis (e.g. Sickle Cell Disease, spherocytosis) Reticulocyte count (increased) Haptoglobin (reduced) Coomb's test Cold or warm agglutinins Biliriubin levels Red cell life span (^{51}Cr labelling)
3. Deficiencies	Serum ferritin, iron and total iron binding capacity Serum B_{12} and folate (and red cell value)
4. Bone marrow	Sternal puncture – aspiration Iliac crest: aspiration and/or Trephine
5. Red cell mass	Differentiation between primary or secondary polycythaemia
6. Immunoglobulins	Serum IgG, A, M, E (Benign gammopathies, myeloma, lymphomas)
7. ESR, Plasma viscosity, C-reactive protein	increased non-specifically in chronic inflammatory conditions
8. Urine Bence–Jones protein	myeloma

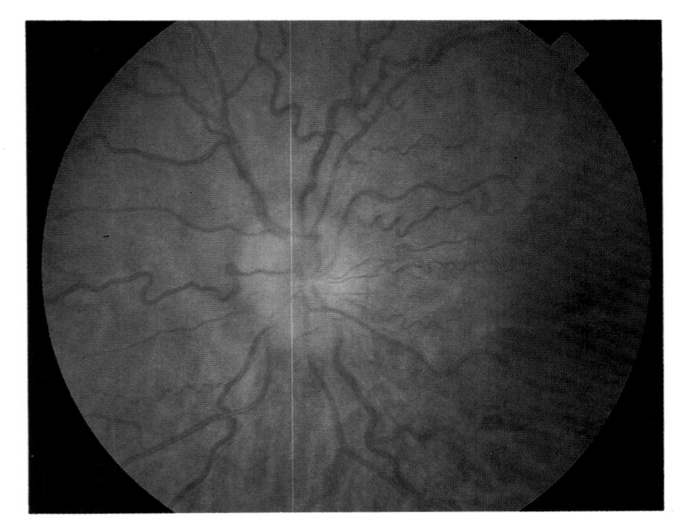

Fig. 11.2 Fundus appearance in polycythaemia.

11.4 LEUKAEMIAS

Retinopathy is a common manifestation of the leukaemias (Figs 11.3, 11.4) and may be the presenting feature of the disease. It has been estimated that about 90% of all cases of leukaemia will develop intraocular manifestations. These ocular manifestations may be caused by:

1. haematological disorders, associated with the leukaemia, such as thrombocytopenia, anaemia and hyperviscosity of the blood with associated ischaemia;
2. by direct infiltration of neoplastic cells into the retina or choroid;
3. by opportunistic infection.

The ocular manifestations are not limited to the retina. There are reports of leukaemic infiltration

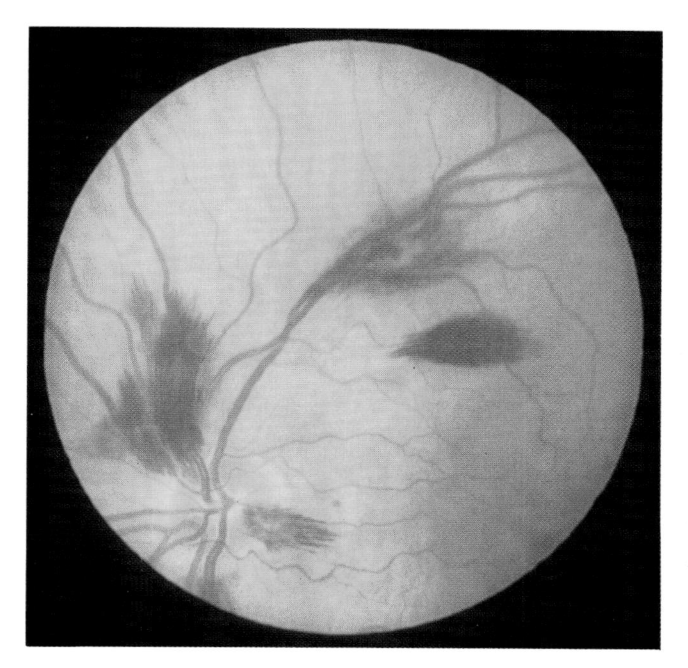

Fig. 11.3 Fundus appearance in chronic lymphatic leukaemia.

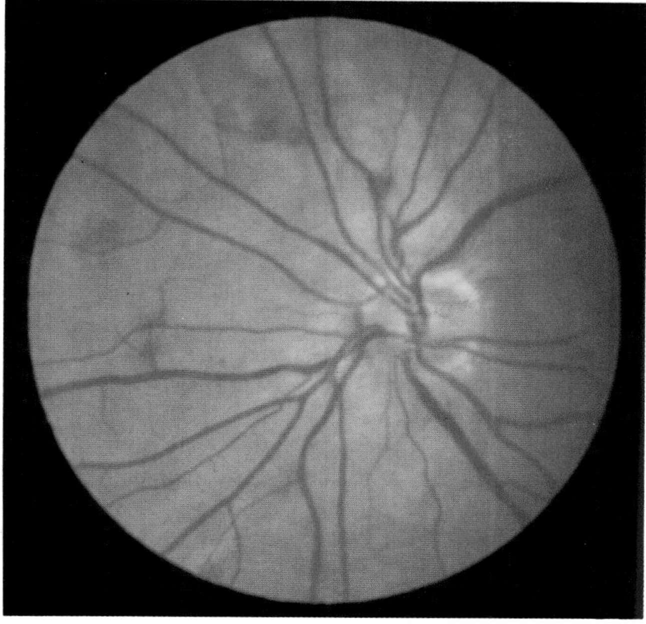

Fig. 11.4 Fundus appearance in chronic myeloid leukaemia.

occurring in the anterior chamber, iris, optic nerve and choroid. Sub-conjunctival and anterior chamber haemorrhages (hyphaemas) also occur.

Leukaemic retinopathy is the term commonly used for the fundal manifestations of anaemia, ischaemia and increased blood viscosity. Retinopathy is more commonly seen and more florid in the acute leukaemias. The features of leukaemic retinopathy are:

1. Retinal haemorrhages:
   these are often seen as large flame-shaped haemorrhages around the retinal vascular arcade vessels. In acute leukaemias huge sheet-like preretinal haemorrhages may occur, as well as smaller intraretinal and subretinal haemorrhages. Haemorrhages probably arise as a result of ischaemic changes in combination with anaemia and thrombocytopenia. Thrombocytopenia may be the most important factor in the formation of retinal haemorrhages as there is a relationship between platelet count and intraretinal haemorrhage.
2. Cotton wool spots:
   these may be the presenting sign of leukaemia and are usually caused by ischaemia secondary to anaemia and hyperviscosity. Rarely they have been attributable to leukaemic infiltration.
3. Hyperviscosity:
   high blood viscosity, which may occur in the leukaemias, can cause a number of characteristic signs that have been described:
   (a) Dilatation and tortuosity of retinal veins. Beading of the veins may be seen, similar to pre-proliferative diabetic retinopathy.
   (b) Central retinal vein occlusion.
   (c) Peripheral retinal microaneurysms.
   (d) Peripheral retinal neovascularization, usually associated with ischaemic areas in the retina due to capillary bed closure. Optic disc neovascularization has also been reported.

Other findings in leukaemic patients are:

1. Retinal and choroidal infiltration:
   leukaemic retinal infiltrates have been reported in cases of myelogenous leukaemia, but are much rarer than choroidal infiltration. The choroid, which is highly vascular, is the most commonly involved part of the eye, but signs of choroidal infiltration may be subtle. The infiltrates may appear as solid choroidal masses or have an overlying serous retinal detachment. Such cases have been reported in patients with acute and chronic lymphocytic and myelogenous leukaemias. 'Leopard-spot' pigmentation in the peripheral fundus has been described and has a quite striking appearance. It probably represents clumping of the pigment epithelium, and may be caused by choroidal infiltration.

2. Vitreous gel infiltration:
   the vitreous humour is composed of a high molecular weight gel which is almost inert. However, vitreous infiltrates can occur in severely ill patients and appear on direct ophthalmoscopy as multiple dark opacities overlying the retina. This may make examination of the retina difficult and 'murky'. Vitreous infiltration can occur in the leukaemias but is more characteristic of reticulum cell sarcoma, Burkitt's lymphoma, multiple myeloma and Hodgkin's disease, which are sometimes called the 'masquerade diseases' as this appearance can masquerade as uveitis.
3. Optic nerve infiltration:
   leukaemic infiltration of the optic nerve (Fig. 11.5) may occur in patients with acute lymphocytic leukaemia, and may cause a reduction in visual acuity. If the optic disc is swollen it may be difficult to differentiate between optic disc oedema secondary to leukaemic infiltration and papilloedema caused by raised intracranial pressure. It should be remembered that visual loss is usually unaffected in the early stages of papilloedema, and it is usually bilateral. In these situations a CT scan of the brain and ventricles and a lumbar puncture (once raised intra-cranial pressure is excluded) are usually necessary to differentiate the two conditions.
4. Opportunistic infections:
   these occur in patients with leukaemia in whom the immune system is compromised by the disease and/or the immunosuppressant treatment. The following infections have been reported:
   (a) cytomegalovirus retinitis (Fig. 11.6);
   (b) herpes viruses causing retinitis;
   (c) *Toxoplasma* retinitis;
   (d) intraocular fungal infections.

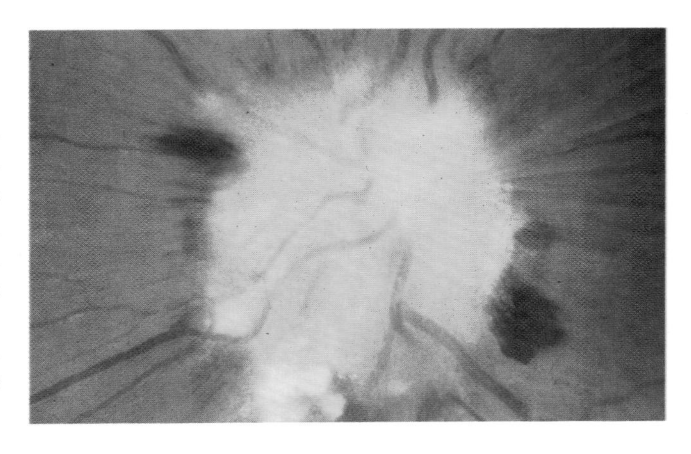

Fig. 11.5 Leukaemic infiltration of optic nerve.

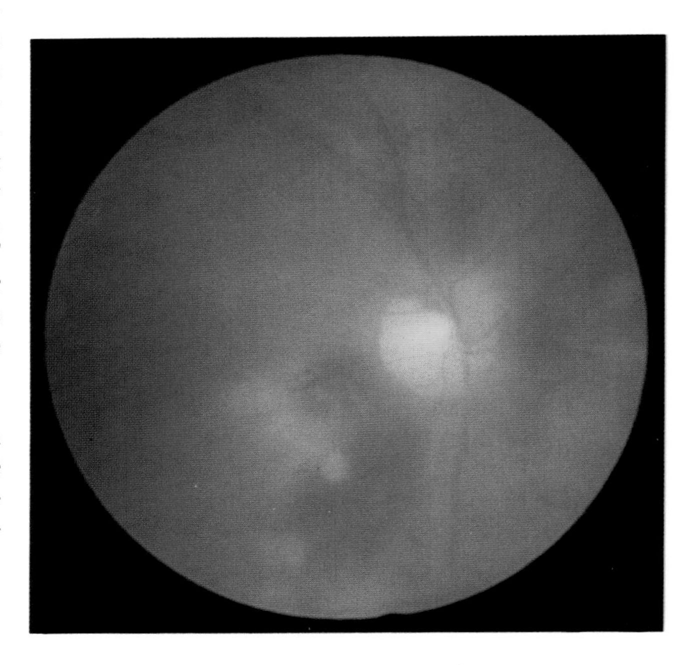

Fig. 11.6 CMV retinitis in leukaemic patient.

11.4.1 Prognosis and treatment

Leukaemic retinopathy (i.e. manifestations of anaemia, thrombocytopenia and hyperviscosity) are said not to be of prognostic significance in leukaemic patients, but as they are related to abnormal blood indices they are usually a sign of relapse of the disease. Retinal and choroidal infiltration, together with vitreous infiltrates, are usually only seen in terminal disease. Retinal and choroidal infiltrates may also be associated with central nervous system involvement.

The classification and management of the many forms of leukaemia are out of the scope of this book, but two excellent reviews are cited for further reading.

The medical treatment of the leukaemias may have a profound effect on the fundal appearance, as haemorrhages and cotton wool spots may disappear in time with remission. Intraocular manifestations of leukaemia are not treated directly, but are treated with systemic chemotherapy in order to control the underlying disease. It is not known how well chemotherapeutic agents get into the eye, and this has led in rare cases to other routes of entry being tried, such as subconjunctival injections.

11.5 THE LYMPHOMAS

The classification of lymphomas is complex and controversial; for the purposes of considering the ocular manifestations they will be considered as: (1) Hodgkin's lymphoma; (2) non-Hodgkin's lymphomas and (3) multiple myeloma. The medical aspects can be found in the reviews cited for further reading.

11.5.1 Hodgkin's disease

Ocular involvement in Hodgkin's disease is uncommon and has been reported in only a few cases. Opportunistic infections, particularly retinitis associated with herpes virus infections, may occur.

11.5.2 Non-Hodgkin's lymphomas

In this subgroup will be included reticulum cell sarcoma, lymphocytic lymphoma and Burkitt's lymphoma.

Reticulum cell sarcoma (histiocytic lymphoma) is predominantly a disease of middle-aged and elderly persons, that only occasionally involves the eye. However, there does seem to be a subgroup of the disease in which the ocular and central nervous system is primarily involved. This disease is important because it is one of the 'maquerade diseases' that mimic posterior uveitis, and ocular involvement may precede central nervous system disease.

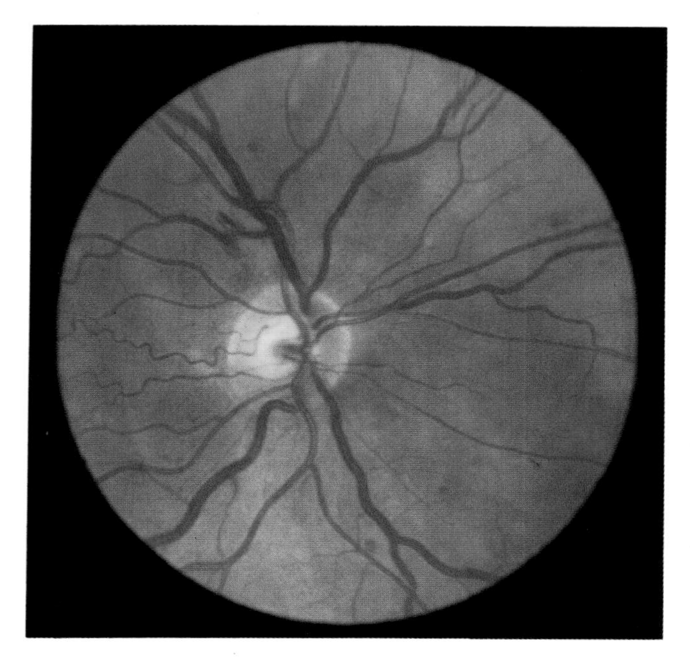

Fig. 11.7 Fundus in multiple myeloma.

Typically patients with this condition present complaining of seeing floaters, caused by vitreous infiltration with the tumour and which is usually bilateral. Fundus examination is often difficult because of the hazy media, but multiple, discrete lesions usually develop under the retinal pigment epithelium. These lesions are said to be characteristic of this condition, they have sharply defined borders and are yellowish-white. Atrophic or disciform scars are left behind if the lesions resolve. Vitreous biopsy for cytological diagnosis may be helpful and treatment is with radiotherapy.

In lymphocytic lymphoma and Burkitt's lymphoma intraocular involvement rarely occurs. Orbital involvement commonly occurs in Burkitt's lymphoma and secondary involvement of the eye can occur.

11.5.3 Multiple myeloma

Multiple myeloma (Figs 11.7, 11.8) is a neoplasm of the plasma cells. It is related to other plasma cell dyscrasias such as Waldenström's macroglobulinaemia, primary amyloidosis and systemic light chain deposition disease, which will also be briefly discussed.

Multiple myeloma typically presents in patients in their sixties, with only a 2% of cases occurring in patients less than 40 years of age. Studies indicate that the malignant change occurs in an early haemopoietic myeloma stem cell.

The presenting features of myeloma include:

Bone pain		70%
Symptoms of hypercalcaemia		30%
Fever		15%
Anaemia	Symptoms of	15%
Renal failure	Symptoms of	10%
Hyperviscosity	Symptoms of	10%
Haemorrhage		7%

Less common presentations are those of amyloidosis, compressive paraplegia, skin involvement and osteosclerosis. To allow the diagnosis of myeloma, two of the following three criteria must be fulfilled:

1. An increase in bone marrow plasma cells (>20% of total marrow nucleated cells).
2. Lytic bone lesions in a full skeletal survey.
3. A paraprotein must occur in serum and/or urine (note, rarely there are a small number of non-synthesizing myelomas in which paraproteins are not found).

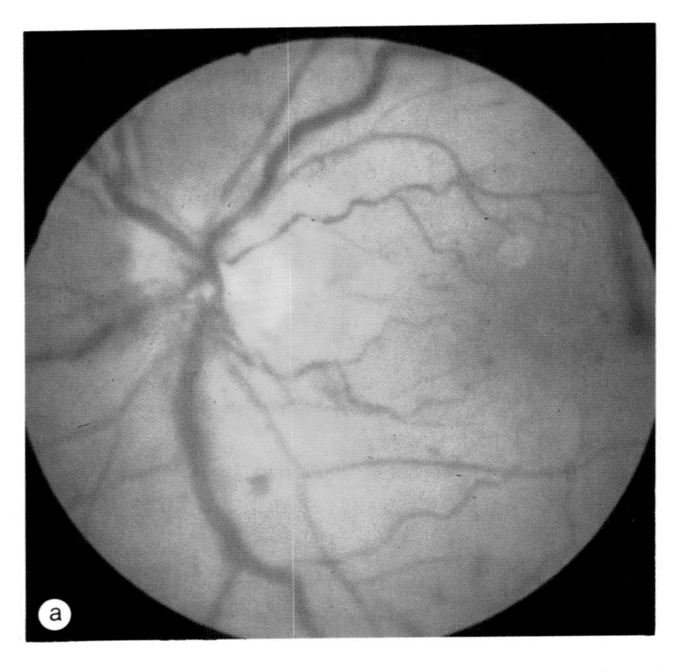

Fig. 11.8 Multiple myeloma. (a) Before plasmaphoresis. (b) Following plasmaphoresis.

The evolution of myeloma leads to three different clinical entities, with monoclonal gammopathy (benign: asymptomatic), indolent myeloma (usually asymptomatic, marrow plasmocytosis increased, monoclonal serum protein levels), and typical multiple myeloma.

Diagnosis is established with the use of investigations which include:

- Full blood count
- ESR
- Renal function, Serum creatinine
- Serum calcium
- Protein electrophoresis
- Serum paraprotein and Immunoglobulin estimation
- Urinary Bence–Jones proteins
- Bone marrow examination
- Skeletal survey

Factors associated with a poorer prognosis are:

- Urine Bence–Jones proteinuria >200 mg/dl
- Serum urea >13 mmol/L
- Haemoglobin <7.5 g/dl
- Serum albumin <30 g/dl
- Albuminuria >40 mg/dl

In multiple myeloma, bony involvement of the orbit may cause proptosis, which may be a presenting feature. Retinal haemorrhages, cotton wool spots and Roth spots occur and are manifestations of anaemia and thrombocytopenia. Micro-aneurysms and increased tortuosity of the retinal veins may occur, as a manifestation of hyperviscosity. The retinopathy often resolves quickly with treatment of the myeloma, and the presence of retinopathy is not thought to have any prognostic significance. Pars plana cysts occur in this condition and may become quite large.

HYPERVISCOSITY SYNDROMES

These syndromes occur most commonly with increased IgA, IgG and IgM (Waldenströms macroglobulinaemia) levels. Hyperviscosity does not usually cause clinical problems but in the severe state, neurological (vertigo, headaches, fits), haematological (mucosal, intracranial haemorrhage) and cardiovascular systems (cardiac failure) are affected. The fundus appearance of hyperviscosity may be very similar to a central retinal vein occlusion, although in this case it is bilateral. Peripheral neovascularization and micro-aneurysms may occur but the signs are usually reversible once the viscosity returns to normal.

In primary amyloidosis loss of vision may occur from accumulation of amyloid in the vitreous, with an appearance similar to asteroid hyalosis but with more cobweb-like veils present. The condition is usually inherited in a dominant fashion and vitreous or rectal biopsy may be necessary to confirm the diagnosis. Vitrectomy may be necessary to restore the vision.

Recently there has been a case report of a patient with another rare type of plasma cell dyscrasia, systemic light chain deposition disease. In this report the patient developed a retinopathy mimicking a retinal vasculitis, which was diagnosed only after serum and urine electrophoresis and special staining of biopsy material from kidney, bone marrow and rectum.

TREATMENT OF MYELOMA

Treatment is currently aimed at the tumour and specific complications. Oral Melphalan is an effective drug in the induction phase of treatment although combination chemotherapy regimes may produce improved results in patient survival. This drug is administered daily at a dose of 0.15 mg/kg for seven days, with courses repeated every six weeks.

Renal impairment is the most common complication, requiring correction of dehydration, and in some patients, hypercalcaemia with biphosphonates (Pamidronate, Etidronate and Clodronate) or corticosteroids. Spinal cord compression may be present during the disease course, and requires an immediate neurological opinion with regard to surgical decompression. Hyperviscosity syndromes with significant clinical signs or symptoms may require plasmapheresis using a cell separator and this can be life saving.

In general, none of the current treatments are curative but newer approaches to treatment being evaluated include interferon, high dose Melphalan, and bone marrow transplantation.

11.6 HAEMOGLOBINOPATHIES

Sickle cell (SC) disease is the most common condition caused by an abnormal haemoglobin. It was first described in 1910 and is now known to be due to a substitution of valine for glutamic acid in the beta chain of the haemoglobin molecule. This substitution causes the haemoglobin to polymerize under conditions of hypoxia, causing erythrocytes to deform and become more rigid, so reducing their ability to traverse the microvascular circulation. This 'sickling' of red blood cells under adverse conditions of hypoxia and acidosis causes infarcts to occur throughout the body. Important systemic manifestations are bone marrow infarcts, aseptic necrosis of the head of the femur, painful joints, abdominal pain, dyspnoea and neurological symptoms.

The term 'sickle cell disease' includes the homozygous sickle cell anaemia (HbS–HbS) but also mixed syndromes in which sickling occurs due to HbS in combination with another haemoglobin such as HbC (HbS–HbC) or beta thalassaemia (HbS–Hbthal). The term sickle cell trait is reserved for the usually clinically silent heterozygous state HbA–HbS.

Initially the disease was described in the indigenous population of West and Central Africa, where in some areas, the prevalence of the abnormal gene is as high as 1 in 3. There is a lower but significant prevalence in Mediterranean countries, the Middle East and in India. In the United Kingdom, the prevalence of the gene in the Afro-Caribbean community is estimated to be about 1 in 10.

11.6.1 Ocular manifestations

The sickle cell haemoglobinopathies can affect all parts of the eye. In the anterior segment important signs are comma-shaped capillary segments in the conjunctiva, iris atrophy, anterior and posterior synechiae as well as anterior chamber flare and cells.

The most severe and important manifestations are those that occur in the posterior segment of the eye, which are sight threatening. Sickle cell retinopathy has been classified by Goldberg (1971) into five stages:

Stage 1. Background changes:
- salmon patches (Fig. 11.9);
- black sunbursts (Fig. 11.9);
- iridescent spots;
- occluded peripheral arterioles.

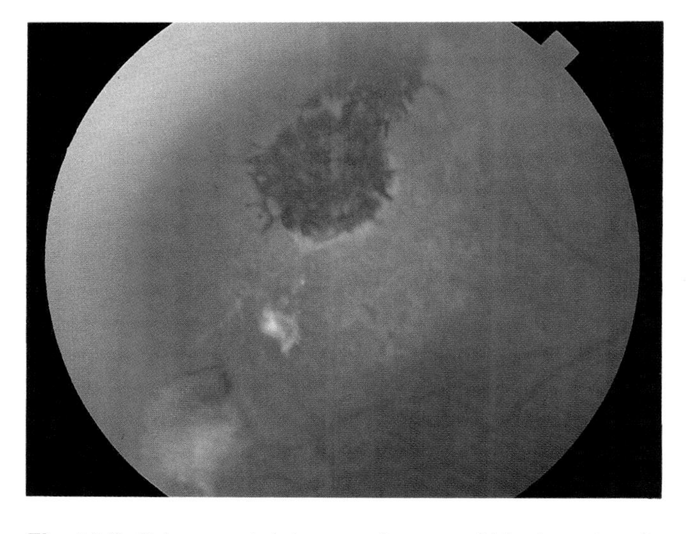

Fig. 11.9 Salmon patch haemorrhage and black sunburst.

Stage 2. Arteriolar-venous anastomoses;
shunt vessels between arterioles and veins in mid-periphery,
silver wire arterioles in far periphery.
Stage 3. Neovascular changes (proliferative sickle cell retinopathy);
sea fans: These new vessels are initially flat, between the neurosensory retina and internal limiting membrane. If this becomes elevated, vitreous movement can cause traction and haemorrhage.
Stage 4. Vitreous haemorrhage.
Stage 5. Retinal detachment.

Perhaps an easier way of remembering these changes is to divide them into background and proliferative sickle cell retinopathy (PSR).

(a) BACKGROUND SICKLE RETINOPATHY

These changes in the retina include characteristic signs such as 'salmon patch haemorrhage', 'iridescent spots' and 'black sunbursts' (Fig. 11.9). The salmon patch haemorrhages occur at the junction of perfused and non-perfused retina, they may be intraretinal or subretinal and can be several disc diameters in size. They are so called because initially the fresh haemorrhage is bright red but after a period of time becomes more pinky-orange (salmon pink). As these haemorrhages resolve they may leave iridescent spots of haemosiderin which are yellow or copper-coloured. If the blood extends under the retina, a black patch of pigmentation or 'sunburst spots' are formed. These latter spots are caused by retinal pigment epithelial changes. An example of inactive sickle cell retinopathy is shown in Fig. 11.10.

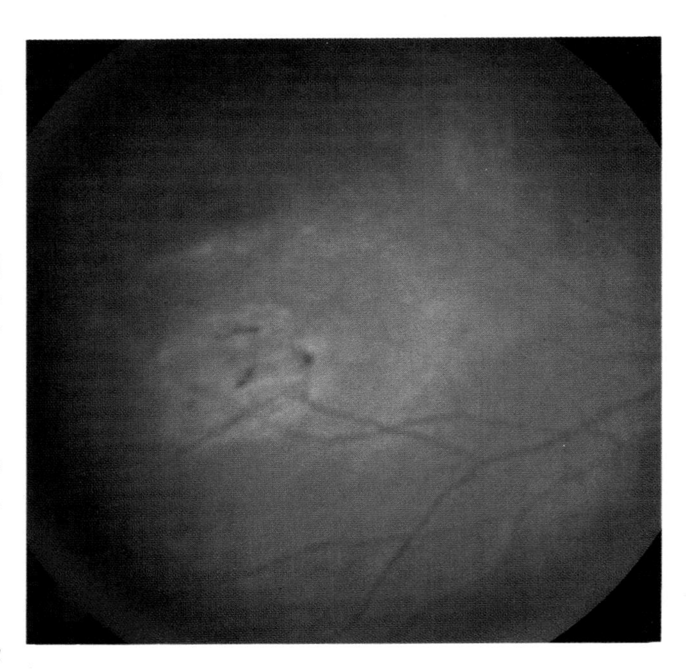

Fig. 11.10 Inactive sickle cell retinopathy.

(b) PROLIFERATIVE SICKLE CELL RETINOPATHY (PSR)

The formation of peripheral neovascular 'sea fans' marks the entry into the proliferative phase of retinopathy. These sea fans are so called because of their resemblance to marine creatures found in tropical seas. The sea fans grow between the neurosensory retina and the internal limiting membrane and at this stage appear to be flat. Any small movement of the vitreous body can potentially cause haemorrhage. Eventually the neovascular fronds can grow into the cortex of the vitreous gel, when they appear elevated and are particularly liable to haemorrhage. Fluorescein angiography can be helpful in identifying the position of sea fans which are bleeding, as the neovascular fronds leak profusely. They can therefore be readily detected and if necessary treated.

The sight-threatening complications of the neovascular sea fans are:

- vitreous haemorrhage;
- vitreous traction;
- retinal traction and detachment;
- epiretinal membrane formation.

Proliferative sickle cell retinopathy is the main sight-threatening complication of sickle cell retinopathy. Its prevalence is reported as affecting 3% of homozygous HbS–HbS patients, compared to 32% in HbS–HbC disease.

(c) OTHER CAUSES OF VISUAL LOSS

There are several other causes of visual loss that occur in sickle cell disease:

- rhegmatogenous retinal detachment;
- exudative retinal detachment;
- macular ischaemia;
- arteriolar occlusions;
- macular hole formation;
- angioid streaks and subretinal neovascularization.

Angioid streaks are thought to occur in about 22% of patients with homozygous disease, and less commonly with SC disease. Despite this, loss of vision from subretinal neovascularization is relatively uncommon. A mottling of the fundus is sometimes seen in association with angioid streaks and this is termed peau d'orange, after its similarity to the skin of an orange. The significance of this change is unknown, but it may be seen before the development of angioid streaks.

11.6.2 Treatment

The natural history of sickle cell retinopathy runs a variable course and there is a tendency for proliferative retinopathy with even quite large sea fans to regress spontaneously. Therefore, treatment is usually only recommended when vision is threatened as shown by the presence of vitreous haemorrhage from sea fans, or large numbers of peripheral sea fans. In recent years there has been a divergence of opinion from the aggressive treatment of all neovascularization regardless of the risks inherent in the treatment, to the opposite policy of serial observation with treatment as a last resort.

Current opinion takes into account that up to 70% of visual loss in sickle cell disease is due to PSR, and that if detected early enough for treatment, the majority of visual loss may be preventable. Treatment modalities available are laser and xenon photocoagulation, as well as cryotherapy.

(a) PHOTOCOAGULATION

Photocoagulation with xenon or more usually laser has been shown to be an effective treatment of the neovascular fronds. Two techniques have been used: (1) direct treatment of the feeder vessels, (2) indirect scatter laser treatment around the sea fans.

Direct photocoagulation of the feeder vessels of the sea fans is effective in causing their regression. The technique requires high power burns to be placed on the feeder arteriole so that segmentation of the vessel occurs and bloodflow stops. After that the main draining vein is also occluded. Unfortunately this technique has been associated with complications, mainly because of the high energy settings that have to be used to obtain sufficiently intense burns. Complications reported include ruptures in Bruch's membrane with choroidal neovascularization, vitreous haemorrhage, pre-retinal membrane formation and subretinal fibrosis. If direct treatment is attempted it may be safer to use longer exposures in a 'slow cooking' method to attempt to close the vessels rather than turning the power higher and higher to produce a 'fast frying' of the feeder vessels.

An alternative, and safer, method is to place gentle scatter laser burns around the neovascular fronds. The rationale for this treatment is that by treating the associated ischaemic areas of retina the neovascularization will regress, in a similar fashion to diabetic patients. If there are multiple neovascular fronds, then 360 degree scatter treatment should be given. In the event that neovascularization fails to regress, further scatter treatment can be applied or at this stage direct feeder vessel closure can be attempted.

(b) RETINAL CRYOPEXY

Retinal cryopexy (use of a freezing probe) can be given under either local or general anaesthesia, and may be most easily facilitated by first removing the conjunctiva. Cryopexy is a simple and effective way of treating peripheral sea fans, but as it produces a larger area of choroidoretinal scarring, is not without risk. Vitreous haemorrhage, epiretinal membrane formation and retinal detachment can all follow over-exuberant cryotherapy for PSR, and for these reasons it is probably better to reserve cryotherapy for those cases in which laser photocoagulation is either not effective or not possible.

Vitreous haemorrhages are treated by observation for a period of six months, as there is a good chance that most will clear during this period. If no view of the retina is possible, it is important to examine with ultrasound to confirm that the retina is flat. Following vitreous haemorrhage fluorescein angiography is helpful in identifying sea fans which can be treated by either cryotherapy or, if the vitreous is clear enough, by laser. Persistent or recurrent vitreous haemorrhages can be treated by vitrectomy.

(c) RETINAL DETACHMENT SURGERY

Retinal and vitreous surgery can be performed for tractional and rhegmatogenous detachments in the same way as for other conditions. Unfortunately there are important, special considerations for the surgeon and anaesthetist in operating on patients with HbSS or HbSC disease:

1. There is a risk of the general anaesthesia itself. This can be lessened by an exchange transfusion pre-operatively although this is a major procedure itself and somewhat controversial. Pre- and post-operative oxygenation are important considerations. If local anaesthesia can be used, this is preferable although not all patients are suitable.
2. The surgeon must be aware of the risk of anterior segment ischaemia, and so encircling bands are contraindicated. The rectus muscles are left intact

and the posterior ciliary vessels are avoided. High intraocular pressure rises are prevented if at all possible, as these will compromise ocular perfusion.

11.6.3 Angioid streaks in other haemoglobinopathies

Angioid streaks have been reported in a variety of types of haemoglobinopathy. The list includes homozygous sickle cell disease, sickle cell trait, haemoglobin SC disease, sickle cell–thalassaemia disease, haemoglobin H disease and beta thalassaemia major. This association between haemoglobinopathies and angioid streaks could be just a chance finding but it seems that this is a significant association. The pathogenesis of angioid streaks in these conditions might be related to chronic iron deposition in Bruch's membrane which makes it brittle, or it might be some inherent defect in the membrane related to the defective haemoglobin molecule. In view of the wide occurrence of these abnormalities in haemoglobinopathy patients it would seem sensible for fundus examination to be carried out.

FURTHER READING

Chopra, R. (1992) Management of acute leukaemia. *Br. J. Hosp. Med.*, **48**(7), 363–75.

Davies, S. (1993) Bone marrow transplantation for sickle cell anaemia. *Br. J. Hosp. Med.*, **49**(4), 229.

Foulds, W.S. (1987) Blood is thicker than water. Some haemorrheological aspects of ocular disease. *Eye*, **1**, 343–63.

Gass, J.D.M. (1987) *Stereoscopic Atlas of Macular Disease*, 3rd edn, C. V. Mosby Company, St Louis.

Gibson, J.M., Ray Chaudhuri, P. and Rosenthal, A.R. (1983) Angioid streaks in a case of beta thalassaemia major. *Br. J. Ophthalmol.*, **67**, 29–31.

Goldberg, M.F. (1971) Classification and pathogenesis of proliferative sickle retinopathy. *Am. J. Ophthalmol.*, **71**, 649–65.

Holt, J.M. and Gordon-Smith, E.C. (1969) Retinal abnormalities in disease of the blood. *Br. J. Ophthalmol.*, **53**, 145–60.

Isaacson, P.G. (1992) Pathology of malignant lymphomas. *Current Opinion in Oncology*, **4**(5), 811–20.

Jampol, L.M., Farber, M., Rabb, M.F. and Serjeant, G. (1991) An update on techniques of photocoagulation treatment of proliferative sickle cell retinopathy. *Eye*, **5**, 260–3.

Kincaid, M.C. and Green, W.R. (1983) Ocular and orbital involvement in leukaemia. *Surv. Ophthalmol.*, **27**, 211–32.

Moriarty, B.J., Acheson, R.W., Condon, P.I. and Serjeant, G.R. (1988) Patterns of visual loss in untreated sickle cell retinopathy. *Eye*, **2**, 330–5.

Nash, G.B. (1991) Blood rheology and ischaemia. *Eye*, **5**, 151–8.

Rennie, I.G. (1992) Ocular manifestations of malignant disease. *Br. J. Hosp. Med.*, **47**(3), 185–91.

Richards, J.D.M., Singer, C.R.J. and Tobias, J.S. (1987) Management of multiple myeloma. *Br. J. Hosp. Med.*

Rogers, S. and Russel, N. (1992) Current trends in the management of chronic myeloid leukaemia. *Br. J. Hosp. Med.*, **47**(11), 816–23.

Ryan, S.J. (ed.) (1989) *Retina*, C.V. Mosby Company, St Louis.

Virella, G. (1993) Malignancies of the immune system. *Immunology Series*, **58**, 517–41.

Winfield, D.A. (1992) Multiple myeloma. *Br. J. Hosp. Med.*, **47**(1), 30–7.

12 *Optic nerve disorders*

Clinical Retinopathies. Paul M. Dodson, Jonathan M. Gibson and Erna E. Kritzinger.
Published in 1995 by Chapman & Hall, London. ISBN 0 412 35930 8

Abnormalities of the optic disc may reflect disorders of the neuroretina, the optic nerve head itself, or of the retrobulbar part of the optic nerve, behind the cribriform plate.

12.1 THE NORMAL OPTIC DISC

Four features of the optic disc, as seen ophthalmoscopically, are employed in the clinical assessment and diagnosis of optic nerve disorders. These are: colour, shape, the appearance of the neural rim and the relationship between the neural rim and optic cup.

In the normal optic disc the neural rim is pinkish in colour and its margin is clearly defined. The central part of the disc takes the form of a funnel-shaped depression, the physiological optic cup, which is almost white in appearance (Fig. 12.1). The difference in colour reflects differences in vascularity; the neural rim has a rich capillary network while the optic cup is almost avascular.

The normal optic disc is elongated in the vertical plane whereas the normal physiological cup is elongated horizontally. The diameter of the disc and the cup:disc ratio, measured along the vertical axis of the disc, vary considerably between normal individuals (ratio range 0.1 to 0.5) (Fig. 12.1). However, a cup:disc ratio 0.6 or greater is used as a clinical indicator of a possible abnormality (Fig. 12.2). As well as an increase in the size of the physiological optic cup (i.e. pathological cupping, as in glaucoma), other signs of abnormality include loss of definition of the outer margin of the disc caused, for example, by hyperaemia and swelling (as in papilloedema), or by optic disc drusen. Loss of the physiological cup, flattening and pallor of the disc occur in optic atrophy, the end-stage of many optic nerve disorders (Fig. 12.3).

12.2 GLAUCOMA

Abnormalities in the circulation or drainage of aqueous fluid result in increased intraocular pressure and the atrophy of neural tissue in the optic nerve head. These in turn lead to typical visual field defects.

A cardinal sign of glaucoma is pathological cupping, an indicator of which is a cup:disc ratio >0.6 (Fig. 12.2). This change in the relationship between the two parts of the optic cup is brought about by the atrophy of neural tissue within the neural rim, which consequently narrows. Splinter haemorrhages, indicative of the early stages of neural atrophy, may be present in the neural rim, where patches of pallor may subsequently develop. Other features of glaucomatous cupping are an enlargement or 'excavation' of the physiological optic cup, which also becomes elongated in the vertical plane. As a result, the central retinal blood vessels emerge from the enlarged cup in a hook-like manner, curving up from beneath the neural rim. The sieve-like cribriform plate may be visible at the base of the enlarged cup.

In advanced glaucoma, the neural rim may be-

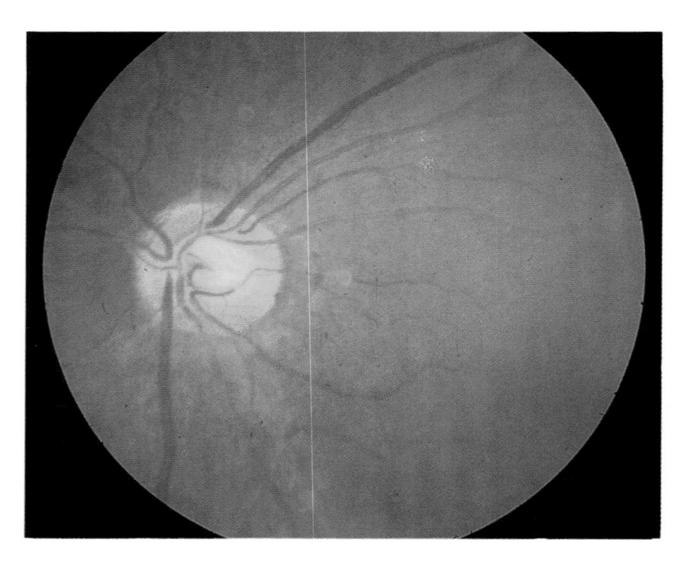

Fig. 12.1 Normal optic disc (note normal cupped disc ratio <0.5).

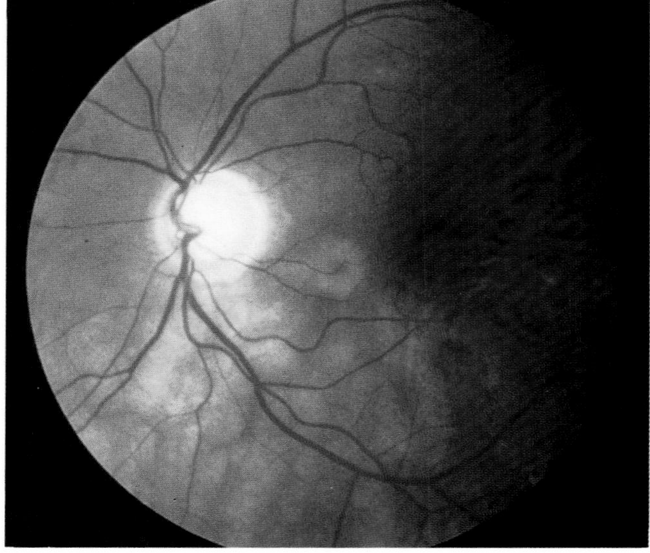

Fig. 12.2 Cupping due to glaucoma.

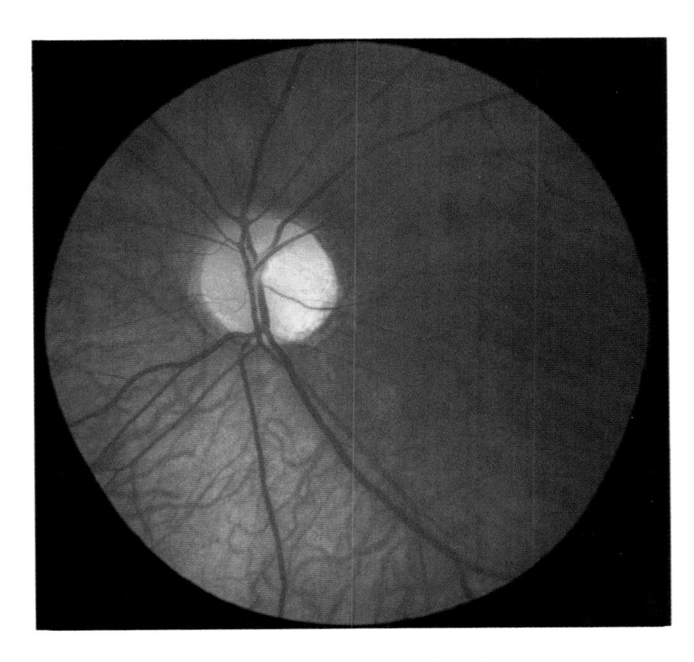

Fig. 12.3 Optic atrophy – no deep pit as in cupping.

come narrowed to such an extent that the pale optic disc, comprised almost entirely of the enlarged cup, appears spuriously flat. This may lead to a false diagnosis of optic atrophy.

Although glaucoma is frequently bilateral, it usually develops asymmetrically, and hence asymmetry of the optic discs is a common finding. A difference in the cup:disc ratio of >0.2 between the two eyes is considered significant.

There are three types of glaucoma.

12.2.1 Primary open-angle glaucoma (chronic glaucoma)

Here the abnormality arises in the drainage angle of the eye (trabecular meshwork), so that the aqueous fluid does not drain as it should. Because the consequent rise in intraocular pressure occurs very slowly, the condition is painless and the constriction of the peripheral visual field may pass unnoticed by the patient. Central vision is maintained, even at a late stage. On clinical examination, intraocular pressure is elevated and ophthalmological examination reveals cupping and asymmetry of the optic discs.

Medical assessment of patients with open-angle glaucoma seems worth while. Hypertension, usually essential, is associated, as well as diabetes mellitus, hyperlipidaemia and smoking. The exact contribution that these might make to the aetiology of open-angle glaucoma is unclear, although they would support a vascular aetiology.

The condition is initially treated medically by the administration of eye drops. These may contain either beta-adrenergic blocking agents (e.g. Timolol) which act specifically on the eye and decrease the production of aqueous fluid, or adrenergic drugs (e.g. adrenaline or adrenaline producing) to increase drainage. Alternatively, miotics (e.g. pilocarpine) may be used; they cause constriction of the ciliary body muscle which helps to open the drainage channels in the trabecular meshwork. Orally administered carbonic anhydrase inhibitors (e.g. acetazolamide) may also be used to decrease the production of aqueous fluid; this drug is unsuitable for long term treatment, however, since it may cause potassium depletion and the formation of renal stones.

If medical control is found to be unsuitable, surgical intervention at the drainage angle is required, i.e. trabeculectomy or, if carried out by laser, trabeculoplasty.

12.2.2 Primary angle-closure glaucoma (acute glaucoma)

This most commonly arises in hypermetropic eyes, in which the anterior chamber is shallow and there is a narrow drainage angle. An attack may be induced by the introduction of mydriatic eye drops, to dilate the pupil in preparation for ophthalmoscopy.

Onset is characteristically rapid, with loss of vision and pain, which may be acute and sufficiently severe to induce vomiting. Treatment has to be provided urgently: eye drops containing miotic agents (e.g. pilocarpine) are administered to constrict the pupil and carbonic anhydrase inhibitors are given intravenously in order to reduce intraocular pressure. Surgical treatment is by peripheral iridectomy or, now more commonly, by laser iridotomy.

12.2.3 Secondary glaucoma

This is brought about by some other disease process in the eye. It may result from obstruction of the drainage angle, e.g. by malignant tumours of the iris or ciliary body, by the accumulation of inflammatory exudates (hypopyon), or by the development of abnormal blood vessels on the iris (rubeosis); the latter occurs, for example, in association with diabetic retinopathy or central retinal vein occlusion. Although laser retinal panphotocoagulation can be used to inhibit neovascularization, the condition (neovascular glaucoma) is difficult to treat once the vessels have developed, and invariably progresses to a painful, blind eye. Occlusion of the pupil may be brought about by inflammatory conditions, such as iritis, which causes the iris to adhere to the lens with the formation of posterior synechiae.

12.3 OPTIC NEUROPATHY AND OPTIC NEURITIS

These terms refer to disorders of the optic nerve, or the blood vessels that supply it. The term optic neuropathy is used to refer to disorders involving ischaemia or toxicity, and optic neuritis for demyelinating or inflammatory conditions. Ophthalmoscopic features differ according to the region of the optic nerve that is affected, and the stage of the disorder; changes affecting the optic disc are characterized as papillopathy or papillitis (Fig. 12.4), with progression to optic atrophy.

The disorders that affect the anterior visual pathways and optic nerve are numerous. The differential diagnosis of optic neuropathy and neuritis comprises:

Demyelination:
- idiopathic
- multiple sclerosis
- encephalomyelitis

Vascular:
- ischaemic optic neuropathy
- giant cell arteritis
- hypertension
- diabetes mellitus
- systemic lupus erythematosus
- syphilis

Compressive:
- orbital tumour
- meningioma
- pituitary adenoma
- parasellar lesions
- aneurysms

Infiltrative:
- carcinoma
- lymphoma
- Tolosa-Hunt syndrome
- orbital pseudotumour

Inflammatory:
- granulomatous
- pyogenic

Hereditary:
- Leber's optic neuropathy
- spinocerebellar degeneration

Toxic:
- nutritional
- tobacco
- alcohol
- drugs, e.g. ethambutol, isoniazid, streptomycin

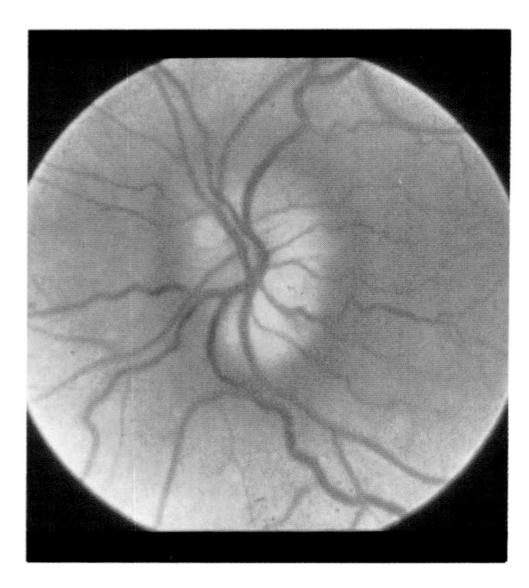

Fig. 12.4 Changes in the optic disc suggestive of papillitis or papillopathy.

The most common in clinical practice include demyelinating, vascular and compressive lesions.

12.3.1 Optic neuropathy

(a) ISCHAEMIC OPTIC NEUROPATHY

This is a disorder associated with damage to the posterior ciliary arterial supply to the optic nerve head. It is characterized by sudden loss of vision (altitudinal defect or central scotoma) brought about by vascular occlusion. Although the ocular symptoms may present unilaterally, the fellow eye invariably becomes affected. On ophthalmoscopic examination, the optic disc appears pale and swollen and the retinal vessels are attenuated (Fig. 12.5).

Table 12.1 shows the common underlying medical conditions. Approximately 5–30% of patients presenting with ischaemic optic neuropathy will have giant cell arteritis (arteric form) (Section 9.11), but a significant proportion will have underlying major cardiovascular risk factors, e.g. diabetes mellitus and hypertension and hyperlipidaemia with no evidence of arteritis (non-arteritic form). The disease process predominantly affects an elderly population and thus few studies are available on a cross-sectional basis with a comparison group. Recent studies on

Table 12.1 Medical conditions underlying anterior ischaemic optic neuropathy

	% of patients	*(n)*
Giant cell arteritis	5.7	(12)
Non-Arteritic Form		
Hypertension	34	(72)
Idiopathic	27	(57)
Presumed atherosclerosis	14	(29)
Hypertension and diabetes mellitus	7	(14)
Migraine	2	(4)

(Data from study of 217 patients)

long-term follow-up suggest that morbidity and mortality from stroke and myocardial infarction are significantly increased. After 5 years of follow-up, 50% of patients showed few changes in the affected eye, whereas 24% had involvement of the second eye (mean time 2.9 years). Treatment to prevent this recurrence is unclear. It is our policy to treat underlying risk factors with the addition of anti-platelet drugs in order to prevent deterioration in the fellow eye.

The disease may also occur in a retrobulbar form with sudden loss of vision. However, because the retrobulbar portion of the optic nerve is primarily affected, the optic disc appears normal in the acute phase, with subsequent progression to primary optic atrophy.

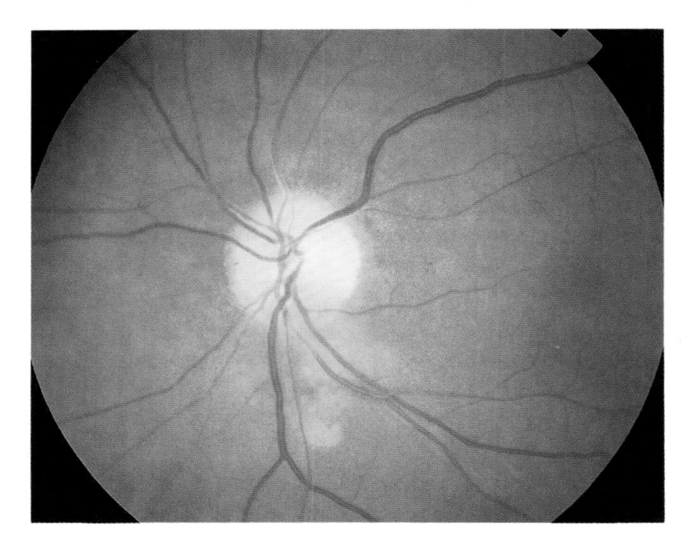

Fig. 12.5 Changes in the optic disc suggestive of ischaemic optic neuropathy.

(b) OPTIC NEURITIS

This is a common cause of sudden visual impairment in young adults. The differential diagnosis is included in Section 12.3. A history and neuro-ophthalmological examination should be helpful in distinguishing the many causes.

Although the conditions listed in Section 12.3 may affect any part of the optic nerve, particular disorders show a regional predilection, for example, multiple sclerosis tends to affect the retrobulbar portion of the optic nerve.

12.3.2 Multiple sclerosis

This may present with retrobulbar neuritis in which there is pain above or behind the eye, aggravated by movement, particularly upward. It is uniocular in 90% of patients. Central visual loss follows over several days, with pain subsiding when visual loss is greatest. Other symptoms may occur:

- central visual loss (absolute central scotoma);
- loss of subdued colours (particularly red–green);
- poor toleration of bright light;
- difficulty in judging distances;
- light flashes (phosphenes) on eye;
- afferent pupillary defect.

Although total blindness may occur, more usually the visual deficit ranges from 6/18 to 6/60. Recovery occurs in 90% of patients within 4–6 weeks.

In the acute phase of retrobulbar neuritis the optic disc may be normal. In papillitis, the optic disc is swollen and hyperaemic in the acute phase and splinter haemorrhages may be present (Fig. 12.4). Optic disc pallor and atrophy will develop on long-term follow-up in 70% of patients, irrespective of the site of the lesion in the optic nerve.

12.3.3 Pathology

The symptomatic lesion is usually a single plaque, usually occurring in the orbital or intra-canalicular portion of the optic nerve. These plaques consist of zones of myelin loss, due to migration of phagocytic macrophages.

12.3.4 Diagnosis

Diagnosis can often be made on the clinical history and examination. Support is added by spontaneous recovery in the majority of patients. The routine investigations on patients with optic neuropathy are:

History:
- smoking;
- alcohol;
- family history.

Examination:
- visual loss;
- optic disc appearance;
- afferent pupillary defect.

Investigations:
- full blood count (MCV);
- ESR;
- blood glucose, liver function tests (γGT);
- syphilitic serology;
- vitamin B12/B1 estimates;
- CAT scan – brain, orbit, optic nerves;
- MRI scan – demonstration of plaques;
- visual evoked potential (VER);
- electroretinography (ERG);
- lumbar puncture (oligoclonal bands).

The visual evoked potential is a valuable test. The standard pattern-reversal in this technique demonstrates delay and alterations in amplitude in various components (P100), but these changes are not diagnostic.

CAT scanning is of limited value in the diagnosis of retrobulbar neuritis but is helpful in excluding structural or compressive lesions (e.g. optic nerve meningioma). Cranial CT may show plaques as low attenuated areas but modern MRI scanning is more sensitive in this respect, picking up plaques in 60% of patients presenting with isolated optic neuritis.

The presence of oligoclonal bands in the CSF obtained from lumbar puncture may aid diagnosis.

12.3.5 Follow-up and treatment

The risk of developing multiple sclerosis following an episode of optic neuritis is variable. Certain features increase the risk:

- female sex;
- aged >20 years;
- bilateral optic neuritis;
- oligoclonal bands in CSF;
- retinal perivascular sheathing;
- cerebral white matter lesions on MRI scanning;
- certain HLA subtypes.

It must be stressed that one clinical lesion does not permit a diagnosis of MS: clinical follow-up is essential to ascertain the recurrence of neurological involvement essential to the diagnosis. The number of adult patients who will subsequently develop MS after an episode of optic neuritis varies from 30–57% according to country, study, and length of follow-up. The rate in children after bilateral optic neuritis is reported to be lower than adults, between 5 and 17%.

Many patients with optic neuritis will make a full spontaneous recovery. Numerous anecdotal reports have suggested that steroids and corticotrophin are effective, but randomized trials have not demonstrated benefit, primarily because of small sample size.

Despite this, most clinicians still prescribe steroids as treatment for acute optic neuritis to hasten improvement in visual acuity. A recent large multicentre trial has investigated various treatment protocols in terms of visual recovery and recurrence rate of optic neuritis over a six-month period. This concluded that intravenous methyl prednisolone followed by oral prednisolone speeds the recovery of visual loss and results in better visual outcome. Of concern, oral prednisolone alone appeared ineffective and increased the risk of new episodes of optic neuritis.

There is agreement from this and other studies that the use of steroids may hasten the degree of recovery finally attained. Traditionally, ACTH injections have been favoured although with little supporting data. Intravenous methyl prednisolone may become the treatment of choice.

12.4 LEBER'S HEREDITARY OPTIC NEUROPATHY

Multiple sclerosis must be distinguished from this condition which presents with bilateral acute retrobulbar neuritis. It was thought to have a recessive inheritance, with sex linking. More recent studies have suggested it is in fact a mitochondrial cytopathy, associated with deficiency of at least one mitochondrial enzyme.

It is characterized by progressive optic atrophy, usually in males, commencing about the twentieth year. There is commonly a central scotoma, either relative or absolute, which is permanent. During the acute phase, ophthalmoscopy may reveal swelling of the nerve fibre layer, but later there is pallor of the temporal half of the optic disc and atrophy.

12.5 TOBACCO AND ALCOHOL USE AND VITAMIN DEFICIENCY

This optic neuropathy is usually bilateral, painless and progressive. The degree of visual loss and optic disc pallor may be indistinguishable from other causes of optic neuropathy.

The combination of alcohol, tobacco and malnutrition (Vitamin B12 and B1 deficiencies) may have an additive effect on the optic nerve. Although the exact mechanism is not clear, some reports have suggested a role for accumulation of cyanide and its metabolic products. Abstinence from alcohol and smoking, in combination with vitamin supplementation, may lead to regression and improvement of symptoms.

12.6 PAPILLOEDEMA

This condition is characterized by swelling and hyperaemia of the optic nerve head. The swelling is thought to be brought about by an accumulation of axoplasm, due to a disturbance in the normal pattern of flow caused by raised intracranial pressure. The retinovascular circulation is also impeded.

Papilloedema therefore invariably signifies serious underlying pathology such as a space-occupying lesion in the brain (e.g. tumour, haemorrhage); other causes include toxicity due to drugs (e.g. long-term systemic steroids) or poisons (e.g. lead). To summarize, the causes of a swollen optic disc are:

- raised intracranial pressure (papilloedema);
- optic neuritis;
- ischaemic optic neuropathy;
- malignant hypertension;
- central vein occlusion;
- intraorbital lesions and exophthalmos;
- infiltration (e.g. leukaemia, sarcoid);
- drugs and toxins (e.g. chloramphenicol, lead);
- associated with increased cerebrospinal fluid protein (Guillain-Barré syndrome and spinal cord lesions);
- anaemia, polycythaemia;
- chronic respiratory failure;
- hypoparathyroidism, hypoadrenalism.

Papilloedema usually occurs bilaterally. The causes of papilloedema can, for practical purposes, be divided according to the CAT scan result:

Negative CAT scan:
- benign intracranial hypertension;
- other causes of a swollen disc (see above).

Positive CAT scan:
- space occupying lesions (neoplasms, abscess, cysts);
- hydrocephalus;
- vascular lesions (haemorrhage: parenchymal, subarachnoid and infarct);
- venous obstructions (cerebral venous thrombosis, Behçet's disease).

The ophthalmoscopic appearance of the optic disc varies at different stages of this disorder. Initially the disc is swollen and its margin is indistinct (Fig. 12.6). As the swelling progresses, the physiological cup is

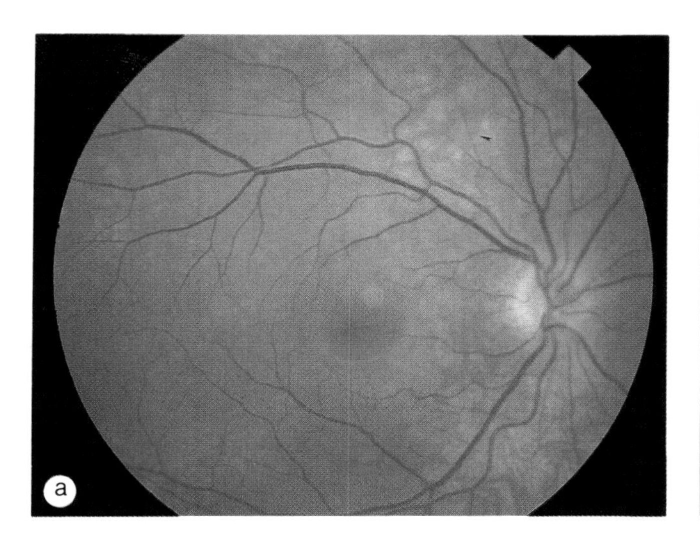

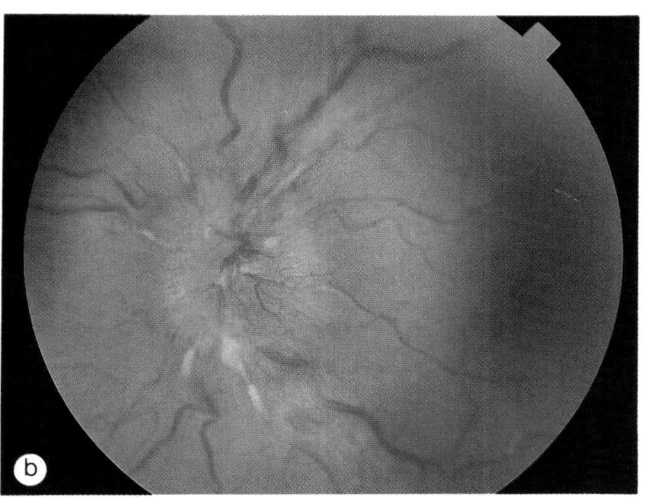

Fig. 12.6 Papilloedema. (a) Early papilloedema with nasal disc swelling. (b) Late stage papilloedema.

obliterated and the disc becomes elevated, arriving at the characteristic 'champagne cork' appearance. The disc is also hyperaemic due to capillary dilatation; splinter haemorrhages may be present. Loss of venous pulsation may be an early sign owing to congestion of the retinal veins, but this sign can occur in 25% of normal individuals. On fundus fluorescein angiography, capillaries on the optic disc are seen to be dilated and leak dye profusely (Fig. 12.7).

Visual acuity usually remains normal or is only slightly affected during the initial stages of the development of papilloedema; the blind spot may be slightly enlarged. These are important clinical clues, and help to distinguish papilloedema from other causes of swelling of the optic disc, such as papillopathy and papillitis, which often present with visual loss.

Since papilloedema is a non-specific, non-localizing sign of raised intracranial pressure, its presence is an indication for urgent referral and neurological investigation. However, it is important to distinguish papilloedema caused by raised intracranial pressure from other conditions in which the optic disc similarly appears hyperaemic and swollen (e.g. pseudopapilloedema; accelerated hypertension), so that patients are spared unnecessary neurological examination.

Papilloedema progresses to secondary optic atrophy. However, in the Foster–Kennedy syndrome, a tumour of the frontal lobe gives rise to primary optic atrophy due to direct pressure of the tumour on the optic nerve, whereas the disc in the fellow eye shows papilloedema caused by raised intracranial pressure.

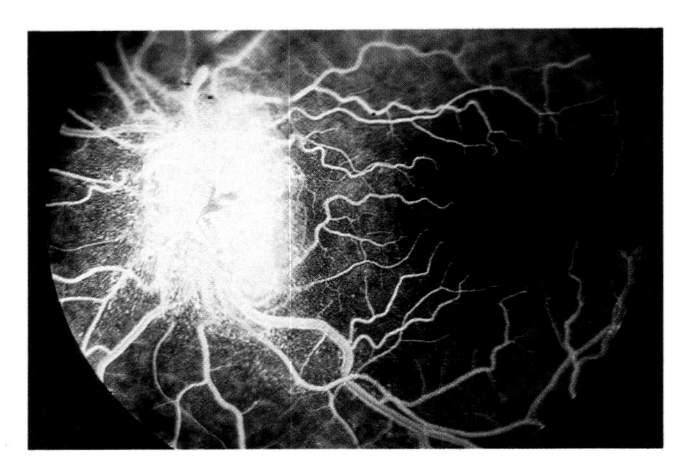

Fig. 12.7 A fluorescein angiogram of papilloedema showing a profuse leakage around the optic disc.

12.7 PSEUDOPAPILLOEDEMA

This is the name given to conditions in which the optic disc is swollen and hyperaemic, tending to mimic papilloedema from which they must be differentiated. They include optic disc drusen (Fig. 12.8a), hypermetropia, medullated nerve fibres (Fig. 12.8b) and diabetic papillopathy. Papilloedema also arises in patients with accelerated hypertension, and has to be distinguished from other causes.

12.7.1 Optic disc drusen (Fig. 12.8(a))

The drusen take the form of swellings on the optic disc. They are thought to be manifestations of a congenital abnormality in which there is a reduction in the size of the cribriform plate, inhibiting axonal flow which predisposes to axonal degeneration and the accumulation of debris on the disc.

The condition is transmitted as a dominant trait

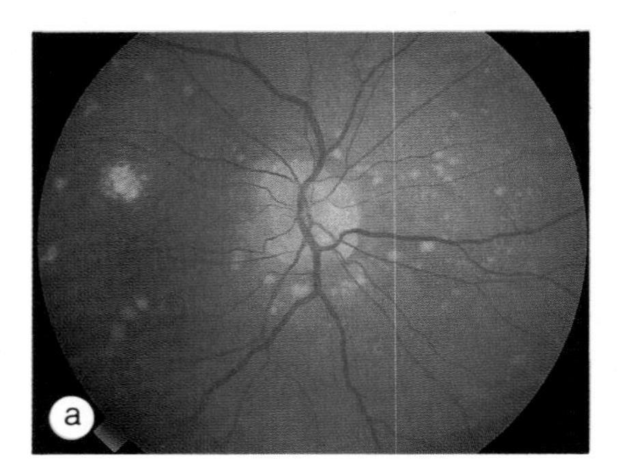

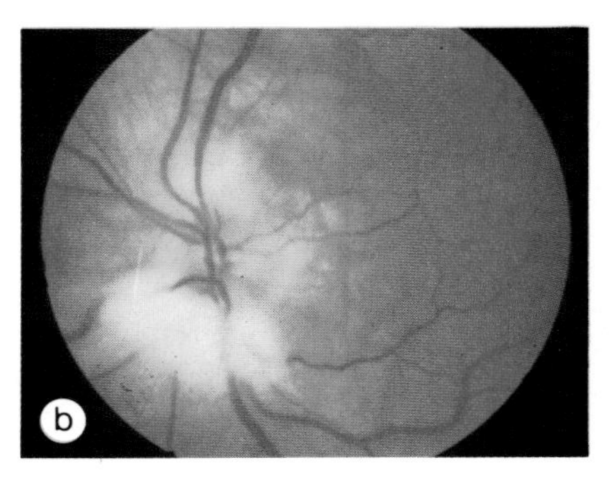

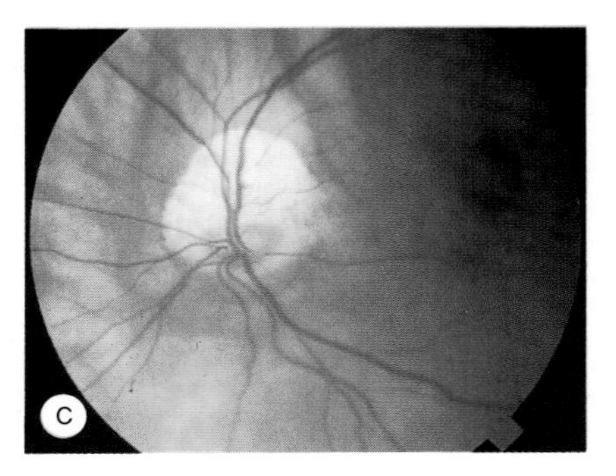

Fig. 12.8 Pseudopapilloedema. (a) Optic disc drusen. (b) Medullated nerve fibres. (c) Tilted optic disc.

with incomplete penetrance; only white races are affected (1% of the population). Drusen generally occur bilaterally (70%).

During childhood, the drusen generally remain 'buried' within the substance of the optic nerve head, although they may cause the margin of the disc to become indistinct. In adolescence and early adult life the drusen present as single or multiple glistening, semi-translucent swellings; these may coalesce to give the disc a yellow-pink appearance. The disc tends to become enlarged and the physiological cup obliterated (cf. papilloedema). There may be splinter haemorrhages on the surface of the disc, and subretinal haemorrhages around its margin.

Fundus fluorescein angiography has an important role to play in differential diagnosis. Drusen pathognomonically show autofluorescence before injection of the dye and are hyperfluorescent during the angiogram. They do not leak dye, or only minimally so (cf. papilloedema). Large drusen become calcified and may show up on computerized tomography or ultrasonography.

Optic disc drusen are usually asymptomatic, although visual acuity may be affected by subretinal haemorrhage and scarring. Compression of the nerve fibres may produce visual field defects. Optic disc drusen should not be confused with retinal drusen, an age-related abnormality.

12.7.2 Hypermetropia (Fig. 12.9)

The hypermetropic eye has a smaller axial length than normal, and a small optic disc. The physiological optic cup is reduced in size in relation to the neural rim, so that the disc appears hyperaemic and spuriously swollen.

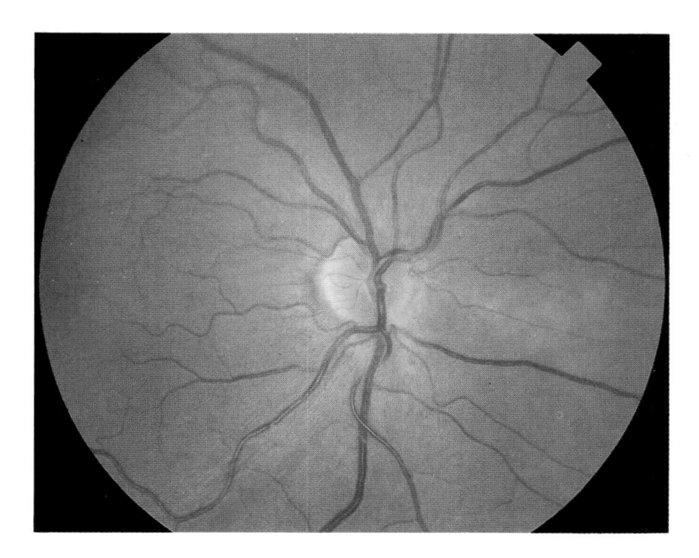

Fig. 12.9 Hypermetropic optic disc.

Features that help to distinguish hypermetropia from true papilloedema are:

- capillaries on the optic disc are not dilated and fundus fluorescein angiography shows that they do not leak dye;
- the central retinal vessels crowd the centre of the small disc; spontaneous venous pulsation is not affected;
- near visual acuity is reduced and the refractive error requires correction with spectacles.

The small size of the eye produces a narrow anterior chamber, predisposing to acute narrow-angle glaucoma. This is particularly likely to arise in the elderly, when the lens increases in size and becomes cataractous.

12.7.3 Diabetic papillopathy

Juvenile onset diabetics are liable to develop this condition during the second or third decade of life. The changes are thought to represent a form of ischaemic papillopathy.

On ophthalmoscopy, the optic disc may be hyperaemic and swollen and its margin indistinct. In severe cases the appearance of the optic disc is similar to that of classic papilloedema.

Clearly, the systemic associations of diabetes mellitus are an important clue to differential diagnosis. Diabetic retinopathy, when present, is limited in extent. Visual loss ranges from mild to moderate in degree, and is frequently transient. It recovers within 6 months of the onset of symptoms, although swelling of the optic disc may take rather longer (up to a year) to resolve; there may be mild secondary optic atrophy. There is, however, no correlation between the changes seen ophthalmoscopically and the eventual visual outcome.

12.8 ACCELERATED HYPERTENSION

The retinal features that characterize accelerated hypertension include papilloedema. The differentiation between this and papilloedema caused by raised intracranial pressure is assisted by the identification of other hypertensive features, visible on ophthalmoscopy (Chapter 5). It is thought that the optic nerve head swelling in accelerated hypertension is commonly due to ischaemic optic neuritis.

12.9 OPTIC ATROPHY

Optic atrophy, characterized by a pale, flat optic disc (Fig. 12.3) and reduced visual acuity, are the result of pathological processes occurring at some point along the course of the optic nerve. Minor degrees of pallor are prey to subjective interpretation. Thus, if disc pallor is suspected, evidence of optic nerve dysfunction should be sought. Clinically this involves changes in visual acuity, afferent pupillary defects, and abnormalities in visual evoked responses. The underlying disorders may be congenital or acquired. Causes of optic atrophy may be summarized:

Primary causes:
- optic neuritis;
- ischaemic optic neuropathy;
- toxins and drugs (e.g. tobacco, ethambutol);
- infections (e.g. herpes zoster, syphilis);
- optic nerve tumour (glioma, sheath meningioma);
- optic nerve compression (e.g. pituitary tumours, meningioma, aneurysm, orbital lesions);
- trauma;
- metabolic (vitamin deficiency);
- hereditary (Leber's optic atrophy and other neurodegenerative disorders).

Secondary causes:
- follows papilloedema

Consecutive causes:
- follows primary retinal disease (e.g. retinitis pigmentosa, choroiditis and glaucoma).

12.9.1 Primary optic atrophy

This arises when the retrobulbar portion of the optic nerve is affected following retrobulbar neuritis or retrobulbar neuropathy.

The optic disc is pale and has a well-defined margin; pallor may be more pronounced on the temporal side of the disc. The neural rim has atrophied and the physiological optic cup is lost, resulting in flattening of the disc.

12.9.2 Secondary optic atrophy

This follows long-standing swelling of the disc. Aetiological factors include papillitis, the ischaemic papillopathies, and papilloedema.

On ophthalmoscopy, the disc is pale and swollen, the physiological cup may be partly or wholly filled in, and the margin of the disc is poorly defined.

12.9.3 Consecutive optic atrophy

This arises as a result of retinal disease, such as retinitis pigmentosa.

Extensive investigation is usually necessary unless there is marked retinal disease or a previously known cause of papilloedema. Tests performed will be as for optic neuropathy (Section 12.3.4).

FURTHER READING

Beck, R.W., Cleary, P.A., Malcolm, M. *et al.* (1992) A randomised, controlled trial of corticosteroids in the treatment of acute optic neuritis. *New Eng. J. Med.*, **366**(a), 581–8.

Beri, M., Klugman, M.R., Kohler, J.A. and Hayreh, S.S. (1987) Anterior ischaemic optic neuropathy: incidence of bilaterality and various influencing factors. *J. Ophthalmology*, **94**, 1020–8.

Clough, C.G. and Dodson, P.M. (1988) Medical aspects of optic nerve disorders. *Update*, 1099–105.

Francis, D.A. (1991) Demyelinating optic neuritis: clinical features and differential diagnosis. *Br. J. Hosp. Med.*, **45**, 376–9.

Katz, J. and Sommer, J.D. (1988) Risk factors for primary open angle glaucoma. *Am. J. Prev. Med.*, **4**, 110–4.

Kritzinger, E.E. and Beaumont, H.M. (1987) *A Colour Atlas of Optic Disc Abnormalities*, Wolfe Medical Publications Ltd, London.

Leber's optic neuropathy (leading article) (1980) *Br. Med. J.*, **I**, 1097–8.

Repka, M.X. *et al.* (1983) *Am. J. Ophthalmol.*, **96**, 478–83.

Wilson, M.R., Hertzmark, E., Walker, A.M. *et al.* (1987) A case-control study of risk factors in open angle glaucoma. *Arch. Ophthalmol.*, **105**, 1066–71.

Sawle, G.V., James, C.B. and Ross-Russell, R.W. (1990) The natural history of non-arteritic anterior ischaemic optic neuropathy. *J. of Neurology, Neurosurgery and Psychiatry*, **53**(10), 830–3.

Talks, S.J., Chong, N.H., Jones, A. *et al.* (1994) Fibrinogen, cholesterol and smoking as risk factors for non-arteritic, anterior ischaemic optic neuropathy. *Eye* (submitted).

13 Other retinopathies

Clinical Retinopathies. Paul M. Dodson, Jonathan M. Gibson and Erna E. Kritzinger.
Published in 1995 by Chapman & Hall, London. ISBN 0 412 35930 8

13.1 INTRODUCTION

This chapter will deal with other retinopathies and retinal changes which may be encountered in clinical practice, although some are rare. These include retinitis pigmentosa, angioid streaks, tumours, and the phakomatoses. Other forms of choroidopathy and retinopathies are included.

13.2 TUMOURS

The most common malignant tumours affecting the eye are metastases and primary tumours situated in other viscera and endocrine glands. Secondary tumours are most common from the breast in females and from bronchogenic carcinoma in males. Both eyes are involved in 20% of cases.

They normally present as choroidal metastases, appearing as pale cream-coloured masses. The overlying retina may have a mottled 'salt and pepper' appearance due to changes in the retinal pigment epithelium (Fig. 13.1).

13.2.1 Choroidal melanoma

This tumour is the commonest primary intraocular malignancy occuring in adults (Fig. 13.2). Tumours are either diffuse or circumscribed in form, the diffuse variety being the more invasive of the two with a worse prognosis. They arise in the uveal tissue, most frequently in the choroid (80%). The condition is generally unilateral occurring in patients over 50 years of age at the time of presentation. The highly malignant nature of the choroidal melanoma may cause the patient to present with metastases particularly in the liver or the lungs. Reduced visual acuity and visual field defects are common early findings. Tumours in the posterior part of the eye are generally painless, but extension of the tumour may occur intracranially either via the subarachnoid space, or along the optic nerve.

13.2.2 Melanocytoma

This is a benign, pigmented tumour, which arises from dendritic melanocytes (Fig. 13.3). It is a form of uveal naevus and occurs where there are cell rests of primitive uveal melanocytes. It most commonly occurs on the optic disc, and is most frequent in pigmented racial groups.

Visual acuity is usually normal and the condition is often discovered at routine eye examination. The tumour is usually stationary but in a small percentage it may slowly increase in size over a timespan of 5 to 20 years.

13.2.3 Phakomatoses

The term phakomatoses originates from the Greek word 'phakos' meaning birthmark. It is used to describe a group of congenital, ectodermal dysplasias, particularly combining hamartomas. These are characterized by abnormalities of the nervous system, skin, eyes, and other organs. Hamartomas are

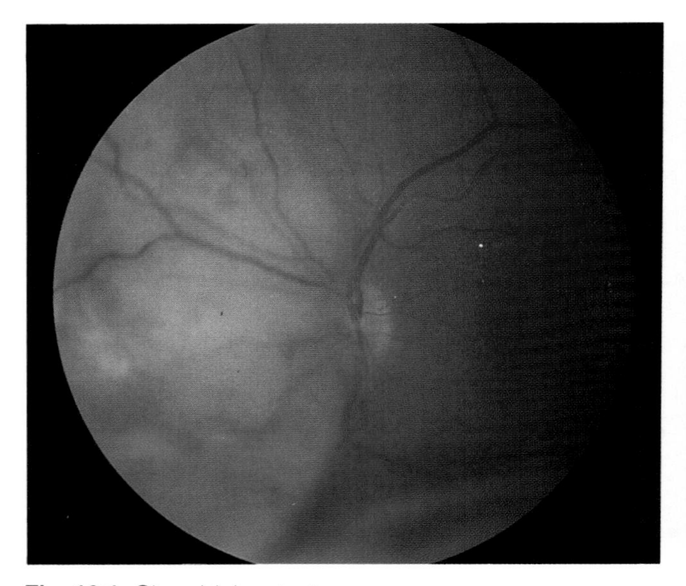

Fig. 13.1 Choroidal metastases.

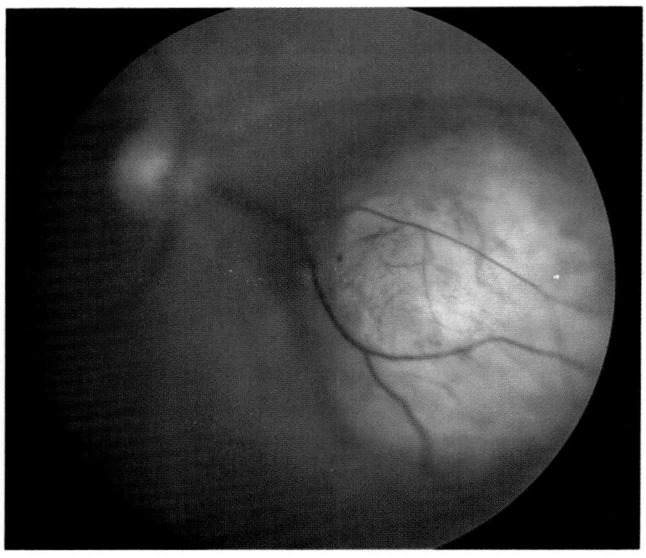

Fig. 13.2 Choroidal melanoma.

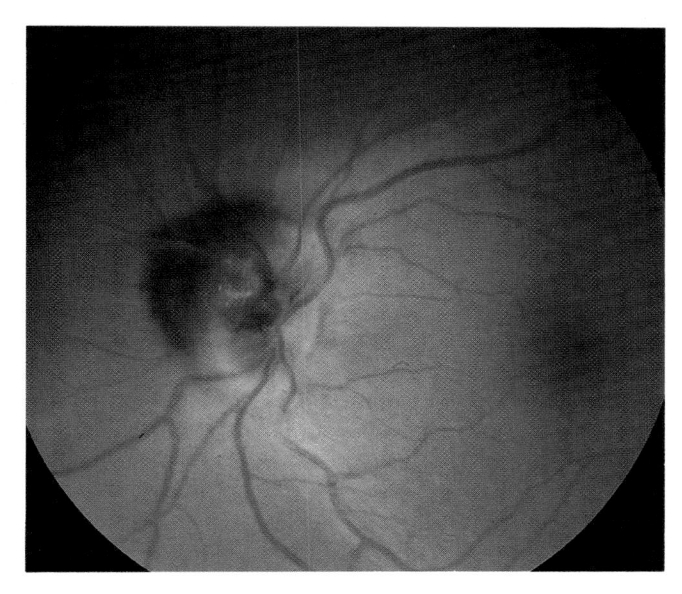

Fig. 13.3 Melanocytoma.

tumour-like malformations which are the outcome of defective maturation within an organ primordium: hyperplasia or over-development. It results in disorganization of this structure, such that the hamartomas contain tissues normal for the site in which they occur, but in a disorganized fashion. Hamartomas of the eye are of three types. The first arise as a result of defective development of supporting elements (astrocytes) and retinal nerve fibre layer. The second involves the retinal pigment epithelium and the third type affects blood vessels of the optic disc and retina. There are five different syndromes currently recognized:

- neurofibromatosis (Von Recklinghausen's disease);
- tuberous sclerosis (Bourneville's disease);
- cerebelloretinal haemangioblastomatosis (Von Hippel–Lindau disease);
- encephalotrigeminal angiomatosis (Sturge–Weber syndrome;
- ataxia telangiectasia (Louis–Bar syndrome).

The types of hamartomas will now be briefly described.

(a) ASTROCYTIC HAMARTOMA

This derives from astrocytes in the optic nerve head and nerve fibre layer of the retina, where it is associated with the ganglion cells. It frequently presents bilaterally and may also be multiple. Astrocytic hamartomas form a tumour-like mask, usually situated near or on the optic disc, but may also present in the peripheral retina. The mature state has a number of striking characteristics, forming a mulberry-like white reflective mass which may become calcified. They are richly vascular and blood vessels can often be seen coursing through their substance. There are important associations with tuberous sclerosis and neurofibromatosis, both of which are transmitted as an autosomal dominant trait. Tuberous sclerosis (Bourneville's disease) is characterized by the classical triad of adenoma sebaceum, mental deficiency and epilepsy, with hamartomas arising in the brain and subungual fibromas. Ocular astrocytic hamartomas occur in approximately 50% of cases with tuberous sclerosis.

In neurofibromatosis (Von Recklinghausen's disease) pigmented skin lesions, known as *café au lait* spots (Fig. 13.4) and multiple neurofibromas (Fig. 13.5) are usually frequent. Flexiform neuromas and multiple fibromas may occur in the nerves and skin

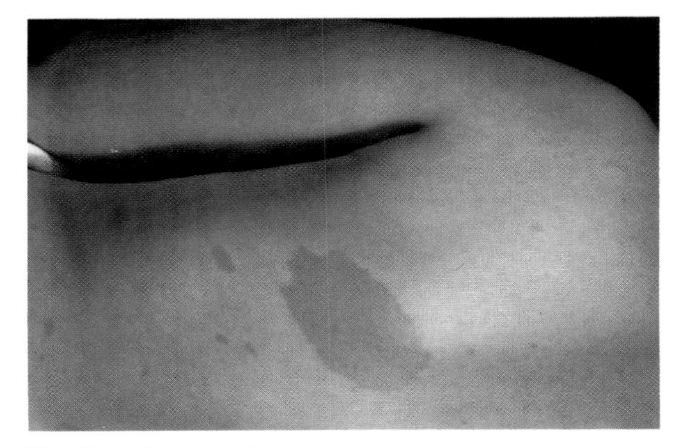

Fig. 13.4 *Café au lait* spots.

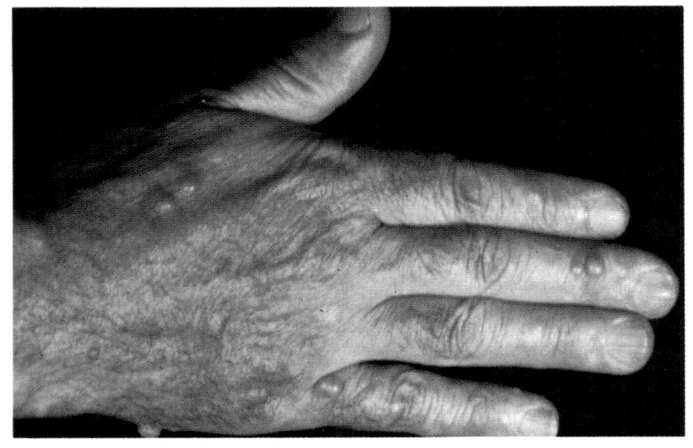

Fig. 13.5 Multiple neurofibromatosis.

respectively. Ocular manifestations include ptosis caused by plexiform neuroma of the eyelid as well as papilloedema and optic atrophy. Myelination of the optic disc also occurs more frequently in cases of neurofibromatosis (Fig. 13.6).

(b) CAPILLARY HAEMANGIOMA

This is a rare condition. Capillary haemangiomas are hamartomas composed of dilated blood vessels which may be found either on the optic disc or in the peripheral retina. Patients with retinal haemangiomas are said to have Von Hippel's disease. Approximately half of these patients may have haemangioblastomas of the cerebellum and other viscera, this latter combination being known as Von Hippel–Lindau disease. The other organ particularly affected is the kidney, which may lead to polycythaemia. The disease is transmitted as an autosomal dominant trait with variable penetrance.

The most obvious visible sign of a retinal angioma in the peripheral fundus is a dilated and tortuous feeding artery and a draining vein (Fig. 13.7). Increase in size and fluid exudation may lead to the exaggerated macular response or an extensive exudative retinal detachment.

(c) CAVERNOUS HAEMANGIOMA

This is a rare hamartoma and involves the retinal venous system. It consists of clusters of thinned wall saccular venous aneurysms similar to bunches of grapes. Capillary or cavernous haemangiomas may also occur in the skin of the face in the dermatome supplied by the trigeminal nerve (Fig. 13.8). A combination with intracranial haemangiomas makes up the encephalotrigeminal angiomatosis (Sturge–Weber syndrome). Coral-like calcification of the underlying cerebral cortex may occur along with epilepsy and mental retardation. The typical facial lesion is the port wine stain.

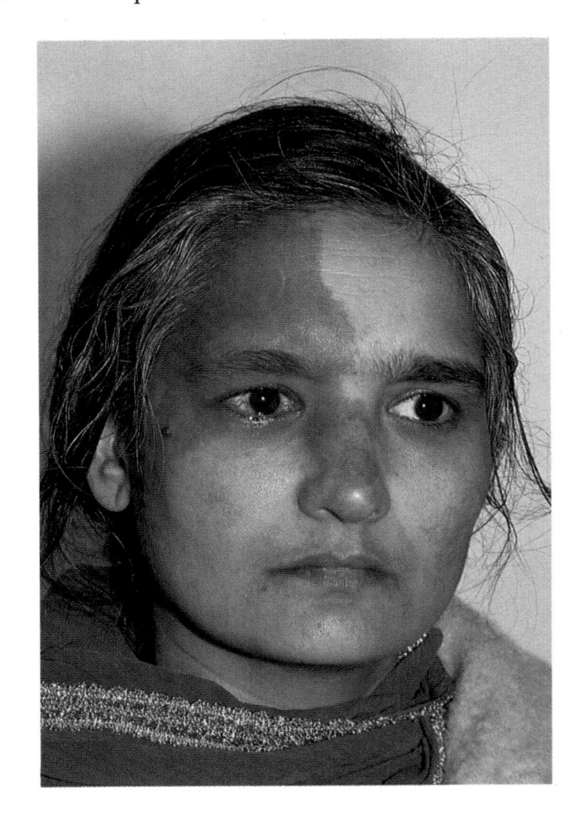

Fig. 13.8 Sturge Weber 'port wine stain'.

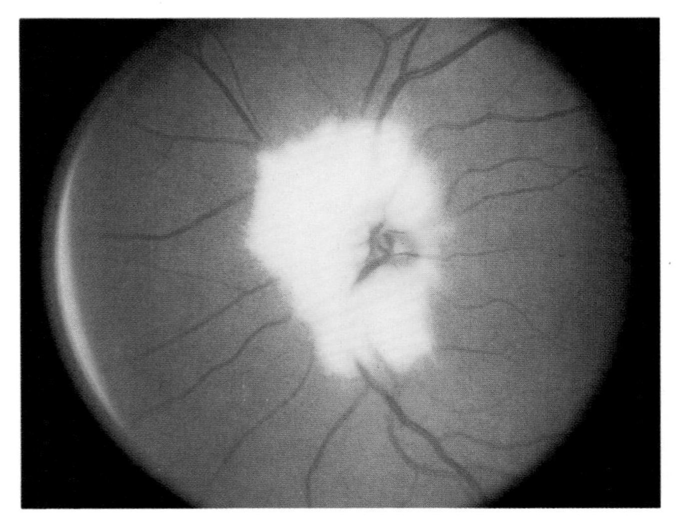

Fig. 13.6 Myelination of the optic disc in neurofibromatosis.

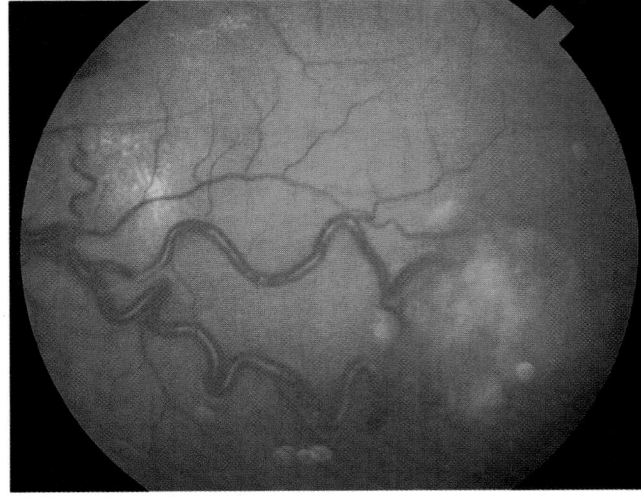

Fig. 13.7 Peripheral retinal angioma in Von-Hippel-Lindau disease.

(d) HEREDITARY HAEMORRHAGIC TELANGIECTASIA (RENDU–OSLER–WEBER DISEASE)

This is an uncommon inherited disorder of blood vessels manifested by haemorrhage from telangiectasia of the skin, mucous membranes and viscera. It occurs as an autosomal dominant trait with complete penetrance, with equal sex contribution. Haemorrhage or vascular malformation may occur in the upper gastrointestinal and respiratory tracts, as well as in the liver, urinary tract, respiratory tract, adrenal gland and central nervous system. Ocular changes are not uncommon. Retinal lesions include telangiectasic tufts and patches adjacent to the retinal arteries or veins. Specific changes include tortuosity and segmental dilatations of the retinal veins, retinal haemorrhages and neovascularization of the retina and the optic disc. Vitreous haemorrhage may occur.

13.3 ANGIOIDS

Angioid streaks arise as a result of breaks in Bruch's membrane, which are due to defects in elastic and collagen tissue. They appear as grey-brown streaks which seem to arise from the optic disc (Fig. 13.9). They are irregular in outline and lie beneath the retinal vessels. Affected eyes are vulnerable to subretinal neovascularization, with subsequent haemorrhage and scarring which may permanently impair vision.

Angioid streaks may occur as an isolated ocular finding in 50% of cases, but should alert the clinician to the possibility of an associated systemic disease:

- pseudoxanthoma elasticum;
- Ehler's–Danlos syndrome;
- Gronblad–Strandberg syndrome;
- acromegaly;
- Paget's disease;
- sickle cell anaemia;
- hypercalcaemia;
- lead poisoning;
- idiopathic thrombocytopenic purpura.

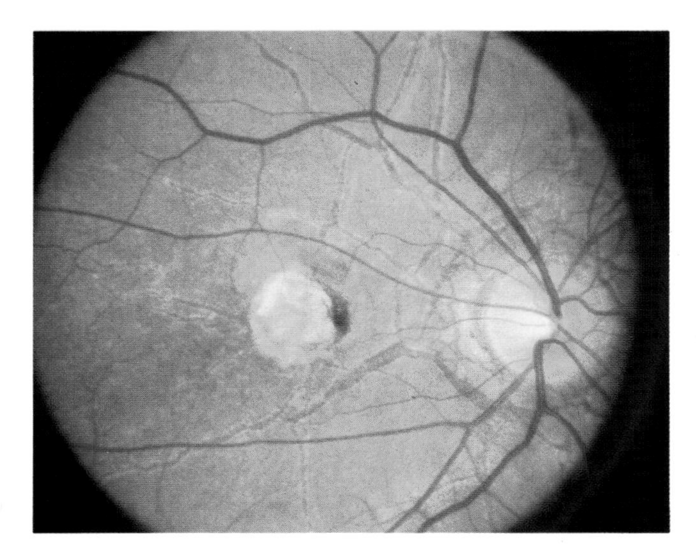

Fig. 13.9 Angioid streaks.

13.3.1 Ophthalmoscopy

Angioid streaks have irregular width and outline. They radiate from an area of peripapillary atrophy and branch in a manner similar to that of the retinal vessels. There may be macular involvement with retinal haemorrhage or scar formation. The peripheral fundus may show a stippled pigmentary change and optic disc drusen may be an associated finding.

13.3.2 Clinical course

The ocular changes are slowly progressive and only present once haemorrhage occurs as a result of retinal destruction. Glaucoma as well as retinal detachment and exophthalmos may occur. The complications of macular involvement and haemorrhage into the macular area, most often occur during the fourth decade of life. Although the condition is generally progressive, plateaus are reached at 55–60 years of age, after which vision remains fairly stable.

13.3.3 Associated medical conditions

(a) PSEUDOXANTHOMA ELASTICUM (Fig. 13.10)

This is a systemic disorder in which the primary defect is production of abnormal elastic fibres. The manifestations of the disease are seen in the skin, cardiovascular system, and the eyes. The defects in the skin elasticity are characterized by rolls of soft, wrinkled, yellow xanthoma-like skin lesions, which are most commonly found in the neck (described like chicken fat). Other skin areas frequently involved include the skin creases of the limbs, axillae and groin and the periumbilical region.

Abnormalities of other elastic tissues, for example in the vascular system, may lead to serious complications from haemorrhage and peripheral vascular disease. Complications include gastrointestinal haemorrhage, premature coronary atherosclerosis, subarachnoid and intracerebral haemorrhage, and progressive intellectual deterioration. Abnormalities of the elastic tissues of the vascular system and hypertension, often due to renal artery narrowing, are the two basic pathological mechanisms responsible for marked vascular disease.

(b) EHLER'S–DANLOS SYNDROME

This is a multisystem genetic disorder which may affect the skin, eyes, vasculature and joints. It may be inherited as either autosomal dominant, autosomal recessive or X-linked recessive. Hyperelasticity of the skin (Fig. 13.11) and hypermobility of the joints are characteristic features and recurrent dislocations of the joints are common. Ophthalmological manifestations include epicanthal folds, blue sclera, keratoconus, ectopia lentis, angioid streaks in the retina and squint.

(c) GRONBLAD–STRANDBERG SYNDROME

This syndrome describes the typical skin features of pseudoxanthoma elasticum in conjunction with angioid streaks of the retina. In this condition 85% of patients with pseudoxanthoma elasticum have angioid streaks, and it is complicated by subsequent loss of central vision in 70% of patients.

13.3.4 Pathological myopia

Patients with high myopia may develop peripapillary atrophy and posterior staphyloma. Degenerative changes within the choroid and retina may cause the formation of lacquer cracks at the posterior pole. These can be associated with the ingrowth of subretinal neovascular membranes and a disciform response. Forster–Fuchs' spot is a dark red, almost black, subretinal haemorrhage occurring at the fovea as a result of a subretinal neovascular membrane. Although central vision is usually compromised, the resulting central scotoma is usually small allowing good visual rehabilitation.

13.4 INFLAMMATORY RETINOPATHY

13.4.1 White dot retinal syndromes

There are several interesting but uncommon conditions that have the common feature of whitish lesions in the retina or choroid. These will be briefly discussed below and are:

- multiple evanescent white dot syndrome (MEWDS)
- presumed ocular histoplasmosis syndrome (POHS)
- punctate inner choroidopathy (PIC)
- multifocal choroiditis
- bird-shot choroidoretinopathy

(a) MEWDS

Multiple evanescent white dot syndrome (MEWDS) typically occurs in young females and is unilateral. Patients may complain of blurred vision and be found to have a central scotoma on the Amsler chart. Fundus examination shows the presence of multiple tiny white dots merging into patches, affecting the posterior pole of the eye. The lesions appear to be at the level of the retina or choroid and fluorescein angiography is helpful in determining

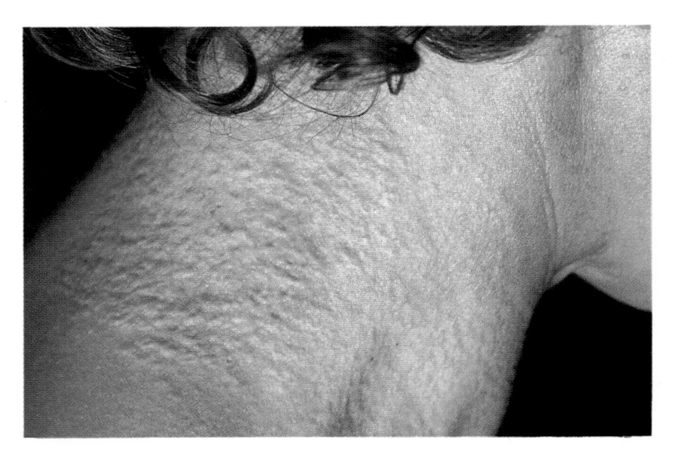

Fig 13.10 Pseudoxanthoma elasticum.

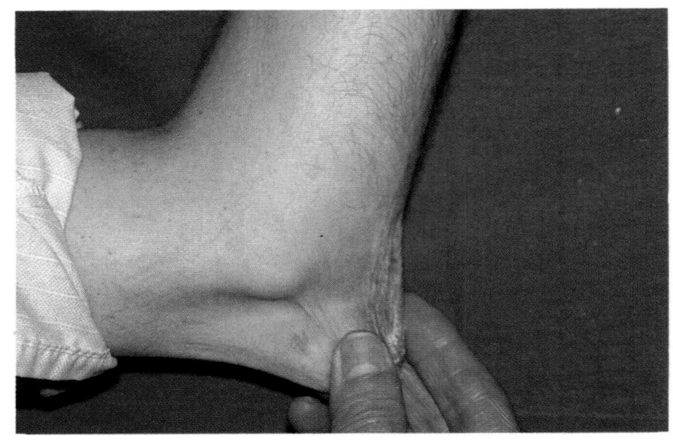

Fig. 13.11 Ehlers-Danlos – skin mobility, hyperelasticity.

their extent. Changes in the ERG have been described in this condition. The prognosis is good, with full visual recovery being normal.

The aetiology of this unusual condition is unknown and there do not seem to be any systemic medical associations.

(b) PRESUMED OCULAR HISTOPLASMOSIS SYNDROME

The presumed ocular histoplasmosis syndrome (POHS) has already been described in Chapter 9. The clinical appearance of POHS is of multiple, small punched-out choroidoretinal scars in the mid-periphery and posterior pole (so-called 'histospots'), peripapillary atrophy and scarring, but no vitreous cellular activity. Some patients exhibit more peripheral, curved areas of linear scarring. Visual loss occurs because of the strong association of subretinal neovascular membranes (SRNVM) with POHS, although the Macular Photocoagulation Study has shown the benefit of treating extrafoveal SRNVM.

The epidemiological evidence for *Histoplasma capsulatum* being the causative agent for POHS is very strong in areas of the United States where the organism is endemic and POHS highly prevalent. However similar clinical pictures are seen in countries where *Histoplasma* is not endemic, including the UK, and this has caused other syndromes to be described. These can broadly be classified as 'pseudo-POHS syndromes'.

(c) PSEUDO-POHS SYNDROMES

Punctate inner choroidopathy (PIC) is a condition in which there are similar fundal lesions to POHS, including the absence of vitreous cells. The condition occurs in patients from areas where *Histoplasma capsulatum* is not endemic, and who have no other clinical evidence of suffering from histoplasmosis. The condition seems preferentially to affect young, myopic females and like POHS has a high association with SRNVM.

(d) MULTIFOCAL CHOROIDITIS

This syndrome is similar to POHS except that there is evidence of vitreous cells on examination and it may be associated with anterior uveitis. The evidence for an inflammatory cause of this condition has led to systemic steroids being used in the acute phase, with some reports of success. Most patients affected are young, myopic females and it has a high association with SRNVM formation.

The similarity of POHS, PIC and multifocal choroiditis in their clinical appearances has led several authors to speculate that they probably represent different manifestations of a common underlying condition.

(e) BIRD-SHOT CHOROIDORETINOPATHY

This condition is characterized by a sudden onset of floaters, blurred vision and photophobia, occurring most commonly in healthy, middle-aged females. There is a strong association with HLA-A29, suggesting that it might have a genetic predisposition.

Fundus examination shows multiple areas of diffuse grey-white lesions of depigmentation, occurring at the level of the choroid or retinal pigment epithelium. The optic disc may be swollen but the most striking feature is the severe vitreous inflammation, which often makes detailed fundus examination very difficult.

Loss of central vision can occur from cystoid macular oedema, and as the condition is usually bilateral, it can be a difficult condition to manage. The disease tends to run a chronic course and responds only poorly to systemic corticosteroids. Eventually the condition burns out leaving extensive scarring in the retina and choroid but often useful vision in at least one eye.

13.4.2 Acute multifocal posterior placoid pigment epitheliopathy (AMPPPE)

AMPPPE is an uncommon but important condition. Typically it occurs in young adults, often with a history of a preceding, influenza-like illness. Patients present with sudden onset of blurred vision usually in one eye, and fundus examination shows characteristic multiple, whitish plaques at the level of the retinal pigment epithelium (RPE) or choroid. The plaques are usually up to one disc diameter in size and scattered throughout the posterior pole. Vitreous cells may be visible on slit-lamp examination, but the anterior segment is characteristically quiet. In some cases optic disc oedema may occur.

Fluorescein angiography shows initial blockage of the choroidal flush by the lesions, followed by staining of those lesions that are active. The lesions gradually resolve over a period of up to six weeks, leaving behind a permanent atrophic area in the RPE with areas of pigment clumping. The visual prognosis is good in most cases unless permanent RPE change occurs at the fovea. There is unfortunately no evidence that systemic corticosteroid treatment is of benefit.

The aetiology of AMPPPE is unknown. Some

authors suspect it is due to a primary inflammation of the RPE whilst others suspect that it is caused by an obstruction to the choroidal circulation, with secondary RPE changes.

13.4.3 Serpiginous choroidopathy

Serpiginous choroidopathy (also known as geographic or helicoid choroidopathy) is a progressive, usually bilateral condition, affecting older adults. Patients present with blurred vision and have a characteristic fundus appearance. The disease is usually limited to the posterior pole of the eye, which is disrupted by a contiguous pattern of lesions spreading outwards, which are similar to pseudopodia in their distribution. Active areas of the lesions appear whitish-grey and are slightly blurred and seen at the leading edge of the lesions. These active areas slowly form atrophic scars as they become inactive and it is this mixture of different generations of lesions, some active, some inactive, which gives this condition its characteristic appearance.

The overall effect of this process is that there is a slow, insidious and often inexorable involvement of most of the posterior pole, with resulting loss of central vision. Corticosteroids and immunosuppressive treatment have been tried but with no firm evidence that they help.

13.5 EALES' DISEASE

Eales' disease nowadays is synonymous with primary retinal perivasculitis, and describes patients, usually young men, with retinal vasculitis, retinal neovascularization and recurrent vitreous haemorrhages. The condition is usually bilateral, and the aetiology may be idiopathic, although important causes of retinal vasculitis must be excluded:

- TB
- sarcoidosis
- polyarteritis nodosa
- temporal arteritis
- systemic lupus erythematosus
- Behçet's disease
- syphilis
- toxoplasmosis
- cytomegalovirus
- herpes zoster
- AIDS
- multiple sclerosis
- pars planitis

13.6 COATS' DISEASE

Coats' disease is usually unilateral and occurs more commonly in males. The findings are of an exudative retinal detachment with massive amounts of fluid and lipid leaking from vascular abnormalities, including telangiectasic vessels and microaneurysms. The peripheral retina is typically involved but the extensive leakage that occurs is often seen at the macula, the so-called 'exaggerated macular response'. It is important always to examine the peripheral retina in any cases of macular disease.

In some patients the vascular abnormalities are limited to the small, paramacular capillaries. This is probably the same condition as Coats' disease, but at a different end of the spectrum, and is usually termed 'Leber's miliary aneurysm'.

Treatment is necessary to preserve vision in severe cases and ranges from laser photocoagulation and cryotherapy, to complicated retinal detachment surgery.

13.7 RETINAL ARTERIAL MACROANEURYSMS

Retinal arteriolar macroaneurysms are an acquired retinal vascular abnormality with a marked association with systemic hypertension. The aneurysms develop on retinal arterioles, and may suddenly bleed causing haemorrhages in all layers of the retina and often a vitreous haemorrhage. Slow decompensation of the aneurysms can occur, when lipid-rich serum slowly leaks out of the aneurysm and accumulates within or under the retina. The aneurysms may be single or multiple and several can occur on the same vessel.

Laser photocoagulation is indicated if the central retina is threatened by exudation and the macroaneurysm can be encouraged to seal off with either directly or indirectly applied laser, the latter to surround the lesion. The natural history of the aneurysms is that they tend eventually to thrombose, often after bleeding, and laser treatment is not required in many cases.

13.8 PIGMENTARY RETINOPATHIES

13.8.1 Retinitis pigmentosa

This is the name for a group of inherited disorders, characterized by night-blindness and constricted visual fields. Although the exact pathogenesis is not known, it appears to be a disease of the photoreceptor and pigment epithelial complex in the outer retina. The rod system is preferentially affected; there is also evidence of cone dysfunction with progressive disease.

Typically the disease is a diffuse, usually bilateral and symmetrical retinal dystrophy. The age of onset, the amount of eventual visual loss, the rate of progression and the presence or absence of associated ocular features are frequently related to the mode of inheritance. These include the patterns of autosomal recessive, autosomal dominant and X-linked recessive. The most common form, and often the more severe, is the autosomal recessive. This is associated with reduction in night vision, visual field loss and cataract. The next most frequent is the autosomal dominant variety which may have a benign course with night blindness and visual field loss not developing until adult life. Equally, cataract may not be a problem until the age of 60. The least common variety is the X-linked recessive in which the female carriers may have normal fundi. The severity of this disease is similar to the autosomal recessive variety.

(a) CLINICAL FEATURES

A typical triad consists of:

- bone spicule pigmentation;
- arteriolar attenuation;
- waxy optic disc pallor (usually a late feature).

In the peripheral retina, pigmentary changes are usually perivascular and have a bone spicule appearance (Fig. 13.12). This may occur in only one segment of the retina. It is often observed initially in the mid-retina and the pigmentary changes tend to extend both posteriorly and anteriorly giving rise to ring-like scotoma in the visual field. Subsequently there is progressive contraction of the visual fields, but later there is atrophy at the chorio-capillaris. This may give rise to the tessellated appearance in association with arteriolar attenuation (Fig. 13.13).

Drusen of the optic disc is a well-recognized association with retinitis pigmentosa. Maculopathy may occur in the cystoid, atrophic or cellophane form. Other ocular features include an association with open-angle glaucoma, posterior subcapsular cataract, keratoconus, myopia, and posterior vitreous detachment.

(b) ATYPICAL FORMS OF RETINITIS PIGMENTOSA

There are four types that fit into this category. The first is retinitis pigmentosa pine pigmento. In this form pigmentary changes appear late and the degree of retinal pigmentation reflects the duration of disease. On investigation, there are typical ERG abnormalities. The second form is retinitis punctata albescens. This is characterized by the retinal appearance of white dots centrally between the posterior pole and the equator. There is subsequent bone spicule development in the retina and the other typical features of retinitis pigmentosa. The two final forms are with sector and pericentric involvement. In these, there is involvement of only one quadrant, usually nasal, or the pigmentary changes are confined to the pericentric region respectively.

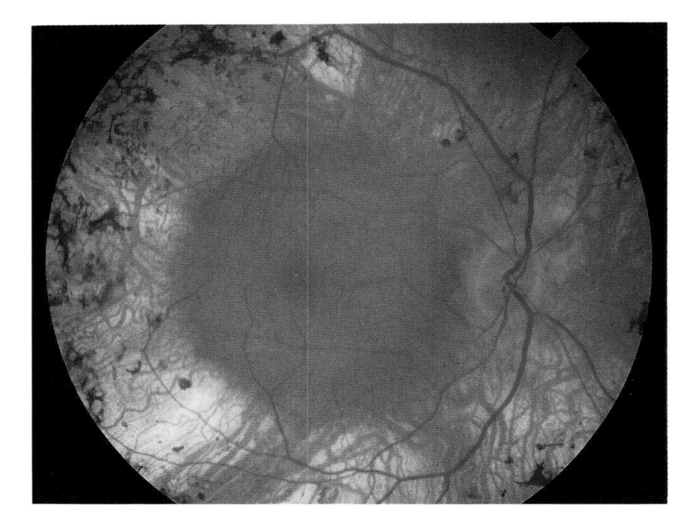

Fig. 13.12 Bone spicule appearance of retinal pigmentary changes.

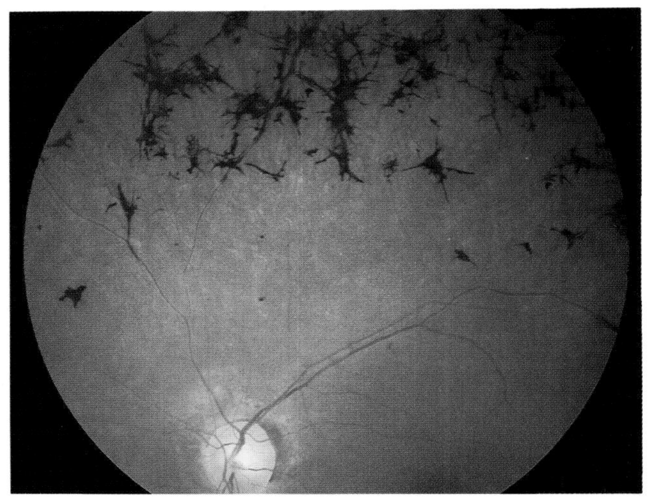

Fig. 13.13 Scattered areas of pigment. Retinal vessel attenuation and optic atrophy in retinitis pigmentosa.

13.8.2 Investigations

The triad of typical fundus changes with clinical background and a family history often makes the diagnosis of retinitis pigmentosa certain. If there is doubt, fundus photography and fluorescein angiography may be helpful. Visual function testing is important. In the electroretinogram (ERG) (scotoptic) amplitude is markedly subnormal, whereas the photopic ERG response is often relatively unaffected. The electro-oculogram (EOG) normally shows an absence of light rise.

13.8.3 Pigmentary retinopathy associated with systemic disease

Types and associations of retinitis pigmentosa are:

Familial:
- autosomal recessive;
- autosomal dominant;
- X-linked recessive.

With systemic diseases:
- Abetalipoproteinaemia (Bassen–Kornzweig syndrome);
- Refsum's syndrome;
- Usher's syndrome;
- Kearns–Sayre syndrome;
- Cockayne's syndrome;
- Friedreich's ataxia;
- Laurence–Moon–Biedl syndrome;
- Mucopolysaccharidoses (Hurlers, Hunters and San Filipino).

The subsequent syndromes to be described in this section are very rare.

(a) BASSEN–KORNZWEIG SYNDROME (abetalipoproteinaemia)

This is a condition comprising spino-cerebellar ataxia, acanthocytosis, abetalipoproteinaemia and fat malabsorption. This is extremely rare but occurs in Ashkenazi Jews and is inherited as an autosomal recessive disease. The typical fundal appearances of retinitis pigmentosa occur in the first decade of life associated with clumps of pigment and peripheral white clumping. This is ultimately fatal but early vitamin A treatment may be helpful.

(b) REFSUM'S SYNDROME

This condition is associated with peripheral neuropathy, cerebellar ataxia, deafness and ichthyosis. There is an elevated cerebrospinal fluid protein. It is inherited as an autosomal recessive condition and is thought to be due to a defect in phytamic acid metabolism. Clinically it presents as night blindness and the fundus appearance shows a 'salt and pepper' type of pigmentary retinopathy. Treatment is with a phytamic acid-free diet but plasma exchange may prevent progression.

(c) USHER'S SYNDROME

This is a congenital, non-progressive condition. Fifty per cent of patients presenting with combined blindness and deafness have Usher's syndrome. Clinical features include a sensori-neural deafness. Retinitis pigmentosa develops prior to puberty. It has a recessive form of inheritance.

(d) COCKAYNE'S SYNDROME

This syndrome comprises dwarfism, cachexia, premature ageing, long hands and limbs. Features may include deafness, nystagmus, ataxia and mental retardation. Retinal appearances include the 'salt and pepper' type of pigmentary disturbance and waxy optic atrophy. It generally has a recessive form of inheritance and is fatal by the third or fourth decade.

(e) KEARNS–SAYRE SYNDROME

This form is associated with chronic progressive external ophthalmoplegia, heart block and retinitis pigmentosa. Occasionally there is short stature, cerebellar ataxia, deafness, mental retardation and delayed puberty. Ocular features include pigmentary retinal changes occurring centrally and often sparing the periphery. It usually presents prior to the age of 20. Some cases are believed to have autosomal dominant transmission, but another interesting possibility is that it may transmit maternally through mitochondrial DNA.

(f) OTHER ASSOCIATIONS

Pigmentary retinopathy is associated with spinocerebellar degenerations, including Friedrich's ataxia. A pigmentary retinopathy is sometimes seen in patients with the dominantly inherited disorder of dystrophia myotonica. Other groups of diseases include the Laurence–Moon–Biedle syndrome, which comprises pigmentary retinopathy, mental retardation, polydactylism, obesity and hypogonadism. Mucopolysaccharidoses are also associated in the forms of Hurlers, Hunters and the San Filipino varieties.

13.9 EPIRETINAL MEMBRANES

Epiretinal membrane formation may occur as a primary event or may be secondary to uveitis, retinal vascular occlusion, trauma and surgery. Primary or idiopathic membranes are usually associated with a posterior vitreous detachment, and it is thought that this stimulates the distribution and proliferation of glial cells on the retinal surface.

Patients with this condition present with blurring of vision and metamorphopsia, caused by the distortion of the photoreceptors in the affected part of the retina. The appearance is similar to a wrinkling up of the retina, hence the alternative name of 'cellophane retinopathy'.

Visual acuity may be only slightly affected and in most cases no treatment is required. In more severe cases vitrectomy surgery and peeling of the membrane can be performed, but this is reserved for those cases with a demonstrable deterioration.

13.10 CENTRAL SEROUS RETINOPATHY

Central serous retinopathy, or chorioretinopathy (CSR), is a condition in which focal leakage of fluid from the retinal pigment epithelium occurs, which causes a serous detachment of the neurosensory retina. CSR most commonly affects males aged between 20 and 40 years and is not apparently associated with any underlying cause, although psychological stress has been implicated by some authors.

Typically patients with CSR suffer a sudden onset of blurred central vision, with metamorphopsia and micropsia. Patients often experience a browny yellow discolouration of the central vision which corresponds to the area of serous detachment of the retina, which can be mapped out by astute patients. Occasionally the condition is symptomless, if the macula is not involved.

The patient should be assessed with visual acuity measurements and the scotoma can be accurately plotted on the Amsler chart. A useful tip when testing the vision is to put a small plus lens in the trial frame over the affected eye which may improve the vision dramatically because the serous retinal detachment has in effect made the eye artefactually hypermetropic. The macular photostress test can be useful in plotting the visual recovery of the retina.

Fundus examination shows a serous detachment of the neurosensory retina, and occasionally these can be so large as to mimic a rhegmatogenous retinal detachment. Fluorescein angiography is useful with the most common finding a small, discrete leakage of fluorescein from the RPE into the subretinal space in a classical smokestack appearance. Multiple leaks are sometimes present and there may be underlying small detachments of the retinal pigment epithelium.

Generally, patients with CSR have a good prognosis, with resorption of the fluid and resolution of symptoms within one to six months. Laser photocoagulation of the leaking area of the RPE causes rapid resolution of the fluid but is generally reserved for those cases where spontaneous improvement is not occurring. An important association with CSR is the presence of a congenital, optic disc pit and in this situation the prognosis is considerably worse.

CSR is typically a condition of young patients and only rarely occurs in the elderly. Care should therefore be taken in diagnosing it in older patients (>45 years) who have similar symptoms and findings because they may have early age-related macular degeneration with the formation of a subretinal neovascular membrane.

13.11 DRUG-RELATED RETINOPATHIES

Several drugs in common usage can cause retinopathy, which may result in permanent loss of vision in some cases. The most important drugs are:

- Chloroquine: associated with bull's eye maculopathy. (Cumulative dose important.)
- Hydroxychloroquine: as above; in practice association with retinopathy much rarer.
- Phenothiazines: associated with pigmentary changes in the RPE.
- Tamoxifen: associated with superficial crystalline deposits at macula. Frequency of retinopathy and visual loss at present unknown.
- Digoxin: interferes with cone function and may cause xanthopsia. (Reversible once drug withdrawn.)
- Desferrioxamine: maculopathy and visual loss may occur suddenly following intravenous administration.
- Quinine: associated with optic atrophy and severe arteriolar narrowing. Visual loss may be profound.

The reader is recommended to consult the larger retinal or pharmacological textbooks for guidance on these.

In trying to assess patients with a possible drug-induced retinopathy, a history of all medications is obviously important, with an idea of the total, cumulative dosage. Visual acuity testing, Amsler chart and colour vision assessment are important, and electrodiagnostic tests can be helpful. Fundus photography is useful in documenting the presence (or absence) of fundal abnormalities, with fluorescein angiography when necessary.

It is important for the doctors involved in detecting drug-related retinopathies to have a clear idea as to who is responsible for organizing and performing screening of those patients at potential risk. This usually involves the ophthalmologist and physician coming to some local arrangement!

FURTHER READING

American Academy of Ophthalmology (1991) *Basic and Clinical Science Course; Retina and Vitreous*. American Academy of Ophthalmology., San Francisco.

Anon. (1981) Retinitis pigmentosa (leading article). *Br. Med. J.*, **282**, 1736–7.

Gass, J.D.M. (1987) *Stereoscopic Atlas of Macular Disease*, 3rd edn, C.V. Mosby Company, St Louis.

Jampol, L.M., Sieving, P.A., Pugh, D. *et al.* (1984) Multiple evanescent white dot syndrome 1. Clinical findings. *Arch. Ophthalmol.*, **102**, 671.

Kritzinger, E.E. and Wright, B.E. (1984) *A Colour Atlas of the Eye and Systemic Disease*. Wolfe Medical Publications Ltd, London, pp. 60–5.

Morgan, C.M. and Schatz, H. (1986) Recurrent multifocal choroiditis. *Ophthalmol.*, **93**.

Rennie, I.G. (1992) Ocular manifestations of malignant disease. *Br. J. Hosp. Med.*, **47**(3), 185–91.

Watzke, R.C., Packer, A.J., Folk, J.C. *et al.* (1984) Punctate inner choroidopathy. *Am. J. Ophthalmol.*, **98**, 572.

Woods, A.C. and Whalen, H.E. (1960) The probable role of benign histoplasmosis in the etiology of granulomatous uveitis. *Am. J. Ophthalmol.*, **49**, 205.

Index

Numbers appearing in **bold** refer to figures and numbers appearing in *italic* refer to tables.